Sciences Basic to Orthopaedics

Sciences Basic to Orthopaedics

Edited by

Sean PF Hughes MS, FRCS, FRCSI, FRCS(Ed)Orth

Professor of Orthopaedic Surgery
Head of Surgery, Anaesthetics and Intensive Care
Chief of Orthopaedic Service, Hammersmith Hospitals NHS Trust
Past Chairman, Intercollegiate Board in Orthopaedic Surgery

and

Ian D McCarthy PhD

Senior Lecturer (Non-Clinical) in Orthopaedic Surgery

Department of Orthopaedic Surgery
Imperial College School of Medicine
London

WB Saunders Company Limited
London   Philadelphia   Toronto   Sydney   Tokyo

W.B. Saunders Company Ltd 24–28 Oval Road
London NW1 7DX

The Curtis Center
Independence Square West
Philadelphia, PA 19106-3399, USA

Harcourt Brace & Company
55 Horner Avenue
Toronto, Ontario, M8Z 4X6, Canada

Harcourt Brace & Company, Australia
30–52 Smidmore Street
Marrickville, NSW 2204, Australia

Harcourt Brace & Company, Japan
Ichibancho Central Building, 22-1 Ichibancho
Chiyoda-ku, Tokyo 102, Japan

A catalogue record for this book is available from the British Library

ISBN 0-7020-1973-9

Typeset by Paston Press Ltd, Loddon, Norfolk
Printed and bound in Great Britain by The Bath Press, Bath

Contents

Contributors

Andrew A Amis PhD, FIMechE, CEng, Reader in Orthopaedic Biomechanics, Imperial College, London, UK

Susanna Benvenuti PhD, Endocrine Unit, Department of Clinical Physiopathology, University of Florence, Florence, Italy

Stephen R Bloom MA, MD, DSc, FRCP, Professor of Endocrinology, Imperial College School of Medicine, London, UK

Maria Luisa Brandi MD, PhD, Associate Professor of Metabolic Disease, Endocrine Unit, Department of Clinical Physiopathology, University of Florence, Florence, Italy

Mark F Brown MA, PhD, FRCSEd(Orth), Consultant Orthopaedic and Spinal Surgeon, North Staffordshire Hospital, Stoke-on-Trent, UK

Euro Ing **Edward RC Draper** PhD, BSc, MIMechE, CEng, MIPEM, Principal Research Fellow in Bioengineering, Department of Orthopaedic and Trauma Surgery, London, UK

Oleg Eremin MD, FRACS, FRCSE, Regius Professor of Surgery, University of Aberdeen, Forester Hill, Aberdeen, UK

John Fisher BSc, PhD, DEng, CEng, Professor of Mechanical Engineering, University of Leeds, Leeds, UK

Andrew Forester BSc, FRCS(Ed) Orth, Senior Lecturer in Orthopaedic Surgery, Imperial College School of Medicine, London, and Consultant Orthopaedic Surgeon, Hammersmith Hospitals and Central Middlesex Hospital NHS Trust, London, UK

Jean WM Gardeniers MD, PhD, Consultant Orthopedic Surgeon, University Hospital Nijmegen, Academisch Ziekenhuis St Radboud Nijmegen, The Netherlands

Samia I Girgis MB, BCH, PhD, MRCPath, Senior Lecturer/Honorary Consultant, Department of Metabolic Medicine, Imperial College School of Medicine, London, UK

Girish Giridhar PhD, Medical Sciences Research Institute, Herndon, Virginia, USA

Michael A Glasby BM, BCh, MA, MSc, CBiol, MIBiol, FICS, FRCSE, FRCS, Reader in Anatomy, University of Edinburgh Medical School, Edinburgh, UK

Allen E Goodship BVSc, PhD, MRCVS, Professor of Orthopaedic Sciences, Royal Veterinary College and Institute of Orthopaedics, UCL, University of London, London, UK

Anthony G Gristina MD, Medical Sciences Research Institute, Herndon, Virginia, USA

Andrew C Hall PhD, Lecturer, Department of Physiology, University of Edinburgh Medical School, Edinburgh, UK

Luise Harrison BVSc, Cert EO, MRCVS, Research student with Allen Goodship

Christopher L-H Huang MA, PhD, DM, MD, DSc, ScD, Reader in Cellular Physiology, Physiological Laboratory, University of Cambridge, Downing Site, Cambridge, UK

Sean PF Hughes MS, FRCS, Professor of Orthopaedic Surgery, Imperial College School of Medicine, London, UK

Mika Hukkanen BSc, PhD, Lecturer in Histochemistry, Department of Histochemistry, Imperial College School of Medicine, London, UK

Latif Khan FRCS (Ed), Senior Surgical Registrar, Department of Surgery, University of Aberdeen, Forester Hill, Aberdeen, UK

Timothy J Lawes BEng (Hons), Research assistant with Allen Goodship

Iain MacIntyre MD, PhD, DSc, FRCPath, FRCP, FRS, Professor and Research Director, William Harvey Research Institute, St Bartholomew's Hospital, Medical College, London, UK

Denis RW May BSc (Hons), PhD, CEng, MIMechE, Regional Head of Clinical Science and Rehabilitation Engineering, Queen Mary's University Hospital, Roehampton Rehabilitation Centre, London, UK; Visiting Senior Research Fellow in Clinical Biomechanics, University of Surrey, Guildford, UK

Laura Masi MD, Endocrine Unit, Department of Clinical Physiopathology, University of Florence, Florence, Italy

Ian D McCarthy PhD, Senior Lecturer (Non-Clinical), Department of Orthopaedic Surgery, Imperial College School of Medicine, London, UK

Karim Meeran BSc, MRCP, MBBS, Consultant Endocrinologist, Hammersmith Hospital, London, UK

Julia M Polak MD, DSc, FRCPath, MRCP, Professor of Endocrine Pathology and Head of the Department of Histochemistry, Imperial College School of Medicine, London, UK

Peter A Revell BSc, MBBS, PhD, FRCPath, Professor of Histopathology, Department of Histopathology, Royal Free Hospital School of Medicine, London, UK

Thomas C Schuler MD, Northern Virginia Spine Institute, Reston, Virginia, USA

Elizabeth Tanner MA, DPhil, MIPEM, FIMechE, FIM, CEng, Reader in Biomaterials and Biomechanics, Interdisciplinary Research Centre in Biomaterials, Queen Mary and Westfield College, London, UK

Annalisa Tanini PhD, Endocrine Unit, Institute of Internal Medicine and Immunoallergology, University of Florence, Florence, Italy

Preface

This new book on the basic sciences related to orthopaedics has been written for orthopaedic surgeons in training.

Basic sciences in orthopaedics are fundamental to clinical practice and there are few books available on this topic. Also, the subjects are changing rapidly as new advances are made in one of the exciting and expanding areas of surgical practice.

This multi-author book attempts to cover the main subjects that are fundamental to orthopaedic surgery. The chapters are written by authorities in their fields who bring up-to-date information that should be easily understood by the clinician and that prepares trainees for the Intercollegiate Examination in Orthopaedic Surgery.

The purpose of this book is to be part of a series of books on orthopaedics which are current and relevant and provide the full range of topics covered in the examination. As more information becomes available, so the books may become dated. Hence, it is the intention to publish new editions of these books at regular intervals in order to discuss and present contemporary practices.

In the first of the series, Dr McCarthy has brought together a number of experts in the field who present up-to-date knowledge on the basic sciences as applied to orthopaedics – a subject that is essential for all trainees and also for all surgeons who wish to take part in a challenging and important aspect of orthopaedic and trauma surgery.

Sean PF Hughes
London, May 1997

Section I

Tissues of the Musculoskeletal System

1

Bone Structure

Peter A Revell

INTRODUCTION

In a typical standard man, the skeleton weighs approximately 2 kg and is made up of 206 individual bones. Bone consists of cells and extracellular matrix; the latter comprises both organic (35%) and inorganic (65%) parts. The organic component includes type I collagen (90%), the γ-carboxyglutamic acid-rich protein osteocalcin (1–2%), osteonectin, proteoglycans, glycosaminoglycans and lipids. The inorganic component consists mainly of calcium and phosphate in crystals of hydroxyapatite. The skeleton stores more than 99% of the calcium in the body, and is also a store for sodium and magnesium. In each bone, these component parts are organised at both a macroscopic and microscopic level to support the two functions of the skeleton, those of mechanical support and mineral homoeostasis.

GENERAL ANATOMY OF BONES

Bones may be divided into different categories for the purposes of their general description. Tubular or long bones have an outer tube of dense cortical bone, which is thickest at the mid-point of the tube (mid-shaft). The inside of the tube is filled with branching trabecular or cancellous bone together with bone marrow and fat. The amount of marrow and fat is greatest at the bone ends. The tubular bones can be subdivided, somewhat artificially, into long and short tubular bones, the humerus, radius, ulna, femur, tibia and fibula comprising the former, whereas the metacarpals, metatarsals and phalanges make up the latter. Each tubular bone is divisible into three main regions: the epiphysis, the metaphysis and

the diaphysis. These are illustrated in *Figure 1.1*. While this is basic, knowledge of these areas is important to the understanding and recognition of particular pathological processes. For example, osteomyelitis occurs in the metaphysis in the highly vascular growth-plate region of the long bones of young children, and particular bone tumours such as osteosarcoma usually arise in the metaphysis, whereas others occur in the epiphysis (chondroblastoma, giant cell tumour).

The ribs, sternum, scapula and most of the cranium comprise the 'flat' bones, which are made up of inner and

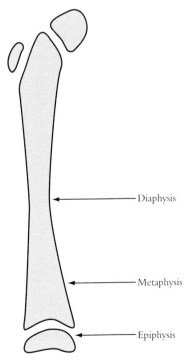

Figure 1.1 Diagram of developing femur to show the localisation of the diaphysis, metaphysis and epiphysis.

outer flattened tables of cortical dense bone betwee
which there is spongy cancellous bone, usually containin
bone marrow.

Other bones do not fit easily into either of thes
categories. The small bones of the hands and feet in th
wrist and ankle are sometimes known as epiphysioi
bones because they develop by ossification of cartilag
nous models from a central point outwards, just like a
epiphyseal ossification centre. They have only a thi
cortical rim of bone and are predominantly cancellou
The vertebrae are difficult to fit into a particular categor
The vertebral bodies are like short, fat, tubular bones bι
have flattened bone with dense cortices (flat bone:
joined together to make the arches and spinous processe:

TYPES OF BONE

There are two main types of bone, lamellar and non-
lamellar, the latter also sometimes known as 'coarse-
fibred' or 'woven' bone. The collagen fibres in lamellar
bone are arranged in parallel layers, whereas non-lamellar
bone shows the presence of randomly oriented criss-
crossing coarse fibres. These two collagen patterns are
clearly visible by polarisation microscopy (*Figures 1.2* and
1.3). Both cortical and cancellous adult bone are lamellar
whereas woven bone is seen in the foetus, young children
and during the early stages of healing in bone. The bone
cells (osteocytes) in woven bone are larger and more
closely arranged than those in lamellar bone. Wover
bone is mechanically weaker than lamellar bone and is
usually replaced and remodelled to a lamellar structure
soon after its formation, under normal circumstances.

Cortical bone has the familiar structure of Haversian
systems or osteons, being made up of central canals
surrounded by concentric lamellae containing circumferentially arranged osteocytes (*Figure 1.4*). The long axis of
the osteon is in the long axis of the bone, and communication between Haversian canals and the medullary
cavity is by transverse or oblique Volkmann's canals
which represent remnants of previously formed osteons
disrupted by the remodelling process that occurs continually in bone. Each osteon is separated from its
neighbour by a dark haematoxylin-stained cement line.
Irregular indentations in these lines represent sites of new
bone formation following resorption and are referred to
as 'reversal' lines. The outer surface of cortical bone is

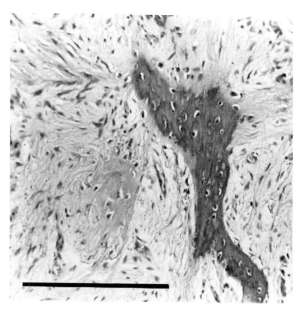

Figure 1.2 High-power photomicrograph of woven
bone showing the presence of numerous large osteocytes
placed close to each other and non-lamellar (woven)
arrangement of collagen fibres. Compare with *Figure 1.3*.
Bar = 100 μm.

covered by the periosteum, which is a thin vascular
membrane-like layer with collagen fibres arranged parallel to the bone surface. This periosteal membrane blends
with the fibres of ligaments and muscle insertions but is
absent at sites of attachment of ligaments directly into

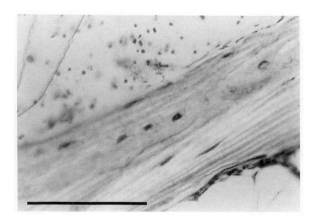

Figure 1.3 High-power view of lamellar (cancellous)
bone showing small osteocytes widely separated from each
other and parallel arrangement of collagen lamellae (partial
polarisation microscopy). Compare with *Figure 1.2*.
Bar = 100 μm.

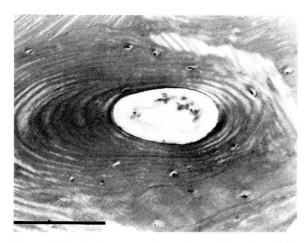

Figure 1.4 High-power photomicrograph of cortical bone showing a Haversian canal with concentric arrangement of collagen lamellae viewed by polarisation microscopy. Bar = 100 μm.

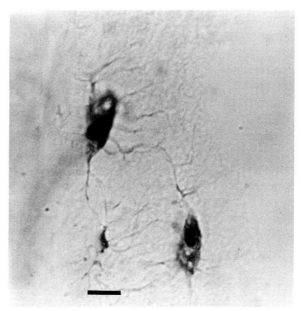

Figure 1.5 High-power view of two osteocytes in their lacunae showing the presence of long processes intercommunicating between cells. Bar = 10 μm.

bone, for example at tuberosities and the linea aspera of the femur.

Cancellous, trabecular or spongy bone is made up of a series of interconnecting plates perforated by holes, although effectively in some sites this produces the appearance of connecting bars or struts. The thickest and strongest trabeculae are oriented in the direction subject to the greatest mechanical forces. The structure of cancellous bone provides mechanical strength without undue weight as well as a large surface area for the cellular activity that is necessary for the metabolic (homoeostatic) functions of bone. Trabecular bone, like cortical bone, contains numerous osteocytes in lacunae which are interconnected but tend to be oriented longitudinally in the direction of the lamellae. An attenuated layer of flattened cells covers the surface of lamellar or trabecular bone. These are the resting or inactive osteoblasts.

THE CELLS OF BONE

The three types of cell normally distinguishable in bone are the osteoblasts, osteocytes and osteoclasts. There is, however, a close relationship between bone-forming cells and the cell lines that produce cartilage and fibrous tissue, so that under changed circumstances a different matrix is produced; for example, chondroid tissue is sometimes seen in fracture callus.

Osteocytes

Osteocytes are small, darkly staining, cells separated from surrounding mineralised bone by a 1–2 μm wide space which forms the osteocyte lacuna. The long cytoplasmic processes of the osteocytes pass through the bone matrix in canaliculi and there is communication between lacunae through these narrow tunnels (*Figure 1.5*).

Electron microscopical examination shows the osteocytes have small nuclei, scanty cytoplasm with few mitochondria, and a small Golgi zone. Osteocytes are formed by the incorporation of osteoblasts at the bone surface, and osteocytes nearer the surface have more endoplasmic reticulum than those more deeply situated. This is thought to be because the more superficial cells are more active. Transformation from osteoblast to osteocyte involves the loss of organelles associated with protein synthesis and the development of long cytoplasmic processes.

It has been suggested that osteocytes are capable of degrading the bone matrix surrounding them in the process of osteocytic osteolysis. This process, if real, must play an insignificant part in bone metabolism (Revell, 1986). It is important, however, to recognise the relationship between bone precursor cells, bone lining cells, osteoblasts and osteocytes. Thus, osteoblasts are now known to produce enzymes (cysteine proteases – the cathepsins) that are capable of breaking down collagen in bone matrix. Because there are no specific cellular markers for osteogenic cells, the relationship between the bone-forming cells and their precursors has to remain conjectural.

Certainly, there are flattened cells forming an attenuated layer at the endosteal surfaces of bone which may be barely discernible by light microscopy. These cells may be referred to as bone lining cells. They form up to 95% of the total normal bone surface and are considered to be in communication with their bone-incorporated relatives, the osteocytes, through processes in the canalicular system. The relationship between bone marrow stromal cells, acting as precursor cells, and the lining cell–preosteoblast–osteoblast lineage has been recognised for some time and is summarised in *Figure 1.6*. That these cells are able to produce other enzymes such as collagenase, as well as mediators like prostaglandins and cytokines, has been demonstrated recently. The role of these mediators in bone cell function will be described in a later chapter. It is considered that the stem cell for these lining cells may become an inducible osteoblast precursor (preosteoblast), then a differentiated preosteoblast; the latter have a commitment to the mediator production mentioned above. Typical osteoblasts are more prominent cells, which may vary from a recognisable layer of cells with plump, if still flattened, nuclei and cytoplasm, to so-called active osteoblasts.

Osteoblasts

Active osteoblasts form a layer of plump polyhedral cells covering the bone surfaces. They are markedly basophilic and show metachromatic staining. Alkaline phosphatase is present in such osteoblasts when they are actively forming bone in apposition to the immediately adjacent osseous protein tissue. These osteoblasts put down this bone matrix or osteoid tissue as a narrow appositional layer, which subsequently becomes mineralised. Osteoid consists of coarse collagen fibres with fine initial focal calcification. The calcification front (mineralisation front) is localised to the interface between the osteoid and the calcified bone. There are various ways in which this has been demonstrated in the past but the most reliable in humans is by the incorporation of tetracycline, which is fluorescent and becomes localised at sites of calcification. More detailed information about tetracy-

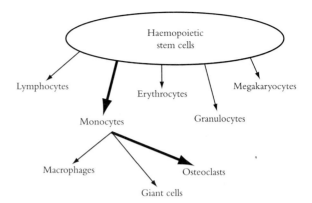

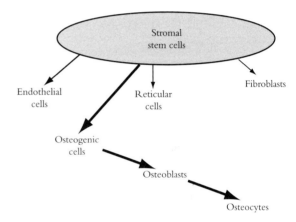

Figure 1.6 Diagram to show the derivation of osteoclasts from haemopoietic cells and that of osteoblasts and osteocytes from bone stromal cells.

cline and other labels in bone is available elsewhere (Revell, 1986). Surfaces of trabecular and cortical bone, where there are active polyhedral osteoblasts and an osteoid layer, represent sites of active bone formation (*Figure 1.7*). Elsewhere, over most of the surfaces in normal bone, the resting cells are flattened to form a thin layer of osteoprogenitor cells (preosteoblasts) and osteoblasts termed the 'endosteum'.

Ultrastructural examination shows that there is abundant endoplasmic reticulum and that free ribosomes and polyribosomes are plentiful in the osteoblast. The Golgi apparatus is well developed and mitochondria are numerous, as befits an actively synthesising cell. Lysosomes and coated vesicles are seen, the latter fusing with the cell membrane. Small numbers of short microvilli are present at the cell surface.

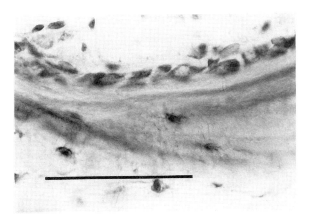

Figure 1.7 High-power view of active osteoblasts (top) forming a layer of osteoid. Recently incorporated cells which are becoming osteocytes can be seen embedded in the bone. Bar = 100 μm.

Osteoclasts

Osteoclasts are multinucleate giant cells found at the surface of bone. They are acidophilic in routinely stained sections, metachromatic with toluidine blue or thionine, and contain acid phosphatase. Active bone resorption is identified by the presence of osteoclasts in relation to a crenated bone surface containing no osteoid in sites known as resorption lacunae (Howship's lacunae) (*Figure 1.8*). Tartrate-resistant acid phosphatase was formerly considered a specific marker of osteoclasts, but is now known to be present in a proportion of macrophages and other cells of the monocyte–macrophage lineage such as macrophage polykaryons (foreign-body giant cells). The receptor for vitronectin (VNR) on the surface of cells has also been claimed as an osteoclast marker, but has recently been shown to be present on various other cell types.

The osteoclasts are considered to belong to the same broad lineage as the macrophages and their polykaryons but opinions differ as to how distinctive these cells are from each other, some workers holding that osteoclasts are predestined to develop from an early stage derived from a multipotential haemopoietic stem cell separate from the macrophage system, whereas others believe that the branching off of osteoclasts from the macrophage line occurs much later in the developmental pathway, so that the relationship is much closer. The mechanism whereby osteoclasts resorb bone is also a matter for discussion, details of which need not be entered into here. In general, it is thought that osteo-

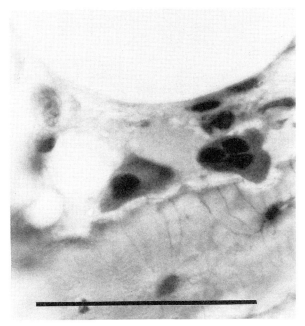

Figure 1.8 High-power view of two osteoclasts that are resorbing mineralised bone. Bar = 100 μm.

clasts can only resorb bone that is mineralised, and it is not certain whether they remove both organic and inorganic components or are responsible for demineralisation alone, phagocytosis of exposed collagen being carried out by macrophages. Osteoclasts contain a moderate amount of rough endoplasmic reticulum, a well-developed Golgi apparatus and plentiful mitochondria at the ultrastructural level. The osteoclast cell surface immediately adjacent to the bone matrix is differentiated into a ruffled border with deep invaginations of the cell membrane formed by numerous microvilli. This is surrounded on all sides by the clear zone, which lacks organelles and has moderately dense granular cytoplasm. The cytoplasm deep to the ruffled border contains smooth and coated vesicles, phagosomes and residual bodies. Active resorption occurs in relation to the ruffled zone and it is the adjacent matrix that shows loss of mineral deposits with detachment of mineral crystals.

ORIGIN OF BONE CELLS

The two main cell types of bone, the osteoclasts and the osteoblasts, are derived from different cell lines (Owen,

1983). Osteoblasts originate from connective tissue cells, and fibroblast-like flattened cells called 'preosteoblasts' are their immediate precursors (see *Figure 1.6*). Bone marrow stromal cells and osteogenic soft tissue are each capable of giving rise to both osseous tissue and marrow stroma. A close relationship exists, therefore, between formation of the bone and of bone marrow stroma. It is of interest in this respect to note that marrow fibrosis in myelosclerosis is often accompanied by osteosclerosis, and that, in turn, marrow stromal changes occur in osteosclerosis. Fibroblasts from other sites form bone only when a suitable inducing agent is present. There are thus 'determined' osteogenic precursor cells, which need no additional stimulus, and 'inducible' precursor cells.

Numerous factors have been recognised as important in bone morphogenesis, including bone morphogenetic protein, osteonectin, osteocalcin and phosphoproteins. These aspects fall into the more basic aspects of bone research and will not be considered further here.

Osteoclasts originate from precursor cells of the mononuclear phagocyte system (see *Figure 1.6*) and are thus derived ultimately from a haematopoietic stem cell. It is considered that various colony-stimulating factors play an important role in this differentiation process, along with other cytokines (Gowen, 1992). Considerable evidence for this close relationship to the macrophage system comes from bone marrow grafting studies in osteopetrotic animals, although there remains some question of the closeness of the relationship between macrophages and osteoclasts (see above) despite the use of modern monoclonal antibody markers.

Table 1.1 Some of the cytokines involved in bone metabolism (adapted from Gowen, 1992).

Cytokine	Bone formation	Bone resorption
IL-1	+	+++
TNF-α	+	+++
TNF-β	+	+++
TGF-α	−	+++
TGF-β	++	++
PDGF	++	++
IGF-1	+++	0
IGF-2	+++	0
FGF	+++	0

IL, interleukin; TNF, tumour necrosis factor; TGF, transforming growth factor; PDGF, platelet-derived growth factor; IGF, insulin-like growth factor; FGF, fibroblast growth factor. +, ++, +++ = stimulatory effect; − = inhibitory effect; 0 = no effect.

DEVELOPMENT OF THE SKELETON

The morphological changes occurring during the development of the foetus at term from a single-celled organism at fertilisation are well described in the embryological literature, although some of the processes may be difficult to conceptualise because they occur in three dimensions. Studies using the modern methods of cellular and molecular biology have greatly enhanced the understanding of events during differentiation of the complete individual from the fertilised ovum. These aspects are available in other sources and will not be described in detail here.

The musculoskeletal tissues arise from the intraembryonic mesoderm, which first appears at the start of the 15th day in human development. By the eighth day the inner cell mass of the developing embryo has two cellular layers, the endoderm and ectoderm, and continues to grow as a disc until the primitive streak appears on the ectodermal surface. Cells derived from the primitive streak invaginate from the surface and migrate to form a third layer, the mesoderm, between the other two layers on the 15th day. A further invagination and caudal migration from the most cephalad part of the primitive streak gives rise to the notochord, which acts both as the central axis around which the somites and the spine form, and as the inducer of the overlying ectoderm to form the neural groove. The mesoderm along both sides of the notochord becomes organised into discrete masses, the somites, which appear in sequence from the cranial to the caudal region (*Figure 1.9*). The axial and appendicular skeletons form at first in cartilage between the fourth and eighth weeks of embryonic life, and the embryo is especially susceptible to the development of malformations if exposed to viruses or teratogens during the first trimester of pregnancy.

The ventromedial parts of the somites make up the 'sclerotomes' from which the axial skeleton is derived. The embryonic connective tissue (mesenchyme) of the sclerotomes undergoes resegmentation and the precartilaginous vertebral body develops from this rearranged mesenchyme, whereas cells in the centre of the original sclerotome form the intervertebral disc (*Figure 1.9*). The mesenchymal vertebral column forms around the framework of the notochord, which itself disappears inside the cartilaginous vertebral bodies, remaining only as the

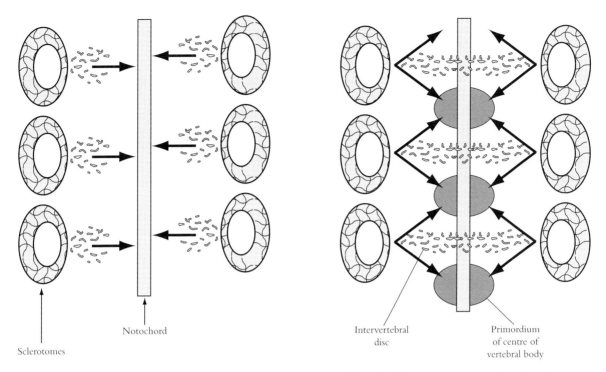

Sclerotomes · Notochord · Intervertebral disc · Primordium of centre of vertebral body

Figure 1.9   Diagram to represent a coronal section of an embryo at the level of the notochord. Cells from the sclerotome migrate towards the midline to form the intervertebral disc in the segmental zone. Other cells migrate from the sclerotomes into the intersegmental zone to form the primordia of the vertebral bodies.

nucleus pulposus in the discs between the vertebral bodies. While the ventral mesenchyme of the sclerotome becomes the vertebral body, the dorsal mesenchyme covers the neural tube and eventually forms the vertebral arches. Three primary centres of ossification appear at the end of the embryonic period, one in the vertebral body and two in the vertebral arches, which are still connected by cartilage at birth, not fusing until 3–6 years of age.

The skull is formed in two distinct parts: the basal chondrocranium and the calvaria. The former arises from a parachordal part containing notochordal remnants and a more anterior prechordal part, whereas the latter forms by intramembranous ossification. Once bone formation in the calvaria has become established in ossification centres, trabecular bone is formed and the intertrabecular spaces become filled with haemopoietic tissue. Closure of the anterior and posterior fontanelles, present at birth and comprised of fibrous tissue, occurs after 2 months in the case of the posterior fontanelle and during the second postnatal year for the anterior fontanelle.

The limbs arise as small buds on the ventrolateral side of the body wall, originating from the lateral somatic mesoderm and covered by ectoderm. The upper limb bud appears at 26 days and the bud for the lower limb at 28 days. A specialised layer of ectoderm, the 'apical ectodermal ridge', influences the underlying mesoderm to promote and control growth. Cartilage models of most of the bones are well formed by 8 weeks. The hands and feet are, at first, like mittens, so tissue between the rays has to disappear for the separate digits to form. Syndactyly results from failure of this process. Each cartilage model of the limb bones is surrounded by perichondrium, which becomes vascularised then ossified to form a ring of bone by endochondral ossification around the middle of the shaft. This cuff of bone advances towards the ends of the bone in both directions, and a transverse band of cartilage becomes delineated towards the end of the bone, forming the epiphyseal plate. The epiphyses develop from the cartilage beyond this plate. The epiphyseal cartilage becomes vascularised from the perichondrium and an ossification centre appears which grows centrifugally at the same time as the epiphysis is enlarged by further cartilage production.

The joints appear as early as 6 weeks and are seen initially as an interzone of densely packed cells forming a disc within the cartilage. These cells differentiate into three parts: (a) the chondrogenic layers from which articular cartilage originates; (b) the synovial mesenchyme which gives rise to the synovial membrane, joint capsule, menisci and intracapsular ligaments; and (c) the central interzone, in which small cavities appear and eventually coalesce to form a single joint cavity containing synovial fluid. Movement of the limb is necessary for the completion of joint development. A major proportion of the cells lining the synovial surface are macrophages and these cells first migrate into the joint during development.

BONE FORMATION

Bone forms either by intramembranous or endochondral ossification. The skull, facial bones, parts of the clavicle and mandible, and all subperiosteal bone form as intramembranous bone, whereas the rest of the skeleton comes into being by the ossification of cartilaginous tissue. Osteoblasts differentiate directly from the mesenchyme in intramembranous ossification and produce fine strands of osteoid (bone matrix) to produce a delicate lattice of trabeculae (woven bone) which becomes mineralised and forms cancellous bone after subsequent remodelling. A pre-existing cartilage model is required for endochondral ossification to take place (see above). Osteoblasts form a collar of bone around the midshaft of each such model, and nearby central chondrocytes hypertrophy and degenerate as vascular tissue penetrates. Following vascularisation, osteoblasts are present and a primary centre of ossification is formed which then spreads in both directions towards the ends of the cartilage model. Vascular invasion at the ends of the bone starts a similar process with the formation of secondary centres of ossification at the epiphyses. A disc of growing cartilage remains between the epiphysis and the metaphysis at the growth plate, and continuing endochondral ossification at this site is responsible for the increasing length of the bone. Intramembranous ossification is responsible for the increase in girth of bones. Detailed accounts of these processes are available in textbooks of histology and embryology.

THE GROWTH PLATE

The growth plate is divisible into different zones according to morphology and state of calcification (*Figure 1.10*). The reserve of resting zone (a misnomer because the cells are not resting) contains small cells singly or in pairs, whereas cells in the adjacent proliferation and hypertrophic zones are arranged in longitudinal columns passing down into the metaphysis. The cells in the upper part of the columns are flattened and make up the proliferation zone. The lower cells in the cartilage

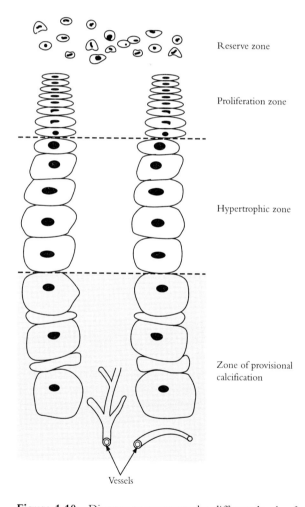

Reserve zone

Proliferation zone

Hypertrophic zone

Zone of provisional calcification

Vessels

Figure 1.10 Diagram to represent the different levels of development in the growth plate from the reserve zone (top) to the zone of provisional calcification (bottom), where there is invasion of the cartilage columns by blood vessels.

columns become progressively larger and spherical in the hypertrophic zone, losing their intracytoplasmic glycogen in the lower half of this zone. The upper part of the hypertrophic zone has the highest content of alkaline and acid phosphatases, glucose-6-phosphate dehydrogenase, lactic dehydrogenase and phosphoglycoisomerase as well as calcium, phosphate, magnesium and lipid. Calcium and phosphorus have been localised to electron-dense granules in the mitochondria of growth-plate chondrocytes by X-ray spectroscopy. There is progressive loss of loading of cells with calcium through the hypertrophic zone, with no calcium present at the bottom of this zone. Accumulated calcium crystals in the longitudinal septa of the matrix between the cells become confluent in what is frequently called the zone of provisional calcification.

The cells in the proliferation zone are flattened and arranged in longitudinal columns (*Figure 1.10*). Like the reserve zone cells, these cells contain glycogen. Tritiated thymidine incorporation studies have shown that these are the only chondrocytes in the growth plate to divide. It is the topmost cell of each column that acts as the source of all the other cells forming the column, and this production of cells is the means by which tubular bones increase in length. Matrix vesicles (see below), which are thought to play a central role in calcification, are in highest concentration in the hypertrophic zone.

There are small vessels in the zone of provisional calcification and the penetration of cartilage by vessels in general is associated with its calcification, as also seen, for example, at the deepest aspect of articular cartilage in the tidemark region.

The growth plate is encircled by a wedge-shaped groove of cells termed the ossification groove and by a band of fibrous tissue and bone known as the perichondrial ring. Oval cells pass from the groove into the cartilage at the level of the reserve zone and so enable increase in girth at the growth plate. The perichondrial ring provides a mechanical support for the bone–cartilage junction of the growth plate (Beighton, 1978; Revell, 1986; Salisbury et al, 1994).

BONE MINERALISATION

The mineral in bone is chemically similar to the geological mineral hydroxyapatite, except that it is relatively deficient in calcium and has an imperfect atomic arrangement, with carbonate, magnesium, fluoride and other ions present. The organic matrix of bone is composed predominantly of type I collagen with a small amount of proteoglycan and other proteins also present. The arrangement of collagen molecules and their relationship to sites of mineralisation are described (Glimcher, 1976) and reviewed (Revell, 1986) elsewhere. Briefly, precursor molecules of collagen (pro-α chains) are made within the osteoblast and exported into the local environment in a form that keeps fibres separate by virtue of the presence of extension peptides. These peptides are removed outside the cell, allowing peptide aggregation to form ordered polymers with cross-links. These collagen molecules, when correctly associated, show a staggered arrangement of $67 \, \mu m$ intervals with hole zones present between them (*Figure 1.11*). The deposition of mineral occurs preferentially in the hole zone of the fibril. After initiation of calcification of collagen fibrils, several rate-dependent processes take place, including nucleation, growth of calcium phosphate particles and the transition of these to crystalline hydroxyapatite. Most of the additional calcium is deposited by secondary nucleation once an initial solid phase has been formed. Bone collagen is laid down by osteoblasts, but there is almost certainly some further influence of these cells on the calcification process as well. References to the various factors that may play a role, such as calcium-binding proteins, proteoglycans and lipids, are obtainable elsewhere (Revell, 1986; Salisbury et al, 1994). Local concentration of calcium in, and export from, mitochondria and the presence of matrix vesicles as buds off the cell membrane containing alkaline phosphatase and pyrophosphatase are important factors. There is a relationship between the disappearance of calcium phosphate particles from mitochondria and the onset of calcification. The concentration of these ions in matrix vesicles also precedes their extracellular deposition. Matrix vesicles are membrane-bound packages containing calcium which are derived from the surface membrane of cells (*Figure 1.12*). The membrane still contains phosphatases such as alkaline phosphatase, inorganic pyrophosphatase and adenosine 5′-triphosphatase (ATPase), which act to raise the phosphatase level locally while the lipids of the membrane concentrate calcium. These locally high concentrations of calcium and phosphate result in crystallisation within the vesicle. Extrusion of the calcium phosphate crystal gives rise to a locally high concentration focus for the propagation of crystal growth.

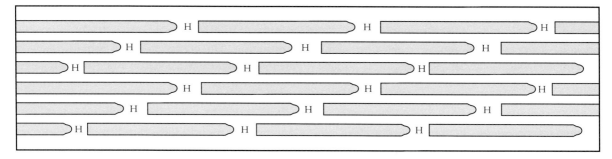

Figure 1.11 Diagram to show the staggered arrangement of the collagen molecules with areas between (hole zones, H). These intermolecular gaps give collagen fibres a characteristic banded pattern when viewed by electron microscopy.

It is not possible to detect sites of calcification in decalcified routine histological sections of bone. In undecalcified sections stained with toluidine blue, thionine or similar methods, the calcification front between osteoid and mineralised bone is a metachromatic purple colour. This method is, however, unreliable as a means of showing where mineralisation is taking place. The most satisfactory technique is to administer a fluorochrome, which is incorporated at sites of active calcification. In humans, the tetracyclines are ethical to use. A much wider range of fluorescent labels is available for studying bone in experimental animals. Visualisation of these labels is by ultraviolet light microscopy.

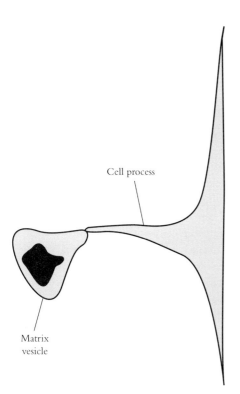

Cell process

Matrix
vesicle

Figure 1.12 Diagram to represent the formation of a matrix vesicle by the pinching off of a long process from the cell membrane. The matrix vesicle acts as a focal point for the concentration of calcium in the process of calcification.

BONE RESORPTION

Calcium homoeostasis does not occur by simple physico-chemical processes but requires the activity of cells, namely resorption of bone by osteoclasts and subsequent replacement by osteoblasts of matrix suitable for calcium deposition. Under physiological conditions, cellular activity is responsible not only for the fulfilment of the metabolic role of bone but also for the maintenance of the skeleton as a supporting structure that is constantly remodelling to suit altering conditions. When bone turnover is low and an adequate supply of calcium is available, changes in calcium levels in the blood and extracellular fluid can be restored by renal and intestinal mechanisms. Physiological control of calcium homoeostasis is mainly through parathyroid hormone, closely linked to vitamin D. Calcitonin is a specific hormonal inhibitor of resorption. Production of a locally low pH is likely to be the mechanism by which bone mineral is removed. Hydrogen ion production from carbonic anhydrase and/or an ATP-driven proton pump in the ruffled border is the likely mechanism, although lactate and citrate may also play a role. The residual unmineralised bone matrix after calcium dissolution then has to be degraded, and extracellular proteinases such as collagenase and other metalloproteinases, as well as lysosomal acid hydrolases, are responsible for this.

REMODELLING OF BONE

Changes that occur in bone structure during development, childhood and adult life comprise growth and initial modelling, remodelling in response to altered mechanical needs, and changes that contribute to the effectiveness of ion exchange between blood and bone. Remodelling is the term used for the continual process of change in response to physiological (mechanical or metabolic) needs. A close relationship exists between bone removal and formation, cellular activity being coupled in what are called the basic multicellular units (BMUs), also sometimes called the bone remodelling unit (BRU) or bone structural unit (BSU) (Frost, 1976; Parfitt, 1982). Remodelling in BMUs follows the sequence *activation–resorption–formation*. In cortical bone the advancing front of osteoclasts forms a structure which is termed the cutting cone. Bone formation follows in the wake of this resorptive activity, with the cells forming the filling cone. The same coupling occurs on the surface of cancellous bone in which it is usual to see osteoclasts in Howship's lacunae, with adjacent osteoblasts filling in the recent resorbed surface defect. Under normal conditions, bone mass remains constant with the rate of osteoclastic resorption equal to the rate of new bone formation. Dissociation of these rates (uncoupling) results in pathological conditions. The coupling of bone cell function is believed to be mediated by soluble chemical mediators, the cytokines. These comprise a group of low molecular weight, usually glycosylated, peptides, which are produced by most cells, notably leucocytes and osteoblasts in the context of bone, and tend to have overlapping biological activities. Bone cell activity is known to be modified by cytokines. A recent source of information on cytokines in bone is provided by Gowen (1992). It is not proposed that a description of this complex area be attempted here. The known effects of some of the cytokines on bone are discussed in Chapter 4.

Electrical potentials can be recorded on the surfaces of bone when they are loaded and changes in bone in response to altered mechanical factors are considered to occur as a result of the effects of these electrical potentials. Stress-generated potential (SGP) is the term used to describe the occurrence of electrical potentials in a material when stress or external forces are applied to it. When a long bone is subject to bending forces along its length, the concave surface is under maximum compression and is electronegative, whereas the convex surface, under maximum tension, is electropositive. Electronegative potentials that are not stress generated are associated with bone formation both at the growth plate and in a healing fracture. More details about endogenous electrical signals in bone may be found elsewhere (Pollack, 1984; Revell, 1986). Cell viability is necessary for non-stress-generated electrical potentials but not for SGPs. SGPs are thought to arise from streaming potentials created by interstitial fluid movement when bones are deformed during loading. Electrical effects and cellular mechanisms, including chemical messages (cytokines, see above) to influence cells, both play a part in the alteration of bone structure in response to altered physical requirements. It was Julius Wolff who first suggested that the functional requirements of a bone determined its structure and who introduced the concept of remodelling of bone to produce an appropriate gross configuration and internal architecture. Wolff's law is still important for a proper understanding of changes occurring in bone.

BLOOD SUPPLY OF BONE

Although aspects of the blood supply to bone are dealt with elsewhere in this book, a brief account will be given here, because a proper understanding of this subject is important in the appreciation of changes that occur in different parts of the skeleton, for example the sites of osteomyelitis and secondary malignancy. The circulation may be divided into afferent, efferent and intermediate parts (Rhinelander, 1980). The afferent system comprises vessels derived from the principal nutrient artery, the periosteal arterioles, which are multiple, and the metaphyseal arteries, which are also multiple. The nutrient artery passes straight through the cortex of the bone without branching and divides in the intertrabecular medullary cavity, sending out descending and ascending branches. These in turn divide into smaller vessels which supply the bone marrow and endosteal surfaces of the bone. Endosteal arteries send off vessels that enter the cortex in the Volkmann canals. Arteries in the intermuscular septae outside the bone give off branches to supply the periosteum and also penetrate the cortex to provide vascularisation to its outer third. The periosteal and endosteal derived vessels anastomose within the cortex. The branches of vessels reaching the end of the bone, which are derived from the nutrient artery, are also met, in anastomosis, by vessels entering on all sides of the metaphysis from the outside of the bone. In the child, the arterioles turn back to enter venous channels, although some vessels penetrate to the epiphyseal region. These vessels crossing into the epiphysis are decreased in number when the epiphyseal ossification centre forms and do not become re-established until closure of the growth plate.

The intermediate parts of the osseous circulation comprise the interconnections between metaphyseal and epiphyseal, and between endosteal and periosteal, vessels. The efferent system comprises an accompanying reversed direction system of veins which eventually collect into a large exiting vein passing through the cortex like the nutrient artery. Further details of the blood supply of bone are available from standard large textbooks of anatomy. A brief mention will be made only of the blood supply to the femoral head, which is still considered by some to be predominantly derived from vessels entering through the ligamentum teres. Although such arteries are patent in a proportion of cases, they supply a relatively small part of the bone. The major sources of supply are through nutrient arteries penetrating the bone on the femoral neck a little below the head–neck junction. There are usually up to six such arteries of large size superiorly and several small arteries entering inferiorly. Radiological studies using radio-opaque contrast medium and injection of vessels (Wertheimer and Fernandes-Lopes, 1971), and our own unpublished serial sectioning histological studies, show that these vessels branch many times as they pass upwards within the intertrabecular space to supply the whole of the femoral head. This vascular supply is, of course, of considerable significance where there is a fracture of the neck of the femur which then results in necrosis of the femoral head.

REFERENCES

Beighton P. *Inherited Disorders of the Skeleton*, 2nd edn. Edinburgh, Churchill Livingstone, 1978.

Frost HM. A method of analysis of trabecular bone dynamics. In: Meunier PJ (ed.) *Bone Histomorphometry*. 2nd International Workshop. Paris: Armour Montague, 1976: 445–476.

Glimcher MJ. Composition, structure and organization of bone and other mineralized tissues and the mechanisms of calcification. In: Aurbach GD (ed.) *Handbook of Physiology – Endocrinology VII*. Baltimore: Williams and Wilkins, 1976: 25–116.

Gowen M. *Cytokines and Bone Metabolism*. London: CRC Press, 1992.

Owen M. Bone cell differentiation. In: Dixon AStJ, Russell RGG, Stamp TCB (eds) *Osteoporosis. A Multidisciplinary Problem*. Royal Society of Medicine International Congress and Symposium Series No. 55. London: Academic Press and Royal Society of Medicine, 1983: 25–29.

Parfitt AM. The coupling of bone formation to bone resorption: a critical analysis of the concept and of its relevance to the pathogenesis of osteoporosis. *Metab Bone Dis Relat Res* 1982; **4**: 1–6.

Pollack SR. Bioelectrical properties of bone. Endogenous electrical signals. *Orthop Clin North Am* 1984; **15**: 3–14.

Revell PA. *Pathology of Bone*. Berlin: Springer, 1986.

Rhinelander FW. The blood supply of the limb bones. In: Owen R, Goodfellow J, Bullough P (eds) *The Scientific Foundations of Orthopaedics and Traumatology*. London: Heinemann, 1980: 126–151.

Salisbury JR, Woods CG, Byers PD. *Diseases of Bones and Joints*. London: Chapman and Hall, 1994.

Wertheimer LG, Fernandes-Lopes SDC. Arterial supply of the femoral head. *J Bone Joint Surg [Am]* 1971; **53A**: 545–556.

2

Blood Flow and Transport in Bone

Ian D McCarthy

INTRODUCTION

Orthopaedic surgery has a different emphasis to some other branches of surgery, in that it is normally more concerned with the functional reconstruction of structures than with ablation. In addition, many of the operative procedures involve the insertion of an artificial material into the skeleton and produce degrees of vascular damage, as occurs, for example, in reaming and insertion of an intramedullary nail. Therefore, it is important to understand how to reconstruct the tissue and how to maintain its viability. There are many unusual features about bone that make it an interesting tissue to study, and there are also many practical reasons for the investigation of bone blood flow by orthopaedic surgeons.

The anatomy of the vasculature in bone is complex, with multiple arterial inputs and venous outflows for a single bone, and frequent anastamoses between these systems. This means that the tissue is difficult to study from a research aspect, but rather more adaptable and forgiving from a surgical perspective. Therefore, a knowledge of the basic organisation of the vascular system in bone helps to understand how reconstructive procedures may be attempted, whilst maintaining viable bone.

While it is appreciated that the structure of bone is related to its mechanical function, it will be suggested in this chapter that the structure of bone is just as important a factor in transport. The vascular tree in bone can be ordered according to size: (1) great vessels; (2) conduit vessels; (3) capillaries; (4) lacunar–canalicular system; and (5) microcanalicular system. This structured porosity, together with the intramedullary pressure, could have a role in controlling transport within the bone, and any modification of this structure would have important consequences for transport, as well as mechanics.

Another important point to be emphasised will be the biochemical importance of endothelial cells in normal and pathological bone. Endothelial cells have been shown to produce substances, such as endothelin, prostacyclin and nitric oxide, that act in a paracrine manner on adjacent cells in bone; additionally, osteoblasts have been shown to produce vascular endothelial growth factors.

Therefore, the vascular system in bone can be regarded as having both physiological and pathological practical significance for orthopaedic surgeons.

ANATOMY OF THE VASCULATURE IN BONE

Appendicular skeleton

Knowledge of the anatomical arrangement of vessels in the skeleton comes from detailed studies by Murray Brookes (1971) and others using techniques of vascular casting. In this section, the general organisation of the blood supply to bone will be discussed. For a detailed atlas of the blood supply from a surgical point of view, the reader should consult the recent atlas by Crock (1996).

The typical organisation of circulation in a long bone is illustrated in *Figures 2.1* and *2.2*. For the cortex of bone, the main supply is the nutrient artery. The nutrient artery traverses the cortex at a very acute angle, and does not branch within the cortex. In the medullary cavity, the nutrient artery divides into ascending and descending medullary arteries. Vessels radiate from these medullary arteries out to the cortex. In normal bone, there is centrifugal flow through cortical bone (Brookes, 1971). Exchange vessels within the haversian canals are parallel to the axis of the bone, and these vessels drain to venules on the periosteal surface of bone.

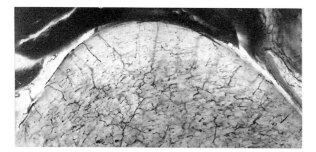

Figure 2.1 Axial section of the shaft of the femur of a young adult, illustrating the periosteal and nutrient artery contributions to cortical bone. From Crock (1996), with permission.

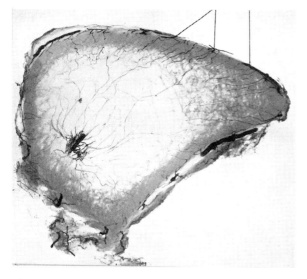

Figure 2.2 Axial section from the upper tibia of an adult (aged over 80 years) showing nutrient artery and periosteal arteries supplying the bone. From Crock (1996), with permission.

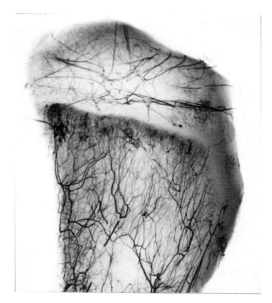

Figure 2.3 Metaphyseal supply of the upper tibia of a child (mid-sagittal section). From Crock (1996), with permission.

depends on the pathophysiological requirement, and the periosteum is acutely capable of responding to injury to the nutrient supply (Reichert et al, 1995) (see also section on vascular response to trauma). The extensive vascularity of the periosteum illustrates the need to maintain periosteal blood supply wherever possible, and the possible ischaemic consequences to subperiosteal bone if this supply is compromised, for example beneath a compression plate.

The arterial supply of the metaphysis is illustrated in *Figure 2.3*, which shows a mid-sagittal section of the upper tibia of a child.

Axial skeleton

For a detailed description of the precise anatomical arrangement in individual bones of the skeleton, the reader is referred to specific textbooks on the subject. However, as has been pointed out by Brookes (1971), 'The pattern of vascularisation comprising a principal nutrient artery in a central position, many small nutrients in the periphery, a capillary net in compact bone substance, and profuse sinusoids in the contained marrow, does not depart significantly from the vascular organisation of a typical long bone.' It therefore seems that this general vascular arrangement is an intrinsic aspect

The periosteum is very vascular, and the outer shell of the cortex is normally supplied by arterioles arising from the periosteum, but in senescent bone and vascularly insufficient specimens the periosteal supply penetrates more extensively and deeply into the cortex (Brookes, 1971). It can be seen from *Figures 2.1* and *2.2* that some periosteal vessels appear to penetrate deeply into the cortex. There are extensive anastamoses between the medullary and periosteal circulations (Trias and Fery, 1979; Skawina et al, 1994), giving an anatomical basis for a flexible blood flow response. It has been suggested that the direction of blood flow in the diaphyseal cortex of bone structure, whatever the particular form of the bone.

Microvascular structure in bone

In cortical bone, capillaries are found within the haversian canals, and are therefore oriented parallel to the long axis of long bones. Capillary structure can be classified as either continuous, fenestrated or discontinuous. Descriptions of capillary structure in dog cortical bone have been made. These studies showed that haversian canals are typically 50–70 μm in diameter, and these canals contained one or two capillaries. The capillaries were continuous in structure, and surrounded with a continuous basement membrane 400–600 Å thick. Nerve fibres were observed in Schwann cells beneath the basement membrane (Cooper et al, 1966).

Microvascular structure in marrow

Capillaries in fatty marrow have also been shown to have a continuous structure, but in haematopoetic marrow the capillaries appear to be discontinuous.

MEASUREMENT OF BONE BLOOD FLOW

Measurement of blood flow to the skeleton is a difficult technical problem and, although several techniques have been used in the experimental animal, there is no generally accepted technique for the measurement of bone blood flow in the clinical situation. The problems of measuring blood flow that are particular to bone are:

- There are over 200 separate bones in the skeleton.
- Each bone has multiple arterial inputs and venous outflows.
- Each bone is heterogeneous, comprising varying proportions of cortical bone, cancellous bone and marrow (both haematopoetic and fatty).

Because of this heterogeneity of the tissue, it is also important to specify precisely the bone or region of bone that is being measured, and this problem accounts for some of the discrepancies between values published in the literature. From a practical orthopaedic perspective,

techniques to measure regional blood flow are normally more informative than determination of total skeletal blood flow.

Several techniques have been used in experimental research on bone blood flow, but most of these are invasive if absolute values of blood flow are required, and are inappropriate for use in a clinical setting. Most of the techniques do involve the use of radioactively labelled tracers.

Research techniques

Isotope fractionation

If an injected tracer is extracted completely during a single passage through the microcirculation, not only in the tissue of interest but in all tissues of the body, then the distribution of tracer within the tissue is proportional to the fraction of the cardiac output going to that tissue.

A special case of the indicator fractionation technique is the use of radioactively labelled microspheres (*Figure 2.4*). This is now generally accepted as the most appropriate technique for experimental studies of bone blood flow. Microspheres are resin particles of uniform cross-section, typically 15 μm in diameter. These are injected into the left ventricle, which has sufficient turbulence to mix the microspheres uniformly in the blood. The microspheres are trapped in the microcirculation, and the number of microspheres trapped per unit weight of tissue is proportional to the proportion of the cardiac output supplying that unit of tissue. If blood is withdrawn at a known rate from a reference artery, then the blood flow to the tissue can be calculated from the equation:

$$\text{Blood flow} = \frac{\text{Microspheres in tissue}}{\text{Microspheres in blood sample}} \times \text{Withdrawal rate}$$

Microspheres are labelled with a radioactive tracer, and so the amount of radioactivity in the tissue and blood samples is proportional to the number of microspheres. Microspheres can be labelled with a variety of isotopes, and so sequential injections can be performed to measure blood flow at different times. The size of the tissue sample that can be investigated is limited by the necessity to inject sufficient microspheres into the ventricle so that the number in the tissue sample is enough to obtain statistical

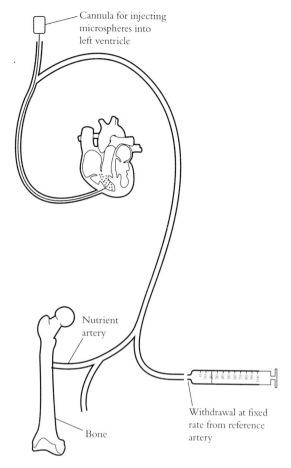

Cannula for injecting microspheres into left ventricle

Nutrient artery

Withdrawal at fixed rate from reference artery

Bone

Figure 2.4   Principle of measurement of bone blood flow using radioactive microspheres; this technique has provided most of the quantitative data on bone blood flow.

precision in the measurement; it is normally assumed that 400 microspheres are required per sample, although experiments have suggested that as few as 150 microspheres per sample can provide sufficient precision (Li et al, 1989).

It is obvious from the description of the technique that it is highly invasive, and suitable only for experimental research purposes. However, this technique has been used extensively in research investigations, and data from microsphere experiments provide most of the information about quantitative values of bone blood flow.

Clearance techniques

Clearance of bone-seeking tracers were one of the earliest techniques used for the estimation of bone blood flow,

when ^{45}Ca was used by Frederickson et al (1955). The technique is based on the Fick principle, that the rate at which tracer accumulates in bone is the difference between the input and output rates, and that the overall deposition in tissue can be obtained from averaging the input and output over time. In principle, any tracer could be used. However, the complexity of venous outflow from bone makes collection of venous blood extremely difficult. Therefore, it has been usual to use tracers with high affinity for bone, and to assume either that these are completely extracted by bone or that the extraction is high and a fixed proportion of the input. Isotopes that have been used include ^{45}Ca, ^{85}Sr and ^{99m}Tc-labelled methylene diphosphonate.

Hydrogen washout

This is a particular application of the washout technique using hydrogen gas. It requires the introduction of a fine platinum electrode into the tissue under investigation. An electrochemical reaction occurs between the platinum and hydrogen, and the measured voltage is proportional to the hydrogen concentration. If the subject breathes some hydrogen, then the washout is proportional to flow. This technique has been used to measure flow in trabecular and cortical bone, and to investigate the contribution of the vertebral endplate on nutrition of the intervertebral disc (Whiteside et al, 1977).

Clinical techniques

Fluorine-18

Fluorine-18 was first used to estimate blood flow in bone by van Dyke and co-workers (1965), and it is a particular use of the clearance technique described above. It had been suggested that fluorine was completely extracted during a single passage through bone. This result has been used to develop techniques to measure bone blood flow by measuring uptake in bone with imaging devices (γ camera, positron emission tomography) and the rate of clearance from plasma. Experiments by Wootton (1974) seemed to confirm that ^{18}F was extracted during a single passage through bone, but later experiments refuted this (Lemon et al, 1980; Tothill and Hooper, 1984). Assuming 100% extraction, Wootton and colleagues went on to develop a technique for estimating overall skeletal blood flow based on measurements of plasma concentration of

[18]F (Green et al, 1987). Apart from the obvious limitations concerning the validity of the assumptions, the technique as described does not measure blood flow to local areas of the skeleton, which is often of more interest in orthopaedic applications.

Bone scanning

Radionuclide bone scanning, using diphosphonates, is now a routine procedure with several applications in orthopaedic surgery. The kinetics of diphosphonate uptake in bone have been investigated by Hughes and co-workers (1977). A quantitative approach to routine bone scanning with [90m]Tc-methylene diphosphonate to assess regional blood flow was described by Deutsch and co-workers (1981). Counts were collected immediately after injection of the tracer, and time–activity curves were plotted for arterial, venous and blood pool phases. Data from each phase were then integrated and divided by the timespan for the phase to give average total counts per unit time. From these values, ratios for normal and diseased tissue were calculated to assess whether blood flow to the diseased bone was decreased or increased. Using this technique, Deutsch and colleagues were able to demonstrate, in a group of patients with Legg–Perthes disease, that measurable flow changes could precede changes in the static image, which in turn would precede structural changes observable in radiographic images. This technique is semiquantitative, in that it does not provide values for blood flow in absolute flow units, but it does provide a quantitative way of determining relative perfusion that provides clinically useful information.

Washout of diffusible tracers

This technique depends on saturating the tissue with a readily diffusible tracer and measuring the rate of removal from the tissue. If a sufficiently diffusible tracer is used, the blood flow is the limiting factor in removal from the tissue. Complications in quantifying blood flow can arise from recirculation of the tracer and from heterogeneity of blood flow within the tissue. In an ideal situation, washout will be in the form of simple exponential decay, with blood flow being proportional to the exponent. If a radioactive tracer is used, then washout can be estimated with an external detector.

Lahtinen et al (1981) used ^{133}Xe to measure blood flow in the femoral head. Xenon is lipid soluble, so cell membranes do not pose an appreciable barrier, and it is relatively insoluble in water, so that it is readily released during passage through the lungs, minimising recirculation.

Laser Doppler flowmetry

Laser Doppler flowmetry is a technique that is very popular in the assessment of skin perfusion. It depends on the reflection of laser light from moving red blood cells. The change in frequency of the reflected light is proportional to the velocity of the cells, and the entire reflected signal can be used to estimate flux within a tissue region. The penetration of the laser light is typically 1–2 mm but, because the volume of tissue under consideration cannot be estimated accurately, it is normal to record the data in terms of flux. The technique is sensitive to movement artefacts, and also to position. The optimum use is to place the probe in position and monitor the relative change in flux in response to some form of intervention. The practical advantages of laser Doppler flowmetry are that it can provide very good temporal assessment of flow changes, but only in a small volume of tissue. Because of the low penetration of the laser light, the probe must be placed on to the tissue being investigated. Therefore, its main use in orthopaedics has been in intraoperative assessment of blood flow (Swiontkowski et al, 1987; Hughes and McCarthy, 1995). It is a useful technique for plastic surgeons in assessing the vascularity of tissue flaps for compound fractures.

Positron emission tomography (PET)

PET is a promising technique for quantitative measurement of blood flow in the clinical situation. Unfortunately, because of the degree of sophistication (i.e. expense) of hardware required to perform these measurements, it is unlikely to become a routine clinical technique.

The basis of PET imaging (*Figure 2.5*) is that positrons (positive electrons), which are emitted by certain types of radionuclide, are absorbed by interaction with an electron, resulting in the simultaneous emission of two γ rays. The two γ rays travel at $180°$ to one another, and can be detected by two photomultiplier detectors opposite each other. The source of the radiation will then be along a line joining the two detectors. Using an array of detectors, this technique allows much more precise spatial

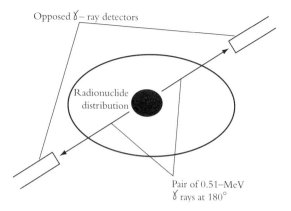

Figure 2.5 Illustration of the principles of imaging using positron emission tomography. Only pairs of γ rays detected simultaneously in opposite detectors are recorded. For clarity, only one pair of detectors is shown; a collimated array of detectors allows reconstruction of the distribution of radioactivity with good resolution, despite relatively well-vascularised soft tissue overlying bone.

resolution of internal isotope distribution than other imaging techniques. Activity in overlying tissues can then be separated from activity arising from bone. Using the latest generation of PET scanners, the resolution of the technique can approach 6 mm.

Only a certain class of radionuclide decays by positron emission. Both ^{11}C and ^{15}O emit positrons, as does ^{18}F. These radionuclides have a short half-life, and it is therefore necessary for the PET systems to be near to the cyclotron producing the radionuclides. The carbon and oxygen nuclides can be used in conjunction with radio-chemistry techniques to produce radioactively labelled molecules, allowing the imaging of many physiological processes apart from blood flow.

Radioactively labelled water has been used to measure blood flow in bone, and the effect of fracture on blood flow to the tibia (Ashcroft et al, 1992). The authors found that there was an increase in blood flow at the fracture site as early as 24 hours after fracture, and that at 2 weeks the peak blood flow response was as much as 14 times normal blood flow. This result is in agreement with that obtained with the microsphere technique in animals (see below).

Normal blood flow values

Most of these data are obtained from experimental studies using radioactive microspheres. There is evidence of

differences in flow between long bones; for example, flow in the humerus is greatest, compared with that in the radius, ulna, femur and tibia (Li et al, 1989). Typical values of blood flow in canine cortical and trabecular bone are 5 and $20 \, \mathrm{ml \, min^{-1} \, 100 \, g^{-1}}$ respectively, although these values can vary by up to 50% depending on the particular bone being assessed.

Quantitative measurements of blood flow have provided supplementary information for the debate about the direction of cortical blood flow, and have shown it to be centrifugal. By occluding the nutrient artery, it can be shown that the nutrient artery supplies at least 62% of the normal diaphyseal cortex (Tothill et al, 1987; Willans, 1987), and recently it has been demonstrated that the periosteum contributes at least 20% (Kowalski et al, 1996).

VASCULAR REACTIVITY OF BONE

Perivascular innervation of bone

Bone and periosteum are innervated by both sympathetic and sensory nerves. As well as noradrenergic sympathetic fibres, peptidergic nerves containing substance P (SP), calcitonin gene-related peptide (CGRP), vasoactive intestinal peptide (VIP) and neuropeptide Y have also been described (Bjurholm et al, 1988). Innervation is more dense near the epiphyseal plate, bone marrow and the periosteum. Many SP and CGRP immunoreactive fibres were observed in association with blood vessels in both periosteum and cortical bone. It has been shown that CGRP is a very potent vasodilator. During fracture repair, periosteal CGRP-containing nerve fibres are very actively proliferating elements, and it has been suggested that vascular control and stimulation of angiogenesis is a major function of CGRP during the fracture healing process (Hukkanen et al, 1993).

Adrenergic control

The most precise measurements of vascular reactivity of bone have been performed in experimental preparations that perfuse the nutrient supply of a long bone, and in which perfusion pressure is monitored continuously to investigate changes in vascular resistance (Dreissens and Vanhoutte, 1979). This technique allows precise physiological assessment of changes in the vascular reactivity of bone as a whole, but does not provide an insight into the anatomical distribution of relative responses, for example major vessels or arterioles, cortical or trabecular bone, or marrow. Using this technique, the response of bone to a wide range of vasoactive substances has been investigated by several groups. It has been shown that, in general, the vasculature in bone responds to most vasoconstrictor and vasodilator substances; however, comparing the vaso-reactive responses in bone with those in other tissues, it has been proposed that bone is relatively hypersensitive to vasoconstrictors and relatively hyposensitive to vaso-dilators (Brinker et al, 1990).

Recently, experiments have been performed on isolated arteries obtained from both animal and human bone. These studies indicate that α_1 receptors are primarily responsible for the constrictive adrenergic response in bone (Lundgaard et al, 1996).

Endothelium-dependent control

Increasing interest has been directed towards the role of the endothelium in controlling vascular tone. In 1980, it was demonstrated that the endothelium was required to produce a vasodilator response from acetylcholine, and it was proposed that a factor, endothelium-derived relaxing factor (EDRF), was released from the endothelium in response to acetylcholine (Furchgott and Zawadzki, 1980). EDRF has subsequently been identified as nitric oxide (NO) (Palmer et al, 1987). Vasodilatation to NO has been demonstrated in bone preparations (Davis and Wood, 1992), and release of NO is diminished significantly by prolonged periods of ischaemia–reperfusion. It is possible that endothelial dysfunction could be an important factor in failure of vascularised bone grafts. In addition, NO could be an important factor in the role of the vascular system in regulating bone biology (Collin-Osdoby, 1995). It has been demonstrated that NO is released from osteoblasts in response to fluid shear (Klein-Nulend et al, 1995), and it is also released after mechanical stimulation of bone for just 15 minutes (Pitsillides et al, 1995).

TRANSCAPILLARY EXCHANGE

Indicator dilution studies

Many studies of the physiology of transcapillary exchange in bone have been published by Kelly's group at the

Orthopaedic Research Laboratories in the Mayo Clinic. Most of the experiments used the technique of multiple tracer indicator dilution. These physiological measurements confirmed the anatomical findings of continuous endothelium, and defined the relationship between blood flow and uptake of bone-seeking tracers in both normal and osteotomised bone (Kelly, 1984).

Transport across the endothelium is by passive diffusion, and at normal physiological flow rates blood flow is not the limiting factor in the rate of uptake of bone tracers such as ^{99m}Tc-labelled methylene diphosphonate.

EXTRAVASCULAR TRANSPORT

Lacuna–canalicula network

Typically, an osteon within cortical bone is approximately 200 μm in diameter. This means that osteocytes within the bone matrix can be up to 100 μm from a capillary. Cortical bone has a very extensive network of channels, allowing communication between plasma and bone matrix. Canaliculi, approximately 0.1 μm in diameter, radiate from the haversian canal and form a complex network connecting osteocytes with the haversian canal and other osteocytes. Radiating from the canaliculi are submicroscopic interfibrillar spaces of bone matrix. The extent of these networks is so great that it has been estimated that the surface area of the canalicular system is approximately 250 mm^2 per mm^3, and that the interfibrillar spaces represent an exchange area of the order of 35 000 mm^2 per mm^3. It has been speculated that, because these distances are relatively large in microvascular terms, diffusion may not be sufficient to supply these cells and that a more rapid turnover of interstitial fluid in bone aids the process of cell nutrition.

The vascular system, canalicular network and bone cells comprise the fluid space of bone. There are precise measurements of the fluid composition of bone. In fact, in mature cortical bone the fluid space amounts to about 30% by volume of the cortex. The distribution of fluid spaces between vascular, cellular and extravascular–extracellular is illustrated in *Figure 2.6*.

It is interesting to do some simple arithmetic, combining these fluid space data with blood flow data presented earlier. Although blood flow to bone is relatively low in absolute terms, it is very high if expressed in terms of cellular mass of the tissue. This suggests that blood flow to

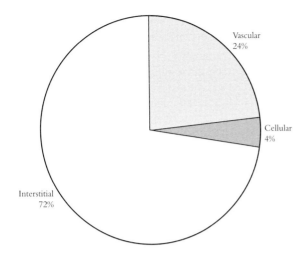

Vascular
24%

Cellular
4%

Interstitial
72%

Figure 2.6   Distribution of fluid spaces in bone between vascular, cellular and extravascular–extracellular spaces.

bone may not have the sole requirement of meeting the metabolic needs of bone cells, and that an important aspect of blood flow is in the homoeostatic control of plasma calcium concentrations, as suggested by Reeve and colleagues (1988).

Extravascular protein movement

Intramedullary tissue fluid pressures were measured in dogs and shown to be unusually high, indicating a transcortical pressure gradient that parallels the general direction of blood flow in the cortical diaphysis, i.e. from endosteum to periosteum (Wilkes and Visscher, 1975). Experimental evidence suggesting that convective flow may contribute to the nutrition of osteocytes comes mainly from studies on the rate of labelled protein molecules through bone. First, the rate at which these molecules move through bone is reported to be too rapid to occur by diffusion only, and second, the appearance of ferritin moving radially from haversian canals has been shown to have a discrete boundary, more typical of bulk volume flow than of a diffusive process (Montgomery et al, 1988). Using mathematical modelling, it has been argued that mechanical loading would enhance perfusion and aid nutrition of osteocytes (Piekarski and Munro, 1977), but Yang and McCarthy (1992) argued that the nutritional requirements of osteocytes were unknown, but presumably relatively low, and that mechanical load may not be required. However, there does appear to be

pressure gradient driving macromolecules through the interstitial fluid of bone.

Control of mineral fluxes

Although the experiments with plasma proteins suggest very rapid and easy transport from blood to bone, other studies have shown that there is a certain degree of control of mineral ion fluxes into and out of bone (McCarthy and Hughes, 1986).

INTERACTIONS BETWEEN THE VASCULAR SYSTEM AND BONE

Endothelial interactions with bone

It has often been recognised that angiogenesis precedes osteogenesis in many practical situations, and this empirical observation has led to the suggestion that the blood vessels play an active role in the process of osteogenesis, and not just a passive role of providing substrates for the process of osteogenesis (Trueta, 1963). Recent laboratory studies have given further direct support to this hypothesis, and also suggested a role for the endothelium in normal skeletal homoeostasis.

Villanueva and Nimni (1990) implanted rat fetal calvarial cells and endothelial cells isolated from rat liver or bovine aorta into diffusion chambers placed subcutaneously in rats. The amount of mineralisation and alkaline phosphatase activity was significantly higher in chambers containing both calvarial and endothelial cells, compared with chambers containing either calvarial or endothelial cells. Endothelial cells alone seemed to enhance angiogenesis around the diffusion chambers. Cell culture experiments have demonstrated that isolated microvessel cells (both endothelium and pericytes) have a mitogenic effect on osteoblast-enriched calvarial cells which is mediated by soluble factors (Jones et al, 1995). It was also shown that the microvessel cells produced a prolonged reduction in the expression of markers of the osteoblast phenotype.

Recent advances in vascular biology show that the endothelium is not a passive barrier between blood and vascular smooth muscle, but an active tissue in its own right, releasing vasoconstrictor and vasodilator substances, and secreting other immunoregulatory factors, and also being a target for circulating hormones and local regulatory factors. It has been shown that vascular endothelial cells produce potential modulators of bone activity such as fibroblast growth factor, interleukins 1 and 6, colony-stimulating factors, prostacyclin, endothelin 1 and NO. Vascular endothelial cells cloned from fetal bovine bone have been shown to respond to parathyroid hormone, progesterone, oestrogen, insulin–like growth factors, platelet-derived growth factor, basic fibroblast factor and endothelial cell growth factor. It has therefore been argued that bone vascular endothelial cells should be considered to be an important part of the bone cell communication network (Collin-Osdoby, 1995).

Venous pressure and bone formation

Several studies have indicated that manipulation of the vascular system to bone can stimulate bone formation and increase the rate of fracture repair. The first reported observation was by Ambroise Pare in 1840, and there have been regular reports in the literature since then.

It has been shown by Kelly and Bronk (1990) that the application of a venous tourniquet proximal to the knee, with a skin pressure of 30 mmHg, can stimulate periosteal new bone formation in the tibia in puppies in 7 days, and by Kruse and Kelly (1974) that it can increase the rate of fracture repair. It was shown that the venous tourniquet increased intramedullary pressure. Direct increase of intramedullary pressure by infusion through a paediatric cannula has been shown to increase the rate of periosteal bone formation in immature goats (Welch et al, 1993).

Interestingly, recent data on bone mass changes during space flight are now also providing data to demonstrate an association between changes in bone mass and pressure changes. Normally, while standing on the surface of the earth, there is a gradient of pressures within the capillaries, the lowest pressures being in the head, and the highest in the feet. When weightless (or when lying down), this gradient disappears, and capillary pressures are uniform throughout the body. Thus, during weightlessness capillary pressures in the head increase, pressures in the feet decrease, and those at the level of the heart remain unchanged. Measurement of bone density after prolonged exposure to microgravity shows that bone is lost mainly from the lower limbs, there is little change in bone mass in the trunk, but bones above the level of the heart increase in mass (Oganov et al, 1992). This is also supported by ground-based studies to simulate weightlessness.

The mechanisms to explain this are not fully under-

stood as yet. It has been shown that circulatory pressure gradients can give rise to streaming potentials (Otter et al, 1990). It is possible that bone responds to mechanical load by some consequence of strain, such as shear forces produced by fluid movement, or by potentials generated by fluid movement, and it is interesting to speculate that the response to pressure changes may be acting via the same mechanism as mechanical loads. However, potentials generated by circulatory pressures are much less than those generated by mechanical loads (Otter et al, 1990). It could be that pH changes, or release of NO by shear forces on osteocytes, could also be involved.

VASCULAR RESPONSE IN FRACTURE REPAIR

Trauma to a bone will always produce a certain amount of vascular damage to the bone. The degree of damage will depend on the degree of injury to the bone. Normally, there will be disruption to the nutrient artery, and there will also be significant vascular damage to the bone if there is a large degree of associated soft tissue damage.

Vascular response to fractures

Measurement of blood flow changes after fracture has been performed in animal models (Wallace et al, 1991), using microsphere techniques, and clinically using PET scanning (Ashcroft et al, 1992). Blood flow is increased by a factor of about 10 at 2 weeks after a fracture or osteotomy. Blood flow decreases after that, but remains raised for many weeks afterwards.

Serum levels of angiogenic factors have been shown to be raised following fractures. Endothelial cell-stimulating angiogenesis factor (ESAF) shows a biphasic response in a normal osteotomy, with peak serum levels occurring at days 4 and 9 after osteotomy, but with a delayed and reduced response in devascularised osteotomies (Wallace et al, 1995). Vascular endothelial growth factor (VEGF) has been observed in the early callus of fractures (Warner and Andrew, 1997).

Recently, nitric oxide synthase (NOS) isoforms have been shown at the fracture site of an experimental model (Corbett et al, 1997). This is, potentially, of major importance as NO has been shown to be not only a potent vasodilator and potential angiogenic stimulus, but also an important second messenger in bone cell metabolism. The demonstration of endothelial NOS in blood vessels around the fracture site suggests that these vessels are active in the production of NO, thereby causing vasodilatation. The NO generated may then also influence the callus formation and ensuing repair process.

Effects of fracture fixation devices

Considering the variety of approaches to fracture fixation that are available, for example conservative treatment, external fixation devices, internal plates and intramedullary nailing with or without reaming, it is clear from the complex vascular anatomy of bone that these will all have different effects on local blood flow.

Several studies were performed at the Mayo Clinic. Comparison of an intramedullary nail, external fixation device and internal compression plate was made in a canine tibia model at times ranging from 4 hours to 90 days after osteotomy. In general, fractures fixed with intramedullary nails had the lowest blood flow, although this was never statistically significant for the fracture as a whole, but was significant at 4 hours and 14 days at the endosteal cortex (Smith et al, 1990).

Recent studies from our laboratory have investigated the response of the intact and osteotomised tibia to intramedullary reaming, using the radioactive microsphere technique. By using this technique, the response of the periosteum could be separated from that of the underlying cortical bone by removing the periosteum from the cortex before measuring the radioactivity in both cortex and periosteum separately. Reaming alone did not result in an overall acute decrease in cortical blood flow, whereas the blood flow to the periosteum increased by a factor of six (Reichert et al, 1995) (*Figure 2.7*). Osteotomy to the tibia did result in a decrease of flow to the cortex, but when an osteotomised tibia was reamed there was no further significant decrease in bone blood flow. These data demonstrate the importance of the periosteum to bone blood flow and the functional anastamoses between the periosteal and nutrient supplies to bone. Further studies need to be performed to investigate whether this periosteal response is only compensation for loss of flow to the cortex from other sources, or whether it represents an

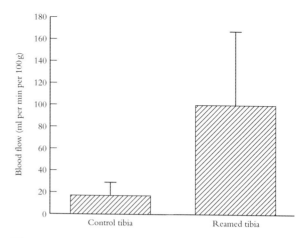

Figure 2.7   Changes in blood flow to the cortex and periosteum as a result of intramedullary reaming and osteotomy. From Reichert et al (1995), with permission.

early indication of the periosteal reaction required for fracture repair.

Studies using a compression plate have demonstrated the degree of avascularity beneath the plate (Perren et al, 1988). Using a combination of intravital staining of blood circulation and polychrome fluorescent labelling of bone remodelling, they concluded that early bone porosis in the vicinity of the implants is the result of internal remodelling of cortical bone that is induced by necrosis rather than unloading due to stress shielding. The data from reaming and osteotomy showed that the periosteum is capable of considerable acute vascular response; it is not known whether such a response would be observed in an osteotomy with plating. However, prevention of unnecessary periosteal damage is obviously of prime importance.

The importance of the periosteum has been further demonstrated in experiments in which the periosteum was removed at the time of osteotomy (Wallace et al, 1991). A silicone rubber sheath was placed over a tibia, extending 2 cm on either side of the osteotomy to produce an avascular osteotomy site. This technique proved to be a good model for non-union. Even after 6 weeks, there was very little healing, and no torsional stiffness could be detected at the fracture site.

It was also shown that in well-vascularised fractures, small changes in external fixator stiffness could have very significant effects on blood flow to the fracture site and to the fracture callus. This observation also means that care must be taken when comparing the vascular response to different types of fixation device, as differences in the mechanical properties of the devices could contribute to the observed differences in vascular response, as well as the degree of vascular disruption caused by the application of the device.

BONE MICROCIRCULATION IN PATHOLOGICAL CONDITIONS

Osteonecrosis

Osteonecrosis, particularly of the femoral head, is a common disorder of bone circulation, and is discussed in Chapter 13.

Reflex sympathetic dystrophy

Reflex sympathetic dystrophy is a clinical condition occurring most frequently in the wrist and hand, or ankle and foot, and is characterised by vascular changes that vary with the stage of the condition (Driessens, 1993). Commonly, the condition is divided into three stages:

- Stage 1: pain, oedema, hyperaemia, redness.
- Stage 2: pain, cyanosis, skin atrophy, joint stiffness.
- Stage 3: reduction or disappearance of pain, continued joint stiffness, possible continuation of skin atrophy.

Radionuclide bone scanning is important in the diagnosis of the condition.

The vascular factors in reflex sympathetic dystrophy have been characterised using human serum albumin scintigraphy (Driessens, 1993). These studies have shown that in stage 1, both the local blood flow and blood volume at the affected site are higher than in the corresponding region on the opposite side. During stage 2, precisely opposite observations are made (i.e. reduced blood flow and volume in the affected site).

Calcitonin has been shown to be an effective therapeutic agent in stage 1 of the condition. Experiments on vascular reactivity (see above) have demonstrated that calcitonin causes prolonged dose-dependent vasoconstriction in the bone vasculature. Rapid improvement in the vascular abnormalities is seen with calcitonin treatment, and there is seldom progression to stage 2.

Paget's disease

Paget's disease of bone is characterised by rapid bone destruction followed by disorganised new bone formation. Histologically, bone is disorganised and there is an increase in osteoclast and osteoblast activity. Measurement of blood flow using the ^{18}F technique described above has shown considerably raised values compared with those in controls (Green et al, 1987). However, given the problems of extraction of fluorine by bone, the extent to which this reflects actual changes in flow must be considered.

Response to ischaemia–reperfusion

Ischaemia is a problem common to all branches of surgery, and the primary aim of every surgeon is to revascularise the tissue as quickly as possible. Paradoxically, it has been observed that reperfusion of ischaemic tissues may result in further injury. The intracellular biochemical changes that take place during ischaemia lead to cellular dysfunction, cellular and interstitial oedema, and ultimately cell death. Reperfusion of the ischaemic tissue worsens the cellular and interstitial oedema, and in the worst case results in progressive cessation of blood flow, due to microcirculatory obstruction, a condition known as the 'no-reflow phenomenon'. Reperfusion injury appears to be primarily endothelial in origin, involving free radicals and particularly xanthine oxidase as a source of these radicals. In orthopaedic surgery, the most common situation in which ischaemia–reperfusion may be a problem is in vascularised bone grafts. Superoxide dismutase (SOD), a free radical scavenger, is effective in reducing the extent of reperfusion injury in bone after 8 hours of normothermic ischaemia (Weiss et al, 1988).

Blood flow in arthritis

Reduced capillary flow and tissue oxygenation, as a result of impaired venous drainage from the synovium and subchondral bone, are significant observations in osteoarthritis. Although the pathogenesis of osteoarthritis is multifactorial, it has been argued that these are the primary factors involved in the pathogenesis of synovial and bone marrow changes, and that these are also indirectly responsible for cartilage degeneration, by inducing changes in the chemistry of the synovial fluid. A significant review of vascular aspects of degenerative joint disorders has been published recently by Arnoldi (1994). Pentosan polysulphate, which mobilises intravascular lipid and thrombi, has been shown to support cartilage repair and modulate synovial inflammation. Recent studies have shown that NO plays an important role in the regulation of blood flow in joints.

Intervertebral disc

The intervertebral disc is the largest avascular structure in the body, but the vertebral endplate contains vessels suitable for solute exchange with the disc (Crock and Goldwasser, 1984). In the experimental animal, bone blood flow to the endplate has been measured, and is comparable in magnitude to normal cortical flow (Hughes et al, 1993). Diffusion via the endplate is the most important nutritional route for the intervertebral disc, and it has been postulated that impairment of blood flow to the endplate may be an important factor in disc degeneration.

REFERENCES

Arnoldi CC, Vascular aspects of degenerative joint disorders: a synthesis. *Acta Orthop Scand Suppl* 1994; **65**: 261.

Ashcroft GP, Evans NTS, Roeda D et al. Measurement of blood flow in tibial fracture patients using positron emission tomography. *J Bone Joint Surg [Br]* 1992; **74B**: 673–677.

Bjurholm A, Kreicbergs A, Brodin E, Schultzberg M. Substance P- and CGRP-immunoreactive nerves in bone. *Peptides* 1988; **9**: 165–171.

Brinker MR, Lippton HL, Cook SD, Hyman AL. Pharmacological regulation of the circulation of bone. *J Bone Joint Surg [Am]* 1990; **72-A**: 964–975.

Brookes M. *The Blood Supply of Bone.* London: Butterworths, 1971.

Collin-Osdoby P. Role of vascular endothelial cells in bone biology. *J Cell Biochem* 1994; **55**: 304–309.

Cooper RR, Milgram JW, Robinson RA. Morphology of the osteon. An electron microscope study. *J Bone Joint Surg [Am]* 1966; **48A**: 1239–1271.

Corbett SA, Hukkanen M, McCarthy ID, Hughes SPF, Polak JM. Upregulation of nitric oxide synthase isoforms in rat tibial fracture callus (abstract). *J Pathol* (in press).

Crock HV. *An Atlas of the Vascular Anatomy of the Skeleton and Spinal Cord.* London: Martin Dunitz, 1996.

Crock HV, Goldwasser M. Anatomic studies of the circulation in the region of the vertebral end-plate in adult greyhound dogs. *Spine* 1984; **9**: 702–706.

Davis TRC, Wood MB. Endothelial control of long bone vascular resistance. *J Orthop Res* 1992; **10**: 344–349.

Deutsch SD, Gandsman EJ, Sparragen SC. Quantitative regional blood flow analysis and its clinical application during routine bone scanning. *J Bone Joint Surg [Am]* 1981; **63A**: 295–305.

Driessens M, Vanhoutte PM. Vascular reactivity of the isolated tibia of the dog. *Am J Physiol* 1979; **236**: H904–H908.

Driessens M. Circulatory aspects of reflex sympathetic dystrophy. In: Schoetens A, Arlet J, Gardeniers JWM, Hughes SPF (eds) *Bone Circulation and Vascularisation in Normal and Pathological Conditions* New York: Plenum Press, 1993: 217–231.

Frederickson JM, Honour AJ, Copp DH. Measurement of initial bone clearance of ^{45}Ca in the rat. *Fed Proc* 1955; **14**: 49.

Furchgott RF, Zawadzki JV. The obligatory role of endothelial cells in the relaxation of arterial smooth muscle by acetylcholine. *Nature* 1980; **288**: 373–376.

Green JR, Reeve J, Tellez M, Veall N, Wootton R. Skeletal blood flow in metabolic disorders of the skeleton. *Bone* 1987; **8**: 293–297.

Hughes SPF, Davies DR, Bassingthwaighte JB, Know FG, Kelly PJ. Bone extraction and blood clearance of diphosphonate in the dog. *Am J Physiol* 1977; **232**: H341–H347.

Hughes SPF, McCarthy ID. Intra-operative measurement of blood flow to dura and nerve root using laser Doppler flowmetry in lumbar spine surgery. *Neuro-orthopaedics* 1995; **17/18**: 191–195.

Hughes SPF, Wallace AL, McCarthy ID, Fleming RH, Wyatt BC. Measurement of blood flow to the vertebral bone and disc. *Eur Spine J* 1993; **2**: 96–98.

Hukkanen M, Kontinnen YT, Santavirta S et al. Rapid proliferation of calcitonin gene-related peptide-immunoreactive nerves during healing of rat tibial fracture suggests neural involvement in bone growth and remodelling. *Neuroscience* 1993; **54**: 969–979.

Jones AR, Clark CC, Brighton CT. Microvessel endothelial cells and pericytes increase proliferation and repress osteoblast phenotypic markers in rat calvarial bone cell cultures. *J Orthop Res* 1995; **13**: 553–561.

Kelly PJ. Pathways of transport in bone. In: *Handbook of Physiology. The Cardiovascular System III.* Bethesda, Maryland: American Physiological Society, 1984: 371–396.

Kelly PJ, Bronk JT. Venous pressure and bone formation. *Microvasc Res* 1990; **39**: 364–375.

Klein-Nulend J, Semeins CM, Ajubi NE et al. Pulsating fluid flow increases nitric oxide (NO) synthesis by osteocytes but not periosteal fibroblasts. *Biochim Biophys Res Commun* 1995; **217**: 640–648.

Kowalski MJ, Schemitsch EH, Kregor PJ, Senft D, Swiontkowski MF. Effect of periosteal stripping on cortical bone perfusion: a laser Doppler study in sheep. *Calcif Tiss Int* 1996; **59**: 24–26.

Kruse RL, Kelly PJ. Acceleration of fracture healing distal to a venous tourniquet. *J Bone Joint Surg [Am]* 1974; **66A**: 730–739.

Lahtinen T, Alhava EM, Karjalainen P, Romppanen T. The effect of age on blood flow in the proximal femur in man. *J Nucl Med* 1981; **22**: 966–972.

Lemon GJ, Davies DR, Hughes SPF, Bassingthwaighte JB, Kelly PJ. Transcapillary exchange and retention of fluoride, strontium, EDTA, sucrose, and antipyrine in bone. *Calcif Tiss Int* 1980; **31**: 173–181.

Li G, Bronk JT, Kelly PJ. Canine bone blood flow estimated by microspheres. *J Orthop Res* 1989; **7**: 61–67.

Lundgaard A, Aslkjaer C, Hansen EB. First report on vascular reactivity in human bone tissue. Seventh International Symposium on Bone Necrosis, Fukuoka, 1996.

McCarthy ID, Hughes SPF. Inhibition of bone cell metabolism increases strontium-85 uptake. *Calcif Tiss Int* 1986; **39**: 386–389.

Montgomery RJ, Sutker BD, Bronk JT, Smith SR, Kelly PJ. Interstitial fluid flow in cortical bone. *Microvasc Res* 1988; **35**: 295–307.

Oganov VS, Grigoriev AI, Voronin LI et al. Bone mineral density in cosmonauts after 4.5–6 month long flights aboard orbital station MIR. *Aerospace and Environmental Medicine* 1992; **26**: 20–24.

Otter MW, Palmieri VR, Cochran GVB. Transcortical streaming potentials are generated by circulatory pressure gradients in living canine bone. *J Orthop Res* 1990; **8**: 119–126.

Palmer RMJ, Ferrige AG, Moncada S. Nitric oxide accounts for the biological activity of the endothelium-derived relaxation factor. *Nature* 1987; **327**: 524–526.

Perren SM, Cordey J, Rahn BA, Gautier E, Schneider E. Early temporary porosis of bone induced by internal fixation of implants. *Clin Orthop* 1988; **232**: 139–151.

Piekarski K, Monro M. Transport mechanism operating between blood supply and osteocytes in long bones. *Nature* 1977; **269**: 80–82.

Pitsillides AA, Rawlinson SCF, Suswillo FL, Bourine S, Zaman G, Lanyon LE. Mechanical strain-induced NO production by bone cells: a possible role in adaptive (re)modeling. *FASEB J* 1995; **9**: 1614–1622.

Reeve J, Arlot M, Wootton R et al. Skeletal blood flow, iliac histomorphometry and strontium kinetics in osteoporosis: a relationship between blood flow and corrected apposition rate. *J Clin Endocrinol Metab* 1988; **66**: 1124–1131.

Reichert ILH, McCarthy ID, Hughes SPF. The acute vascular response to intramedullary reaming. *J Bone Joint Surg [Br]* 1995; **77B**: 490–493.

Skawina A, Litwin JA, Gorczyca J, Miodonski AJ. The vascular system of human fetal long bones: a scanning electron microscope study of corrosion casts. *J Anat* 1994; **185**: 369–376.

Smith SR, Bronk JT, Kelly PJ. Effect of fracture fixation on cortical bone blood flow. *J Orthop Res* 1990; **8**: 471–478.

Swiontkowski M, Ganz R, Schlegel U, Perren SM. Laser Doppler flowmetry for clinical evaluation of femoral head osteonecrosis. *Clin Orthop* 1987; **18**: 181–185.

Tothill P, Hooper G. Invalidity of single-passage measurements of the extraction of bone-seeking tracers in rats and rabbits. *J Orthop Res* 1984; **2**: 75–79.

Tothill P, Hooper G, McCarthy ID, Hughes SPF. The pattern of distribution of blood flow in dog limb bones measured using microspheres. *Clin Phys Physiol Meas* 1987; **3**: 239–247.

Trias A, Fery A. Cortical circulation of long bones. *J Bone Joint Surg [Am]* 1979; **61A**: 1052–1059.

Trueta J. The role of the vessels in osteogenesis. *J Bone Joint Surg [Br]* 1963; **45B**: 402–418.

Van Dyke D, Anger HO, Yano Y, Bozzini C. Bone blood flow shown with ^{18}F and the positron camera. *Am J Physiol* 1965; **209**: 65–70.

Villanueva JE, Nimni ME. Promotion of calvarial cell osteogenesis by endothelial cells. *J Bone Min Res* 1990; **5**: 733–739.

Wallace AL, Draper ERC, Strachan RK, McCarthy ID, Hughes SPF. The effect of devascularisation on early bone healing in dynamic external fixation. *J Bone Joint Surg [Br]* 1991; **73B**: 819–824.

Wallace AL, Makki R, Weiss JB, Hughes SPF. Measurement of serum angiogenic factor in devascularised experimental tibial fractures. *J Orthop Trauma* 1995; **9**: 324–332.

Warner JG, Andrew JG. (1997) Osteoblasts secrete vascular endothelial growth factor (VEGF) in human fracture healing. *J Bone Joint Surg* (in press).

Weiss A, Moore JR, Randolph MA, Weiland AJ. Preventing oxygen free-radical injury in ischaemic revascularised bone grafts. *Plast Reconst Surg* 1988; **88**: 486–495.

Welch RD, Johnston CE, Waldron MJ, Potet B. Bone changes associated with intraosseous hypertension in the caprine tibia. *J Bone Joint Surg [Am]* 1993; **75A**: 53–60.

Whiteside LA, Lesker PA, Simmons DJ. The measurement of regional bone and bone marrow blood flow in the rabbit using the hydrogen washout technique. *Clin Orthop* 1977; **122**: 340–346.

Wilkes CH, Visscher MB. Some physiological aspects of bone marrow pressure. *J Bone Joint Surg [Am]* 1975; **57A**: 49–57.

Willans SM. *Modelling in the exchange of ion between blood and bone.* PhD thesis, University of Edinburgh, 1987.

Wootton R. The single passage extraction of ^{18}F in rabbit bone. *Clin Sci Mol Med* 1974; **47**: 73–77.

Yang L, McCarthy ID. A distributed model of exchange processes within the osteon. *J Biomech* 1992; **25**: 441–450.

3

Local Regulation of Bone Metabolism

Laura Masi, Susanna Benvenuti, Annalisa Tanini and Maria Luisa Brandi

INTRODUCTION

The skeleton stores more than 99% of the body's calcium, and is also a store of sodium and magnesium. Bone consists of cells and extracellular matrix, the latter comprising organic (35%) and inorganic (65%) components. The organic component includes type I collagen (90%), the γ-carboxyglutamic acid-rich protein osteocalcin (1–2%), osteonectin, proteoglycans, glycosaminoglycans and lipids. The inorganic component consists mainly of calcium and phosphate in crystals of hydroxyapatite.

The term 'modelling' has been used to describe the balance of formation and resorption through bone growth, and ceases at adulthood. The term 'remodelling' refers to the process as it continues throughout adult life: it is important for the maintenance of normal bone structure. To maintain the structural integrity of bone, large numbers of new cells must be recruited continuously: osteoblasts, responsible for bone formation, and osteoclasts, responsible for bone resorption.

These two cell types belong to two different lineages; osteoblasts are believed to be derived from undifferentiated mesenchymal cells, which further differentiate into osteocytes and are embedded in calcified tissue. The immediate precursor of the osteoblast is the preosteoblast. The three main types of mature osteoblast are: osteoblasts, bone lining cells and osteocytes. Osteoblasts are cubical cells lying on the matrix they have produced, and are connected to each other by gap junctions, which may also connect them to adjacent bone lining cells and to osteocytes. Osteoblasts have a prominent Golgi apparatus and abundant endoplasmic reticulum, reflecting their capacity for protein synthesis. They are rich in alkaline phosphatase, synthesize type I collagen and osteocalcin, and have receptors for parathyroid hormone. The osteo-cyte is an osteoblast that has become embedded behind the advancing front of growing bone in small cavities within the bone. Osteocytes communicate with each other and with surface osteoblasts and lining cells by a complex system of cell microprocesses within canaliculi, and perhaps contribute to mineral homoeostasis by dissolution and deposition of mineral around their lacunae. Bone lining cells (inactive osteoblasts, endosteal lining cells) cover the surfaces of trabecular and inner cortical (endosteal) bone; they have the aspect of flattened cells that have lost synthetic capability.

Osteoclasts are the major cells responsible for bone resorption. They are large multinucleated cells present only in bone, possessing a 'ruffled border', which is a highly specialized and complex region of the plasma membrane consisting of multiple membrane folds and finger-like projections. Osteoclasts are richly endowed with lysosomal enzymes, especially tartrate-resistant acid phosphatase, which is considered to be specific for osteoclasts. The carbonic anhydrase content of osteoclasts contributes to their ability to produce acid in their environs, which is a factor in their ability to dissolve mineral. It is believed that osteoclast progenitors are of haematopoietic origin, and they are recruited from haematopoietic tissues such as bone marrow and circulating blood to bone. Osteoclast progenitors then proliferate and differentiate into mononuclear preosteoclasts and fuse with each other to form multinucleated osteoclasts. When a mononuclear precursor, most likely of monocyte macrophage series, undergoes a process of differentiation, it develops tartrate-resistant acid phosphatase and expresses the calcitonin receptor. It is now established that the development of osteoclasts from haemopoietic percursors cannot be accomplished unless stromal/osteoblastic cells are present. In fact, the cells of this lineage mediate the effects of both systemic hormones, i.e.

parathyroid hormone and 1,25-dihydroxyvitamin D_3 and locally produced factors that stimulate osteoclast development (Suda et al, 1992).

Cortical (compact) bone represents 80% of the skeleton and is found particularly in the shafts of long bones, providing structural integrity. Only 20% of skeletal mass is trabecular bone, which, having a much greater surface:volume ratio, contributes more to mineral homoeostasis. Remodelling occurs throughout life, and is essential for the maintenance of normal bone structure and for balance of bone formation and resorption. The sequence of formation and resorption is carried out by a group of cells, including osteoblasts and osteoclasts and their progenitors, which represent a basic multicellular unit (BMU) of bone turnover. A bone remodelling sequence is initiated by the appearance of osteoclasts and osteoclast precursors following any of several humoral or local stimuli to resorption. Then the osteoclasts resorb mineralized bone matrix, producing a small resorption pit. The motile osteoclasts move to another site and the resorptive phase is followed by an active reversal phase characterised by deposition of a cement line. The next steps are early formation, when osteoblasts deposit osteoid on the cement line, and late formation, when mineralization occurs between the cement line and osteoid seam. Quiescence is restored at completion of the cycle, with lining cells on the surface. The process of bone resorption followed by an equal amount of formation has been termed coupling.

SYSTEMIC FACTORS

Bone is a highly organized tissue, the structure of which reflects its primary functions of providing support and protection, and the environment for haematopoiesis. The adult skeleton is in a dynamic state, being continually remodelled by the integrated processes of bone formation and bone resorption. Endochondral bone formation and appositional bone formation are also important in bone development. All these processes are influenced by systemic hormonal modulation as well as by local microenvironmental factors. Several factors that regulate bone turnover and the main calcium-regulating hormones are: parathyroid hormones, calcitonin and vitamin D, and oestrogens; these are discussed in detail in Chapter 4.

LOCAL FACTORS

Evidence has clearly established that the bone marrow microenvironment plays an essential role in regulating bone remodelling. In fact, bone cells and cells of the haematopoietic bone marrow produce and respond to a surprisingly large number of cytokines and growth factors that affect bone and cartilage metabolism under physiological as well as pathological conditions (*Table 3.1*).

Interleukin 1

Interleukin (IL) 1 was the first cytokine reported to affect the bone resorption process. Originally, its name referred to its property of causing proliferation of CD4-positive T helper cells via the induction of the autocrine growth factor IL-2. In fact, its first name was lymphocyte-activating factor (LAF). Many other biological activities were later identified when recombinant materials became available, including leucocyte endogenous mediator (LEM), mononuclear cell factor (MCF), osteoclast-activating factor (OAF), catabolin and others. Studies to identify endogenous pyrogen activity from leucocytes permitted identification of IL-1 structure (Auron et al, 1984).

Table 3.1 Local regulators of bone remodelling.

Interleukins (ILs)
IL-1α and IL-1β
IL-2
IL-3
IL-4
IL-5
IL-6
IL-11

Growth factors
Insulin-like growth factors I and II
Fibroblast growth factors α and β
Platelet-derived growth factor
Transforming growth factors α, β_1, β_2 and β_3
Epidermal growth factor

Colony-stimulating factors (CSFs)
Granulocyte–macrophage CSF
Granulocyte CSF
Macrophage CSF

IL-1 refers to two proteins (IL-1α and IL-1β), the acidic and the neutral forms, with molecular weights around 17 kDa. IL-1α and IL-1β concentrations vary in different tissues and species, but their main biological activities seem to be similar and involve induction of fever and the acute-phase response. A murine receptor, a member of the immunoglobulin superfamily, has been cloned for IL-1; this binds both IL-1α and IL-1β and could explain the similar biological activity of these two proteins. In connective tissues, IL-1 stimulates synovial cells, chondrocytes and osteoblast-like cells to produce proteinases such as collagenase and stromelysin, as well as plasminogen activators which contribute to the breakdown of connective tissue matrices.

IL-1 was one of the first OAFs to be characterised and is the most potent bone-resorbing molecule yet identified. IL-1 and other cytokines, such as IL-6, have been postulated to play an essential role in the pathogenesis of postmenopausal osteoporosis. It has been suggested that in the increased bone resorption induced by oestrogen deficiency in women with postmenopausal osteoporosis, circulating monocytes release increased amounts of IL-1 (Dinarello, 1991), which could be prevented by oestrogen replacement. Recent studies have also demonstrated that oestrogen can modulate the secretion of a specific competitive inhibitor of IL-1, IL-1 receptor antagonist: in normal menopausal women, but not in those with osteoporosis, levels of IL-1 receptor antagonist are increased. Moreover, it is now clear that IL-1 modulates osteoclastogenesis and *in vitro* studies have demonstrated that IL-1 together with tumour necrosis factor (TNF) stimulates osteoclast development from haematopoietic progenitors (Pfeilschifter et al, 1989). Further, IL-1 increases the release of calcium from bone explants (Gowen and Mundy, 1986). Such effects on osteoclast cells seem to be mediated through the effects of these cytokines on stromal and/or osteoblastic cells. IL-1 also has a complex effect on the production of matrix components, including collagen, osteocalcin and proteoglycans. Low doses of IL-1 act as a potent co-mitogen for fibroblasts and human osteoblast-like cells.

Interleukin 6

IL-6 is known to be responsible for different biological effects previously ascribed to other factors such as interferon β_2, B cell-stimulating factor 2 and others. IL-6 is a 23–28 kDa protein that can be produced by connective tissue cell types. It acts together with IL-1 and TNF to induce hepatic acute-phase protein synthesis and is probably also an essential mediator of the acute-phase response. Recently, it has been reported that IL-6 is important among the cytokines that affect bone metabolism. Its role in the early stage of haematopoiesis and in osteoclastogenesis has been established. In fact IL-6, co-acting with IL-3, stimulates the formation of the colony-forming unit for the granulocyte–macrophage (CFU-GM) (Girasole and Passeri, 1994) and acts on the formation of osteoclast precursors from cells present in CFU-GM colonies (Girasole and Passeri, 1994); anti-IL-6 antibodies inhibit pit formation by human osteoclasts (Suda et al, 1995).

Recent studies have demonstrated that IL-6 also stimulates osteoclastic bone resorption *in vivo*: transplantation of IL-6-producing tumours into nude mice induces hypercalcemia and, following administration of anti-IL-6 antibodies, serum calcium levels decrease to basal levels (Suda et al, 1995). It has been reported that in IL-6 gene knockout mice bone loss is prevented. Recently it has been proposed that IL-6 alone may not be sufficient to stimulate osteoclast formation in mouse co-culture systems. Recent findings demonstrate that IL-6 acts via a cell surface receptor which consists of two parts: a membrane-bound IL-6 receptor and its signal-transducing 130-kDA glycoprotein called gp130. When IL-6 receptor is bound to IL-6, the complex binds to gp130 to transduce IL-6 signals. Soluble IL-6 receptors transduce via gp130 too, and they have been found in the serum of healthy subjects. In several metabolic bone diseases soluble IL-6 receptor serum levels are increased, suggesting a direct involvement in osteoclast bone resorption induced by IL-6. When soluble IL-6 receptor was added together with IL-6 in mouse co-culture studies, cells were differentiated to mature osteoclasts.

Transforming growth factor (TGF) β

TGF-βs are members of a much larger gene superfamily and are produced by a wide variety of cells and tissues including T cells, macrophages, platelets and bone (Centrella et al, 1995). TGF-β is a disulphide-linked dimer comprising two identical 12 500-Da subunits. From bovine bone matrix five isoforms have been isolated: homodimers of TGF-β_1, TGF-β_2 and TGF-β_3, and two heterodimers containing one type 2 subunit combined with either a type 1 subunit (TGF-$\beta_{1,2}$) or a type 3 subunit (TGF-$\beta_{2,3}$); however, the homodimers are represented more abundantly (Centrella et al, 1995).

TGF-βs are thought to be the most important regulatory cytokines in connective tissue and bone. There are modifications in relative TGF-β isoform potency on bone cell metabolism, but no consistent qualitative differences in the spectrum of biological effects have been reported in skeletal tissue. It is now well known that bone cells secrete various TGF-βs and express several cell surface TGF-β-binding sites. *In vivo* studies have demonstrated a strong increase in bone mass with local and systemic TGF-β administration, but cell biology and biochemistry of TGF-β in bone tissue have been determined with continuous cell lines expressing varying types of osteoblast phenotype. TGF-β weakly enhances replication in undifferentiated foetal rat bone cell cultures, but is a potent mitogen in osteoblast-enriched cultures from fetal tissues. In fact, the effectiveness of TGF-β decreases at high doses, and in some cultures derived from more mature organisms (Centrella et al, 1995). Furthermore, TGF-β inhibits DNA synthesis in clonal bone cell lines and in some osteosarcoma cell lines that were represented by well-differentiated osteoblasts. Systemic hormones, such as parathyroid hormone and 1,25-dihydroxyvitamin D$_3$, stimulate osteoblasts to produce TGF-β, which is released as a latent form. Acidic conditions or proteolysis can activate the growth factor, which can also act directly on osteoblasts as a classical autocrine factor. Moreover, TGF-β increases production of matrix protein including fibronectin, osteopontin, collagen and osteonectin by osteoblast cells (Canalis et al, 1991).

Studies on the role of TGF-β in bone resorption are controversial. Tashjian et al (1985) demonstrated that TGF-β stimulates radiocalcium release in neonatal mouse calvaria, suggesting that TGF-β may also be a potent stimulator of local bone resorption. Using a human bone marrow culture system, an inhibition of osteoclast-like cell formation by TGF-β was demonstrated. Studies in ovariectomized animals showed that TGF-βs decrease the proliferation of osteoclast precursors in a bone marrow culture of oestrogen-deficient mice, but are unable to suppress bone resorption in ovariectomized animals *in vivo*. Fiorelli et al (1994) recently demonstrated an autocrine role for TGF-β in regulating differentiation of a clonal human preosteoclastic cell line towards the osteoclast phenotype.

Insulin-like growth factors

Insulin-like growth factors (IGFs) are growth hormone polypeptides with a molecular weight of 7600 Da. Two IGFs have been characterised: IGF-I and IGF-II. These are synthesised by many tissues, including bone. In fact, IGF-I and IGF-II, together with TGF-β, are the best defined and most abundant growth factors in bone. Osteoblasts are the most important IGF target cells within bone, but IGFs are also required for osteoclast generation and differentiation. IGFs increase transport of glucose and amino acids into osteoblast cells and can stimulate net incorporation of these metabolites into glycogen and protein respectively. In addition, IGFs stimulate osteoblast precursor replication *in vitro*; they are also relatively weak mitogens for normal bone cells (Schmid, 1993). Besides, IGFs play an important role in osteoblast differentiation, as demonstrated by an increase in alkaline phosphatase activity, osteocalcin production and collagen type I synthesis after stimulation with IGFs (Schmid, 1993).

Other cytokines and growth factors

A surprisingly large number of other cytokines and growth factors have effects on bone metabolism, and a major task of the researcher is to determine how all these agents interact and which are the most important in different disease states. It is clear that many of these factors, produced locally and stored within the bone matrix, have to be considered as serious candidates for involvement in the modulation of bone remodelling. These include TNFs, IL-4, interferon (IFN) γ, colony-stimulating factors (CSFs), platelet-derived growth factor (PDGF) and fibroblast growth factors (FGFs).

TNFs, together with IL-1, were the first cytokines identified to affect bone resorption process, and exist in two forms, α and β. Isoforms show a wide homology and similar spectrum of biological activity. The effects of TNF on connective tissue are similar to those of IL-1, and include induction of bone resorption. The two cytokines can act in synergistic fashion, and their importance under physiological conditions depends on which other factors are present, as well as their local concentration. Together with IL-1, TNF increases bone resorption in rodents and osteoclast development from haematopoietic precursors *in vitro* (Pfeilschifter et al, 1989). Constitutively, it is produced by osteoblasts isolated from adult human trabecular bone, neonatal murine calvaria cells or osteo-blast cell lines in very low concentrations. Probably, despite the low levels of release, TNF is important for amplification of the effects of local cytokines and/or systemic hormones.

IL-4 is another cytokine released by cells of immune system that is present in the bone marrow microenvironment. IL-4 inhibits bone resorption via suppression of osteoclastogenesis. Recent findings, in fact, have shown that overexpression of the cytokine in transgenic mice induces osteoporosis histologically similar to that often appearing in postmenopausal women. IL-4 also inhibits the development of osteoblasts from bone marrow.

Among other local factors that inhibit osteoclast formation and bone resorption, IFN-γ is a cytokine that was originally described by its capacity to inhibit viral replication. IFN-γ is now known to have many other effects, particularly on cell proliferation and differentiation. It can be viewed as a potential natural antagonist to IL-1 and TNF. IFN-γ has potent inhibitory action *in vitro* on the formation of osteoclasts stimulated by IL-1 and TNF, but has less effect on resorption stimulated by classical calciotropic hormones, parathyroid hormone or 1,25-dihydroxyvitamin D_3 (Gowen and Mundy, 1986). IFN-γ is also a strong inhibitor of collagen synthesis and, unlike the other cytokines, inhibits DNA synthesis.

Colony-stimulating factors (CSFs), or haematopoietic factors, are peptide hormones that are known to be responsible for the *in vitro* proliferation of bone marrow progenitor cells into mature differentiated cells, and to influence bone cell formation. Granulocyte and macrophage CSFs can increase the formation of osteoclast-like cells from marrow cultures. However, the same effect was not shown in bone organ cultures. Furthermore, osteoblasts are also able to produce the same CSFs that are secreted by stromal cells, suggesting a probable unique stromal progenitor that gives rise to stromal cells for the control of haematopoiesis as well as to osteoblasts.

PDGF was originally isolated from platelets but is known to be produced by various cell types including bone cells. It is a protein that is a dimer of two similar peptide chains, designated A and B. PDGF is one of the most potent growth factors present in serum, and is expressed by bone cells that also exhibit receptors. When PDGF is administered locally over the calvaria of mice *in vivo*, it causes a profound increase in new bone formation.

However, this is accompanied by an increase in osteoclastic bone resorption, which may limit its effectiveness as a potential therapeutic agent.

FGFs are members of a group of related peptides that are mitogenic for many cell types, including fibroblasts and osteoblasts. There are acidic and basic forms of FGF; acidic FGF is derived mainly from neural tissue, and basic FGF is produced by different cell types and is present in bone matrix. Both isoforms stimulate osteoblast proliferation but not differentiation. Only the basic form has been demonstrated to be produced by osteoblasts.

REFERENCES

Auron PE, Webb AC, Rosenwasser LJ. Nucleotide sequence of human monocyte interleukin 1 precursor cDNA. *Proc Natl Acad Sci USA* 1984; **81**: 7907–7911.

Canalis E, McCarthy TL, Centrella M. Growth factors and cytokines in bone cell metabolism. *Annu Rev Med* 1991; **42**: 17–24.

Centrella M, Rosen V, Horowitz MC et al. Transforming growth factor-β gene family members, their receptors, and bone cell function. *Endocr Rev* 1995; **4(1)**: 211–226.

Dinarello CA. Interleukin-1 and interleukin-1 antagonism. *Blood* 1991; **133**: 553–562.

Fiorelli G, Ballock RT, Wakefield LM et al. Role for autocrine TGF β_1 in regulating differentiation of human leukemic cell line toward osteoclast-like cells. *J Cell Physiol* 1994; **160**: 482–490.

Girasole G, Passeri G. Local factors, bone remodelling and skeletal disorders. *Ital J Mineral Electrolyte Metab* 1994; **8**: 153–165.

Gowen M, Mundy GR. Action of recombinant interleukin 2 and interferon gamma on bone resorption *in vitro J Immunol* 1986; **136**: 2478–2482.

Pfeilschifter J, Chenu C, Bird A et al. Interleukin 1 and tumor necrosis factor stimulate the formation of human osteoclast like cells *in vitro*. *J Bone Miner Res* 1989; **4**: 113–118.

Schmid C. IGFs: function and clinical importance. The regulation of osteoblast function by hormones and cytokines with special reference to insulin-like growth factors and their binding proteins. *J Intern Med* 1993; **234**: 535–542.

Suda T, Takahashi N, Martin TJ. Modulation of osteoclast differentiation. *Endocrinol Rev* 1992; **13**: 66–80.

Suda T, Udagawa I, Nakamura C et al. Modulation of osteoclast differentiation by local factors. *Bone* 1995; **17(2)**: 87S–91S.

Tashjian AH Jr. Voelkel EF, Lazzaro M et al. α and β human transforming growth factor stimulate prostaglandin production and bone resorption in culture mouse calvaria. *Proc Natl Acad Sci USA* 1985; **82**: 4535–4538.

4

Hormonal Regulation of Bone Metabolism

Samia I Girgis, Mika Hukkanen, Julia M Polak and Iain MacIntyre

INTRODUCTION

The skeleton is not simply a supporting tissue and a mineral reservoir, but is a metabolically active tissue. It receives about 10% of the cardiac output. The turnover rate of trabecular bone in adults is approximately 25% per year, and that of cortical bone is about 3%.

Throughout life, bone undergoes a continual process of remodelling 'renewal'. In this process, which involves all bone surfaces, resorption by osteoclasts (bone-resorbing cells) is followed by new bone formation by osteoblasts (bone-forming cells). These two closely coupled events are controlled by the numbers and activities of these bone cells. Various systemic and local factors modify the activities and/or numbers of these cells.

This chapter deals with systemic regulators of bone metabolism. Local factors that modulate bone metabolism are considered in Chapter 3. A list of systemic factors that regulate bone metabolism is shown on *Table 4.1*. These factors are grouped into two categories: calcitropic hormones (under feedback control by calcium in the extracellular fluid) and non-calcitropic hormones.

Table 4.1 Hormones that regulate bone metabolism.

Calcitropic hormones	Non-calcitropic hormones
Parathyroid hormone	Thyroid hormone
Calcitriol	Glucocorticoids
Calcitonin	Gonadal steroids
	Growth hormone
	Insulin

CALCITROPIC HORMONES

Parathyroid hormone

Chemistry

Parathyroid hormone (PTH) is an 84-amino-acid single-chain polypeptide. It has a molecular weight of 9600 Da. The structures of bovine, porcine and human PTH are known (Keutmann et al, 1978) (*Figure 4.1*). Human PTH differs at only 11 positions from the bovine and porcine hormones. Full biological activity resides in the amino-terminal portion of the molecule within amino acids 1–34.

Parathyroid hormone-related protein (PTH-rp)

This protein shares considerable functional and structural homology with PTH. PTH-rp shares a significant homology with PTH in the critical amino-terminal region, allowing it to bind to the PTH receptor. Many different cell types produce PTH-rp, including brain, pancreas, heart, lung, placenta, mammary tissue, endothelial cells and smooth muscle. This protein is now regarded as a paracrine or autocrine factor and plays a role in both fetal development and adult physiology. PTH-rp has little to do with calcium homoeostasis, except in disease states when large amounts may be released by tumours into the circulation (Suva et al, 1987; Martin and Suva, 1989).

Biosynthesis, secretion and metabolism

PTH is produced by the chief cells of the parathyroid glands. The PTH gene is a simple gene located on the short arm of chromosome 11. The gene has two introns

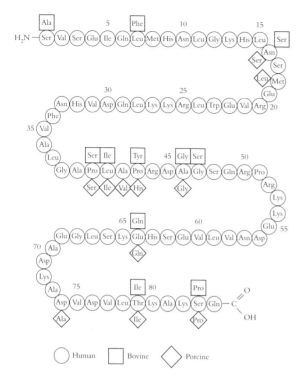

Figure 4.1 The complete amino acid sequence of human parathyroid hormone (PTH). Non-identical amino acid residues of bovine and porcine PTH are indicated beside the appropriate position on the human sequence. From Keutmann et al. (1978), with permission.

and three exons. After processing, the mature PTH messenger RNA (mRNA) is translated into prepro-PTH (a 115-amino-acid polypeptide) and is synthesized by ribosomes bound to membranes of the rough endoplasmic reticulum (Habener et al, 1984). The first 25 amino acids of prepro-PTH are enzymatically cleaved off from the amino-terminus, and the remaining 90-amino-acid peptide (pro-PTH) is then transported to the Golgi apparatus, where a further six amino acids from the amino-terminus are removed, leaving the mature hormone. The hormone is then incorporated in secretory granules which are transported to the periphery of the cell and excreted. In comparison with many peptide-secreting endocrine cells, relatively little PTH is stored.

The parathyroid cells recognise and respond to minute fluctuations in the extracellular ionised calcium (Ca^{2+}) concentration. Thus, hypocalcaemia stimulates

PTH secretion, whereas hypercalcaemia inhibits it (Habener et al, 1984). This negative feedback regulatory effect of calcium on PTH release is exerted via a Ca^{2+}-sensing receptor on the parathyroid gland. This receptor has been cloned by Brown et al (1993) from bovine parathyroid glands. The receptor is a member of the superfamily of G protein-coupled receptors and couples to the activation of phospholipase C via a G protein, resulting in accumulation of inositol 1,4,5-triphosphate (IP_3) and release of Ca^{2+} from intracellular stores.

Although calcium is the most important cation in regulating PTH secretion, magnesium can also affect PTH secretion. Severe hypomagnesaemia due to magnesium depletion may grossly impair PTH secretion. Receptors for calcitriol ($1,25-(OH)_2D$) are also present in the parathyroid cells. Calcitriol has a direct effect on parathyroid function, including inhibition of PTH gene transcription (Ishimi et al, 1990), reduction in parathyroid cell proliferation and perhaps apoptosis of parathyroid cells.

There is little to suggest control of PTH secretion by transcriptional or translational modulation by extracellular calcium. The two major mechanisms that regulate PTH biosynthesis are hyperplasia or atrophy of the gland over long periods of time, and calcium-dependent intracellular degradation of PTH in the short term (Habener et al, 1975). Thus, chronic hypocalcaemia leads to hyperplasia of the parathyroid glands, and acute hypocalcaemia is followed by an immediate increase in secretion due to release of stored hormone, combined with inhibition of intracellular peptide degradation.

Plasma PTH is very heterogeneous. The dominant circulating fragment corresponds to the carboxy-terminal portion of the molecule and has a molecular weight near 6000 Da. There are also amino-terminal fragments as well as the complete 84-amino-acid mature hormone. Both the amino-terminal fragment and the mature hormone have a very short half-life in the circulation, whereas the larger carboxy-terminal fragment has a much longer half-life. The carboxy-terminal fragment is removed by the kidney and, therefore, raised levels of this species are seen in patients with renal failure. The problems inherent in accurate measurements of PTH in blood due to heterogeneity of circulating forms of the molecule are now overcome by the use of double antibody assays that detect only the intact molecule (Nussbaum et al, 1987).

Biological actions of PTH

The principal role of PTH involves preservation of extracellular calcium and elimination of phosphorus.

Effects on kidney. The hormone has three separate effects on the kidney: it increases the distal tubular reabsorption of calcium; it markedly inhibits the proximal tubular reabsorption of phosphate and bicarbonate; and it accelerates the conversion of 25-hydroxycholecalciferol to its active metabolic form 1,25-dihydroxycholecalciferol (calcitriol) by stimulating the 1α-hydroxylase enzyme located in the proximal tubule (Garabedian et al, 1972).

Effects on bone. PTH has a dual action on bone: calcium replacement and bone remodelling effects. PTH transfers calcium and phosphate from bone to the blood using bone as a buffer for extracellular fluid calcium homoeostasis. PTH is a potent stimulator of osteoclastic bone resorption. It produces a rapid increase in both the number and activity of osteoclasts (increase in size and volume of the ruffled border of osteoclasts) both *in vivo* and in organ cultures. This effect is not exerted directly on osteoclasts. It follows a primary action of PTH on osteoblasts (which have receptors for PTH), which then secrete a local activator of osteoclastic activity. The nature of this activator is not established, but prostaglandins and interleukin–1 have been suggested.

In addition to this action, which produces an increased rate of bone destruction, there is some evidence that PTH can have an anabolic effect on bone (Hock et al, 1988). This anabolic effect has been demonstrated when PTH is administered intermittently and at relatively small doses, which may not produce hypercalcaemia. This is the basis of the proposed use of PTH to enhance bone mass in osteoporosis.

Effect on gut. The effect is an indirect one exerted via the increased renal production of calcitriol that causes enhancement of both calcium and phosphorus absorption.

Mechanisms of PTH action

PTH receptors. Cloning of the PTH/PTH-rp receptor (Jüppner et al, 1991) has allowed the characterisation of its properties. The receptor belongs to a novel family of G protein-coupled receptors that have seven transmembrane domains, three extracellular and three cytoplasmic loops, and an intracellular carboxy-terminus. The receptor has a marked sequence homology with that of calcitonin (37% identity) and secretin (42% identity). It is interesting that the receptor binds amino-terminal fragments of PTH and its close relative PTH-rp with equal affinity and is equally activated by both peptides. This is rather surprising, considering that only eight of the first 13 amino acids of PTH-rp are identical to PTH. The region from 14 to 34 residues shares little primary sequence homology with the sequence of PTH, but can displace PTH from binding sites on PTH receptor-bearing cells. The receptor activates both adenosine 3′, 5′-cyclic monophosphate (cAMP) production and IP_3 synthesis.

Pathophysiology

Primary hyperparathyroidism. The clinical and biochemical features of hyperparathyroidism follow from the known actions of the hormone. There is hypercalcaemia, hypophosphataemia and hyperphosphaturia. Circulating levels of PTH (intact 1–84) are either raised or within a normal level inappropriate for the high serum calcium levels. Half or more of patients with hyperparathyroidism have manifestations of the diseases involving the kidneys and bone. The unique bone involvement of osteitis fibrosa cystica is now rare because of early diagnosis. This, histologically, includes a reduction in the number of trabeculae, an increase in the number of osteoclasts, and replacement of the cellular and marrow elements by fibrous tissue.

Secondary hyperparathyroidism. Chronic renal failure is almost always associated with some degree of parathyroid hyperplasia. This is due to hyperplastic drive caused by a combination of low serum calcium and low plasma calcitriol levels.

Vitamin D – endocrine system

The term vitamin D is generally used to describe a number of chemically related compounds with common anti-ricketic properties, but with different potencies.

Chemistry

Vitamin D_3 (cholecalciferol) is a steroid derivative. The parent saturated hydrocarbon from which it is derived

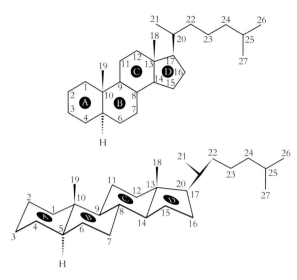

Figure 4.2 Conventional and perspective formulae of 5α-cholestane, parent molecule of vitamin D_3. From MacIntyre et al (1978), with permission.

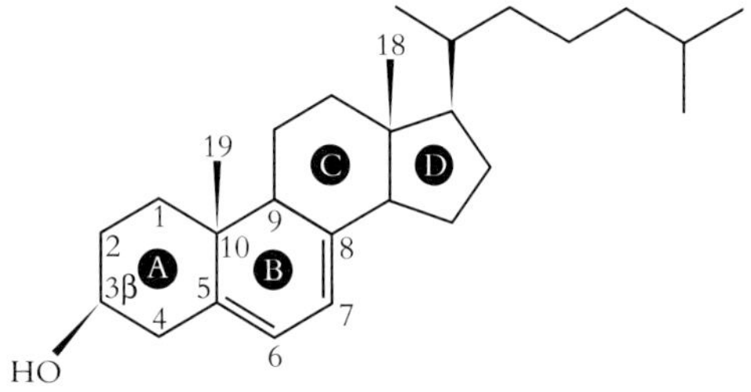

Figure 4.3 7-Dihydrocholesterol. From MacIntyre et al (1978), with permission.

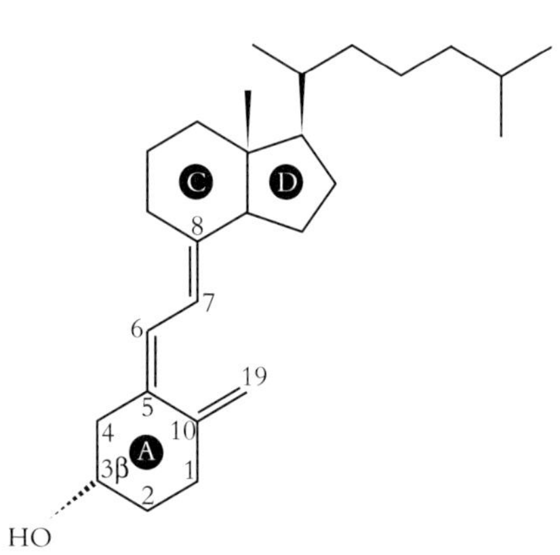

Figure 4.4 Cholecalciferol, vitamin D_3. From MacIntyre et al (1978), with permission.

(5α-cholestane) is shown in *Figure 4.2*. 7-Dehydrocholesterol (*Figure 4.3*) is the immediate precursor of vitamin D_3. It is present in the skin and, under the influence of ultraviolet light, the bond between carbons 9 and 10 in ring B is broken. Ring A then rotates through 180° around the single bond between carbon 6 and 7. A double bond is formed between carbons 10 and 19. This structure (cholecalciferol or vitamin D_3) is a 9,10-seco-steroid (*Figure 4.4*). Vitamin D_2 (ergocalciferol), which is derived from plants, differs from cholecalciferol (vitamin D_3) by having a double bond between carbons 22 and 23 and a methyl group at carbon 24.

Metabolism

Vitamin D produced in the skin or ingested in the diet is almost inactive. It is first transported in the plasma by binding to vitamin D-binding protein. It must undergo two successive hydroxylation reactions before it can assume its physiological role as a major calcitropic hormone (Norman et al, 1982). The first stage is 25-hydroxylation in the liver to produce 25-hydroxy vitamin D (25-OH-D_3), the major circulating form, which has an estimated half-life of 21 days but only modest biological activity. The second hydroxylation reaction takes place in the kidney in a physiologically regulated manner. A mitochondrial enzyme system converts 25-OH-D_3 to either 1α, 25-dihydroxy vitamin D (1,25-$(OH)_2D$), which is highly active, or to 24,25-$(OH)_2D$, which has similar potency to 25-OH D_3 D.

Regulation of vitamin D metabolism. The kidney functions as a classical endocrine organ to produce, under complex hormonal regulation, the two dihydroxylated metabolites. For all factors regulating vitamin D metabolism there is a reciprocal effect on 1,25-$(OH)_2D$ and 24,25-$(OH)_2D$. When the production of one is stimulated, that of the other is inhibited. These factors are: (a) serum calcium and phosphorus – hypocalcaemia by itself stimulates the production of 1,25-$(OH)_2$ vitamin D; hyperphosphataemia has the opposite effect (Boyle et al, 1971; Larkins et al, 1973); (b) PTH – in the presence of hypocalcaemia, PTH stimulates the production of 1,25-$(OH)_2$ vitamin D; however, when secretion of PTH coincides with hypercalcaemia, this stimulating effect may be overcome; (c) growth hormone and prolactin, which have stimulating effects on 1,25-$(OH)_2$ vitamin D production; (d) calcitonin, which directly stimulates the production of 1,25-$(OH)_2$ vitamin D (Galante et al, 1972; Kawashima et al, 1981); (e) vitamin D metabolites – calcitriol exerts a direct inhibitory effect on its own production, but a stimulating effect on 24,25-$(OH)_2D_3$ production.

Although the kidney is the principal endocrine organ that produces calcitriol, a number of other tissues, such as placenta, intestine, and also the immune cells of patients with sarcoidosis, are capable of producing a small amount of 1,25-$(OH)_2$ vitamin D.

Biological effects of vitamin D

The 1,25-$(OH)_2$ vitamin D receptor is fully characterised. It belongs to the superfamily of steroid hormone receptors that are related to the oncogene v-*erb A* (Pike, 1991). The principal target tissues for calcitriol are the intestine, bone and kidney. 1,25-$(OH)_2$ vitamin D passes through the cell membranes and binds to high-affinity nuclear receptors. The binding of the hormone to its specific receptor causes a conformational change, which allows binding to specific DNA-binding sites. This in turn induces the subsequent biosynthesis of new mRNA molecules which code for proteins related to the biological response of 1,25-$(OH)_2$ vitamin D; for example, in the intestine calcium-binding protein is synthesised, and in bone osteocalcin, osteopontin and alkaline phosphatase are produced.

Effect on the gut. The major and most documented action of 1,25-$(OH)_2$ vitamin D is to enhance the absorption of calcium and phosphorus from the gut by active transport. This is due to the synthesis of a calcium-binding protein in the intestinal epithelium.

Effect on bone. With respect to **osteoclasts**, the effects of 1,25-$(OH)_2$ vitamin D on bone are unique. It is a potent bone-resorbing agent. It mobilises calcium stores from bone by inducing the dissolution of bone mineral and matrix. 1,25-$(OH)_2$ vitamin D acts in concert with PTH to induce bone resorption as part of bone remodelling and for the maintenance of serum calcium levels when dietary intake is inadequate. High concentrations of 1,25-$(OH)_2$ vitamin D stimulate bone resorption even in the absence of PTH. It stimulates osteoclastic bone resorption indirectly and increases osteoclast formation. It induces the fusion and differentiation of cells with the characteristics of osteoclast

progenitors into mature cells (Roodman et al, 1985). As the multinucleated cells mature, they lose their vitamin D receptors.

With respect to **osteoblasts**, mature osteoblasts have receptors for vitamin D and respond to it by increasing the synthesis of osteocalcin (a calcium-binding protein produced by osteoblasts), osteopontin and alkaline phosphatase. It also modulates the synthesis of collagen. 1,25-$(OH)_2$ vitamin D is essential for the development and maintenance of mineralised skeleton. However, its role in mineralisation is not clear. It is likely to be an indirect one by increasing the supply of minerals available for the mineralisation process, through its action on gut and bone.

Other actions. Apart from the classical target organs in the gut, bone and kidney, vitamin D receptors are found in the parathyroid gland, C cells of the thyroid, pituitary, β cells of the pancreas, and in skin, ovary, uterus and mammary gland (Norman et al, 1982). 1,25$(OH)_2$ vitamin D also has effects on immune cell function, which could influence local factors regulating osteoclast activity.

Pathophysiology

Rickets in children and osteomalacia in adults are the consequence of an inadequate supply of the active hormonal form of vitamin D. An essential feature is the impaired mineralisation of the protein matrix of bone. Mineralisation of rachitic bone can be achieved, in the absence of vitamin D, by provision of adequate calcium in the diet or by infusion, suggesting an indirect role of vitamin D in enhancing mineralisation. In vitamin D-dependent rickets type II, in which there is target organ resistance to 1,25-$(OH)_2$ vitamin D and the serum levels of this hormone are increased, there are some defects in the receptor protein in the critical regions where the receptor binds to DNA (the zinc fingers).

Inadequate production of 1,25-$(OH)_2$ vitamin D in patients with chronic renal failure is a major factor in the calcium malabsorption, parathyroid hyperplasia and bone disease. Careful administration of 1,25-$(OH)_2$ vitamin D in these patients may inhibit parathyroid hyperplasia and thus prevent further bone disease and the necessity for parathyroid surgery.

Calcitonin

Chemistry

Calcitonin is a 32-amino-acid single-chain polypeptide, with a 1–7 disulphide bond and prolineamide at the carboxy-terminus. The complete sequence of 32 amino acids and the carboxy-terminal prolineamide are required for full biological activity. The amino acid sequences of calcitonin from various species are now known. There is marked interspecies variation, with only eight invariant residues clustered at the amino and carboxy termini, suggesting their importance for biological activity (Girgis and MacIntyre, 1993) (*Figure 4.5*). In humans, calcitonin is produced mainly by the parafollicular or C cells of the thyroid gland. These cells are of neural crest origin (Pearse and Polak, 1971). During embryonic development they migrate to be localised mainly in the thyroid gland. In submammalian vertebrates these cells remain as a separate gland, termed the ultimobranchial body. Submammalian calcitonins (e.g. salmon, eel) have been found to be approximately 20 to 50 times more potent than those of mammals.

Biosynthesis, secretion and metabolism

As with most hormonal peptides, calcitonin is produced as a precursor that is processed by cleavage and amida-tion before secretion. The human calcitonin precursor is a 141-amino-acid peptide in which calcitonin is flanked by two peptides: a carboxy-terminal 21-amino-acid peptide, called katacalcin, and an amino-terminal 82-amino-acid peptide. Calcitonin and katacalcin are co-secreted from the same granules. The calcitonin gene is located on the short arm of chromosome 11 between the genes for catalase and PTH (Przepiorka et al, 1984). It is a simple gene and consists of six exons. It encodes for two precursors, one for calcitonin and the other for a related peptide, calcitonin gene-related peptide (CGRP). The mRNAs for these two precursors are produced, in a tissue-specific manner, by differential processing of a single primary nuclear transcript, by the selection of alternative polyadenylation sites (Rosenfeld et al, 1983). Calcitonin is expressed mainly in the thyroid gland, whereas CGRP is produced predominantly in the neural tissues (Jonas et al, 1985). CGRP is a very potent vasodilator and may serve a neuromodulatory role in the central nervous system. In addition, there is a second CGRP gene (Steenburgh et al, 1985), which is transcribed into mRNA for CGRP in the central nervous system, but is silent for calcitonin. Calcitonin is released in response to an increase in plasma calcium concentration (Copp et al, 1961; Kumar et al, 1963). In addition, C cells have receptors for calcitriol.

```
            1       5         10        15        20        25        30
            *     * * * *     *                               *       *
Human     C G N L S T C M L G T Y T Q D F N K F H T F P Q T A I G V G A P
Rat       - - - - - - - - - - - - - - - - L - - - - - - - - S - - - - - -
Rabbit    - - - - - - - - - - - - - - - - L - - - - - - - - - - V - -

Salmon 2  - S - - - - - - - - K L S - - L H - L Q - - - R - N T - A - V -
Salmon 3  - S - - - - - V - - K L S - - L H - L Q - - - R - N T - A - V -
Salmon 1  - S - - - - - V - - K L S - E L H - L Q - Y - R - N T - S - T -
Eel       - S - - - - - V - - K L S - E L H - L Q - Y - R - D V - A - T -
Chicken   - A S - - - - V - - K L S - E L H - L Q - Y - R - D V - A - T -

Porcine   - S - - - - - V - S A - W R N L - N - - R - S G M G F - P E T -
Bovine    - S - - - - - V - S A - W K - L - N Y - R - S G M G F - P E T -
Ovine     - S - - - - - V - S A - W K - L - N Y - R Y S G M G F - P E T -
```

Figure 4.5   Amino acid sequences of the calcitonins, arranged in order of their similarity to human calcitonin. Amino acid identities with the sequence of human calcitonin are noted by dashes. The eight invariant residues are indicated by asterisks. From Girgis and MacIntyre (1993), with permission.

Biological effects and mode of action

Calcitonin produces a range of effects, the most obvious of which is its effect on bone.

Bone. When calcitonin is injected intravenously into young animals with a high bone turnover, there is a marked fall in plasma calcium concentration (Robinson et al, 1967). A similar effect is observed in patients with Paget's disease following the administration of calcitonin, but it is not seen in normal adults. This calcium-lowering effect of calcitonin is due to acute inhibition of osteoclastic activity, with a marked decrease in the flow of calcium from bone to blood. Abundant, specific, high-affinity receptors have been characterised on isolated rat osteoclasts (Nicholson et al, 1986) and have also been demonstrated by direct *in vivo* autoradiography (Warshawsky et al, 1980). The osteoclast is sensitive to human calcitonin at femtomolar concentrations (Zaidi et al, 1987), which fall well within the reported levels for circulating calcitonin. This suggests that calcitonin probably exerts a tonic influence on osteoclasts, possibly as a physiological regulator of its function (Chambers and Moore, 1983). Chambers and Moore were able to visualise directly an acute effect of calcitonin on osteoclasts (*Figure 4.6*).

Calcitonin has two main actions on the modulation of osteoclast activity: first, in the inhibition of osteoclast recruitment resulting in continued reduction in osteoclast numbers, and second, a direct powerful inhibition of the resorptive activity of mature osteoclasts. Acute inhibition follows binding of calcitonin to a surface receptor belonging to a new family of G protein-coupled receptors (Lin et al, 1991). This family now includes secretin, glucagon-like peptide and PTH/PTH-rp. The subsequent inhibitory action of calcitonin is mediated by two second messengers: cAMP and calcium. The increase in cAMP concentration is consequent on activation of adenylate cyclase via a stimulating G_s protein. The increase in cAMP concentration rapidly inhibits secretion and arrests the ruffling of the secretory membrane. The detailed pathway for increased intracellular calcium activity is not clear.

When calcitonin is administered chronically in patients with Paget's disease or osteoporosis, the number of osteoclasts declines progressively (Haymovits et al, 1977). The chronic effect of calcitonin is most dramatically demonstrated in patients with the osteolytic form of Paget's disease who have been treated with calcitonin. The osteolytic area of bone usually fills in with calcified tissue and may approach normality.

Other effects of calcitonin. Calcitonin has a natriuretic, hypocalcuric and phosphaturic effect on the kidney (Robinson et al, 1966; Williams et al, 1972) (the latter is minor in comparison to that of PTH). It also stimulates 25-hydroxyvitamin D_3- 1α-hydroxylase in proximal tubules of the kidney (Galante et al, 1972; Kawashima et al, 1981). Calcitonin administered intracerebroventricularly produces an analgesic effect (Pecile et al, 1975).

Physiological role of CT

The most reasonable hypothesis is that the major role of calcitonin is to protect the skeleton during periods of calcium stress such as growth, pregnancy and lactation (Stevenson et al, 1979; MacIntyre, 1995).

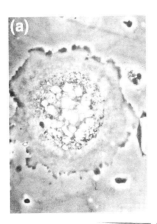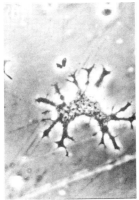

Figure 4.6 (a) An osteoclast, after 2 hours in control medium, showing lobulated periphery, with dense peripheral staining corresponding to pseudopodial motility. (b) Inhibition of motility with a physiological concentration of calcitonin. (Courtesy of Professor T.J. Chambers, Department of Histopathology, St George's Hospital Medical School, London, UK.)

NON-CALCITROPIC HORMONES

These are systemic hormones that influence bone cell function, but are not under negative feedback control by calcium in extracellular fluid.

Oestrogens and androgens

Oestrogens are important inhibitors of bone resorption *in vivo*. Loss of ovarian function, such as at the menopause, results in a dramatic loss of bone that can be prevented by oestrogen replacement (Lindsay et al, 1976, 1980). However, the mechanism by which lack of oestrogen leads to enhanced osteoclastic bone resorption is not entirely clear. In organ culture systems oestrogens have not been shown to have any direct effect (Caputo et al, 1975). However, oestrogen receptors have been identified in human cells with the osteoblast phenotype (Eriksen et al, 1988). It is well recognised that oestrogen regulates bone remodelling by modulating the production of cytokines and growth factors from bone marrow and bone cells (Pacifici, 1996). It has been shown that oestrogen enhances the expression of transforming growth factor (TGF)β by cells with the osteoblast phenotype (Keeting et al, 1989). One possible mechanism to explain the increased bone loss after the menopause is that oestrogen loss results in an interleukin 6-mediated stimulation of osteoclastogenesis (Jilka et al, 1992).

A hypothesis that has not been tested sufficiently is that oestrogen-induced skeletal protection is mediated by oestrogen-induced increases in the release of nitric oxide (NO) from bone vascular endothelium as well as from bone cells. This is supported by the following studies: circulating levels of nitrite and nitrate, the stable end-products of NO metabolism, are raised in postmenopausal women on replacement therapy with 17β-oestradiol (Rosselli et al, 1995); constitutive endothelial isoforms of NO synthase are expressed in osteoblasts, osteoclasts and osteocytes (Hukkanen et al, 1995); *in vivo* experiments in rats showed that NO donors abolish the ovariectomy-induced bone loss (Wimalawansa et al, 1996); osteoclastic bone resorption is potentiated by inhibitors of NO synthase in rats *in vivo* (Kasten et al, 1994); and NO inhibits osteoclastic bone resorption *in vitro* (MacIntyre et al, 1991; Brandi et al, 1995; Ralston et al, 1995). Photomicrographs demonstrating endothelial and inducible isoforms of NO synthase in osteoclast-like cells are shown in *Figure 4.7*.

Androgens have important effects on skeletal development and are needed for the maintenance of adult bone mass. Androgen deficiency acquired in adult life causes bone loss (Stepan et al, 1989; Stanley et al, 1991). The cellular mechanisms by which androgens influence bone metabolism are poorly defined. High-affinity androgen receptors are found in osteoblast- and osteoclast-like cell lines (Colvard et al, 1989). Androgens also increase gene expression and excretion of TGF-β (Kasperk et al, 1990) and decrease prostaglandin E_2 secretion by mixed bone cells *in vitro* (Orwoll et al, 1991).

When used before maturity, oestrogens and androgens stimulate skeletal maturation and closure of the epiphysis, resulting in short stature.

Glucocorticoids

Glucocorticoids have complex effects on bone (Mundy and Raisz, 1974). The major effect of cortisol is to decrease bone formation (Raisz et al, 1993); a less marked effect is to increase bone resorption (LoCascio et al, 1990). The net outcome of cortisol excess can be a marked reduction in bone mass (Reid, 1989; Lukert and Raisz, 1990) and, in children, a reduction in linear growth as well. Several actions contribute to this outcome and include: decreased calcitriol synthesis and interference with its action and, therefore, decreased intestinal absorption of calcium (Klein et al, 1977); increased urinary calcium excretion, so that less calcium is available for mineralisation; inhibition of collagen synthesis by osteoblasts (Oikarinen et al, 1992); and inhibition of the differentiation of mensenchymal osteoblast precursors.

Growth hormone and insulin–like growth factor 1

Growth hormone (GH) has dramatic effects on immature bones. It plays the main role in the modulation of skeletal growth of children from birth until puberty. In the absence of GH, linear growth occurs at about half to one-third of the normal rate. However, the role of GH in the maintenance of skeletal mass in adults is not established. Skeletal growth is stimulated in patients with GH overproduction, such as in acromegaly and gigantism. In the latter there is, in addition, stimulation of cartilage growth before epiphyseal closure.

The effects of GH on the skeleton appear to be mediated largely through the production of somatomedin C, or insulin-like growth factor (IGF)1, in peripheral

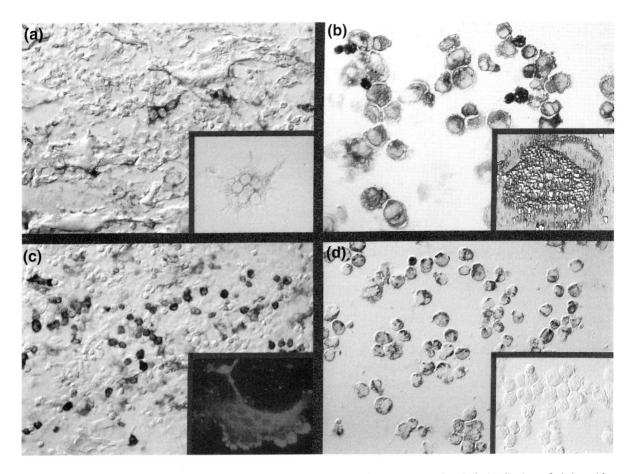

Figure 4.7 Photomicrographs showing examples of histochemical and immunocytochemical visualisation of nitric oxide synthase (NOS) activity and inducible and endothelial isoforms of NOS protein in rat and human osteoclast-like cells. (A) Intense reduced nicotinamide adenine dinucleotide phosphate (NADPH)- diaphorase activity (a histochemical marker for NOSs) is localised in bone trabeculae attached osteoclasts in rat tibia *in situ*. (A, inset) In isolated rat osteoclasts, NADPH-diaphorase activity was found to be expressed only at low levels. (B) Phorbol 12-myristate 13-acetate (PMA)-treated preosteoclastic human FLG 29.1 cells show strong immunoreactivity for the endothelial isoform of cNOS. (B, inset) Three-dimensional image reconstructions of isolated rat osteoclasts reveal a characteristic intracellular distribution of cNOS immunoreactivity, found most abundantly in the thick central perinuclear area and in the pericellular pseudopodes (peroxidase method). (C) Intense immunoreactivity for the inducible NOS isoform in mononuclear and multinuclear cells in lipopolysaccharide (LPS)-treated rat tibia *in situ*. (C, inset) Three-dimensional image reconstruction (laser scanning confocal image) of isolated rat osteoclast treated with LPS plus interferonγ, showing intense inducible NOS immunoreactivity with similar intracellular distribution as for the cNOS isoform (immunofluorescence method). (D) PMA-treated preosteoclastic human FLG 29.1 cells show intense immunoreactivity for inducible NOS after 48 hours of stimulation. (D, inset) In non-treated FLG 29.1 cells, inducible NOS immunoreactivity was expressed only at low levels or was absent. From Brandi et al (1995), with permission.

tissues, particularly in the liver. Therefore, GH acts indirectly on the skeleton as IGF-1 is a necessary intermediate. GH stimulates osteoblasts and skeletal fibroblasts also to secrete IGF-1 (Ernst and Froesch, 1988; Ernst and Rodan, 1990).

Thyroid hormones

Thyroid hormones can produce direct stimulation of bone resorption in organ culture (Mundy et al, 1976). However, the effect is relatively small. In hyperthyroidism there is a marked increase in bone turnover, probably due to an increased frequency of activation of remodelling cycles (Harvey et al, 1990). Hyperthyroidism is associated with osteopenia and occasionally with hypercalcaemia (Mundy and Raisz, 1979). Hypercalcuria is frequently found in normocalcaemic hyperthyroid patients, as well as in hypercalcaemic patients (Aub et al, 1929), and almost certainly represents increased bone resorption. It has also been reported that suppressive doses of thyroxine significantly reduce bone mineral density in elderly and middle-aged women (Diamond et al, 1990).

ACKNOWLEDGEMENTS

This work was supported by the Medical Research Council and the Grand Charity of Freemasons.

REFERENCES

Aub JC, Bauer W, Heath C et al. Studies of calcium and phosphorus metabolism. III. The effects of the thyroid hormone in thyroid disease. *J Clin Invest* 1929; **7**: 97–137.

Boyle IT, Gray RW, DeLuca HF. Regulation by calcium of *in vivo* synthesis of 1,25-dihydroxycholecalciferol and 21,25-dihydroxycholecalciferol. *Proc Natl Acad Sci USA* 1971; **68**: 2131–2134.

Brandi ML, Hukkanen M, Umeda T et al. Bidirectional regulation of osteoclast function by nitric oxide synthase isoforms. *Proc Natl Acad Sci USA* 1995; **92**: 2954–2958.

Brown EM, Gamba G, Riccardi D et al. Cloning and characterization of an extracellular Ca^{2+} sensing receptor from bovine parathyroid. *Nature* 1993; **366**: 575–580.

Caputo CB, Meadows D, Raisz LG. Failure of estrogens and androgens to inhibit bone resorption in tissue culture. *Endocrinology* 1975; **98**: 1065–1068.

Chambers TJ, Moore A. The sensitivity of isolated osteoclasts to mophological transformation by calcitonin. *J Clin Endocrinol Metab* 1983; **57**: 819.

Colvard D, Spelsberg T, Eriksen E et al. Evidence of steroid receptors in human osteoblast-like cells. *Connect Tissue Res* 1989; **20**: 33–40.

Copp DH, Cameron EC, Cheney B, Davidson AGF, Henze KG. Evidence for calcitonin – a new hormone from the parathyroid that lowers blood calcium. *Endocrinology* 1961; **70**: 638–639.

Diamond T, Nery L, Hales I. A therapeutic dilemma: suppressive doses of thyroxine significantly reduce bone mineral measurements in both premenopausal and postmenopausal women with thyroid carcinoma. *J Clin Endocrinol Metab* 1990; **72**: 1184–1188.

Eriksen EF, Colvard DS, Berg NJ et al. Evidence of estrogen

receptors in normal human osteoblast-like cells. *Science* 1988; **241**: 84–86.

Ernst M, Froesch ER. Growth hormone dependent stimulation of osteoblast-like cells in serum-free cultures via local synthesis of insulin-like growth factor I. *Biochem Biophys Res Commun* 1988; **151**: 142–147.

Ernst M, Rodan GA. Increased activity of insulin-like growth factor (IGF) in osteoblastic cells in the presence of growth hormone (GH): positive correlation with the presence of the GH-induced IGF-binding protein BP-3. *Endocrinology* 1990; **127**: 807–814.

Galante L, Colston KW, MacAuley SJ, MacIntyre I. Effect of calcitonin on vitamin D metabolism. *Nature* 1972; **238**: 271–273.

Garabedian M, Holick MF, Deluca HF, Boyle IT. Control of 25-hydroxycholecalciferol metabolism by parathyroid glands. *Proc Natl Acad Sci USA* 1972; **69**: 1673–1676.

Girgis SI, MacIntyre I. The calcitonin gene peptide family: molecular biology, physiology, pharamcology and relations to malignancy. In: Mazzaferri EL, Samaan NA (eds) *Endocrine Tumours*, Boston: Blackwell Scientific Publications, 1993: 671–686.

Habener JF, Kemper B, Potts JT Jr. Calcium-dependent intracellular degradation of parathyroid hormone: a possible mechanism for the regulation of hormone stores. *Endocrinology* 1975; **97**: 431–441.

Habener JF, Rosenblatt M, Potts JT Jr. Parathyroid hormone: biochemical aspects of biosynthesis, secretion, action and metabolism. *Physiol Rev* 1984; **64**: 985–1053.

Harvey RD, McHardy KC, Reid IW et al. Measurement of bone collagen degradation in hyperthyroidism and during thyroxine replacement therapy using pyridinium crosslinks as specific urinary markers. *J Clin Endocrinol Metab* 1990; **72**: 1189–1194.

Haymovits A, Zbuzek V, Ling A, Hobitz H, Fotino M. Studies on short-term therapy with human calcitonin and ultrastructural, immunological and genetic observations on the aetiology of Paget's disease. In: MacIntyre I (ed.) *Human Calcitonin and Paget's Disease, Proceedings of an International Workshop.* Berne: Hans Huber, 1977; 138–154.

Hock JM, Gera I, Fonseca J, Raisz LG. Human parathyroid hormone (1–34) increases bone mass in ovariectomized and orchidectomised rats. *Endocrinology* 1988; **122**: 2899–2904.

Hukkanen M, Hughes FJ, Buttery LDK et al. Cytokine-stimulated expression of inducible nitric oxide synthase by mouse, rat, and human osteoblast-like cells and its functional role in osteoblast metabolic activity. *Endocrinology* 1995; **136**: 5445–5453.

Ishimi Y, Russell J, Sherwood LM. Regulation by calcium and 1,25-$(OH)_2D_3$ of cell proliferation and function of bovine parathyroid cells in culture. *J Bone Miner Res* 1990; **5**: 755–760.

Jilka RL, Hangoc G, Girasole G et al. Increased osteoclast development after estrogen loss: mediation by interleukin-6. *Science* 1992; **257**: 88–91.

Jonas V, Lin CR, Kawashima E et al. Alternative RNA processing events in human calcitonin/calcitonin gene-related peptide gene expression. *Proc Natl Acad Sci USA* 1985; **82**: 1994–1998.

Jüppner H, Abour-Samra A-B, Freeman M et al. A G protein-linked receptor for parathyroid hormone-related peptide. *Science* 1991; **254**: 1024–1026.

Kasperk C, Fitzsimmons R, Strong D et al. Studies of the mechanism by which androgens enhance mitogenesis and differentiation in bone cells. *J Clin Endocrinol Metab* 1990; **71**: 1322–1329.

Kasten TP, Collin-Osdoby P, Patel N et al. Potentiation of osteoclast bone-resorption activity by inhibition of nitric oxide synthase. *Proc Natl Acad Sci USA* 1994; **91**: 3569–3573.

Kawashima H, Torikai S, Kurokawa K. Calcitonin selectively stimulates 25-hydroxyvitamin D_3-1α-hydroxylase in proximal straight tubule of rat kidney. *Nature* 1981; **291**: 327–329.

Keeting PE, Bonewald LF, Colvard TC et al. Estrogen-mediated release of transforming growth factor-beta by normal human osteoblast-like cells. *J Bone Miner Res* 1989; **4**: 655.

Keutmann HT, Sauer MM, Hendy GN, O'Riordan JLH, Potts JT Jr. Complete amino acid sequence of human parathyroid hormone. *Biochemistry* 1978; **17(26)** 5723–5729.

Klein RG, Arnaud SB, Gallagher JC et al. Intestinal calcium absorption in exogenous hypercortisonism. Role of 25-hydroxyvitamin D and corticosteroid dose. *J Clin Invest* 1977; **60**: 253–259.

Kumar MA, Foster GV, MacIntyre I. Further evidence for calcitonin – a rapid-acting hormone which lowers plasma calcium. *Lancet* 1963; **ii**: 480–482.

Larkins RG, MacAuley SJ, Colston KW, Evans IMA, Galante LS, MacIntyre I. Regulation of vitamin-D metabolism without parathyroid hormone. *Lancet* 1973; **ii**: 289–291.

Lin HY, Harris TL, Flannery MS et al. Expression cloning of an adenylate cyclase-coupled calcitonin receptor. *Science* 1991; **254**: 1022–1024.

Lindsay R, Hart DM, Aitken JM et al. Long-term prevention of postmenopausal osteoporosis by oestrogen: evidence for an increased bone mass after delayed onset of oestrogen treatment. *Lancet* 1976; **i**: 1038–1041.

Lindsay R, Hart DM, Forrest C et al. Prevention of spinal osteoporosis in oophorectomised women. *Lancet* 1980; **ii**: 1151–1153.

LoCascio V, Bonucci E, Imbimbo B et al. Bone loss in response to long-term glucocorticoid therapy. *Bone Miner* 1990; **8**: 39–51.

Lukert BP, Raisz LG. Glucocorticoid-induced osteoporosis: pathogenesis and management. *Ann Intern Med* 1990; **112**: 352–364.

MacIntyre I. Calcitonin: physiology, biosynthesis, secretion, metabolism and mode of action. In: DeGroot LJ (ed.) *Endocrinology*, Vol. 2. Philadelphia: WB Saunders, 1995: 978–989.

MacIntyre I, Colston KW, Szelke, Spanos E. A survey of the hormonal factors that control calcium metabolism. *Ann NY Acad Sci* 1978; **3074**: 345–355.

MacIntyre I, Zaidi M, Towhidul Alam ASM et al. Osteoclastic inhibition: an action of nitric oxide not mediated by cyclic GMP. *Proc Natl Acad Sci USA* 1991; **88**: 2936–2940.

Martin TJ, Suva LJ. Parathyroid hormone-related protein in hypercalaemia of malignancy. *Clin Endocrinol* 1989; **31**: 631–647.

Mundy GR, Raisz LG. Drugs for disorders of bones. *New Ethic Med Prog* 1974; **ii**: 165–199.

Mundy GR, Raisz LG. Thyrotoxicosis and calcium metabolism. *Miner Electrolyte Metab* 1979; **2**: 285–292.

Mundy GR, Shapiro L, Bandelin JG et al. Direct stimulation of bone resorption by thyroid hormones. *J Clin Invest* 1976: **58**: 529–534.

Nicholson GC, Moseley JM, Sexton PM, Mendelsohn FAO, Martin TJ. Abundant calcitonin receptors in isolated rat osteoclasts. *J Clin Invest* 1986; **78**: 355–359.

Nussbaum SR, Zahradnik RJ, Lavigne JR et al. Highly sensitive two-site immunoradiometric assay of parathyrin, and its clinical utility in evaluating patients with hypercalcemia. *Clin Chem* 1987; **33(8)** 1364–1367.

Norman AW, Roth J, Orci L. The vitamin D endocrine system: steroid metabolism, hormone, receptors, and biological response (calcium binding proteins). *Endocr Rev* 1982; **3**: 331–366.

Oikarinen A, Autio P, Vuori J et al. Systemic glucocorticoid treatment decreases serum concentrations of carboxyterminal propeptide of type I procollagen and aminoterminal propeptide of type III procollagen. *Br J Dermatol* 1992; **126**: 172–178.

Orwoll ES, Stribrska L, Ramsey EE, Keenan EJ. Androgen receptors in osteoblast-like cell lines. *Calcif Tissue Int* 1991; **49**: 183–187.

Pacifici R. Estrogen, cytokines, and pathogenesis of postmenopausal osteoporosis. *Bone Miner Res* 1996; **11(8)**: 1043–1051.

Pearse AGE, Polak JM. Cytochemical evidence for the neural crest origin of mammalian ultimobranchial C-cells. *Histochemie* 1971; **27**: 96–102.

Pecile A, Ferri S, Braga PC, Olgiati VR. Effects of intracerebroventricular calcitonin in the conscious rabbit. *Experientia* 1975; **31**: 332–333.

Pike JW, Vitamin D_3 receptors: structure and function in transcription. *Ann Rev Nutr* 1991; **11**: 189.

Przepiorka D, Baylin SB, McBride OW, Testa JR, de Bustros A, Nelkin BD. The human calcitonin gene is located on the short arm of chromosome 11. *Biochem Biophys Res Commun* 1984; **120**: 493–499.

Raisz LJ, Bogdanovics E, Taxel P et al. Effect of glucocorticoids on bone formation and resorption. In: Christiansen C, Riis B (eds) *Fourth International Symposium on Osteoporosis 27 March–2 April 1993*. Hong Kong, 1993: 506–508.

Ralston SH, Ho LP, Helfrich M et al. Nitric oxide: a cytokine induced regulator of bone resorption. *J Bone Miner Res* 1995; **10**: 1040–1049.

Reid IR. Pathogenesis and treatment of steroid osteoporosis. *Clin Endocrinol* 1989; **30**: 83–103.

Roodman GD, Ibbotson KJ, MacDonald BR et al. 1,25 Dihydroxyvitamin D_3 causes formation of multinucleated cells with several osteoclast characteristics in cultures of primate marrow. *Proc Natl Acad Sci USA* 1985; **82**: 8213–8217.

Robinson CJ, Martin TJ, MacIntyre I. Phosphaturic effect of thyrocalcitonin. *Lancet* 1966; ii: 83–84.

Robinson CJ, Martin TJ, Matthews EW, MacIntyre I. Mode of action of thyrocalcitonin. *J Endocrinol* 1967; **39**: 71.

Rosenfeld MG, Mermod J-J, Amara SC et al. Production of a novel neuropeptide encoded by the calcitonin gene via tissue-specific RNA processing. *Nature* 1983; **304**: 129–135.

Rosselli M, Imthurn B, Keller PJ, Jackson EK, Dubey RK. Circulating nitric oxide (nitrite/nitrate) levels in postmenopausal women substituted with 17β-estradiol and norethisterone acetate. *Hypertension* 1995; **25(4)**: 848–853.

Stanley HL, Schmitt BP, Poses RM et al. Does hypogonadism contribute to the occurrence of a minimal trauma hip fracture in elderly men? *J Am Geriatr Soc* 1991; **39**: 766–771.

Steenburgh PH, Höppener JWM, Zandberg J, Lips CJM, Jansz HS. A second human calcitonin/CGRP gene. *FEBS Lett* 1985; **183**: 403–407.

Stepan JJ, Lachman M, Zverina J et al. Castrated men exhibit bone loss: effect of calcitonin treatment on biochemical indices of bone remodelling. *J Clin Endocrinol Metab* 1989; **69**: 523–527.

Stevenson JC, Hillyard CJ, MacIntyre I et al. A physiological role for calcitonin: protection of the maternal skeleton. *Lancet* 1979; **ii**: 769.

Suva LJ, Winslow GA, Wettenhall REH et al. A parathyroid hormone-related protein implicated in malignant hypercalcemia: cloning and expression. *Science* 1987; **237**: 893–896.

Tregear GW, Van Rietschoten J, Greene E et al. Bovine parathyroid hormone: minimum chain length of synthetic peptide required for biological activity. *Endocrinology* 1973; **93**: 1349–1353.

Warshawsky H, Goltzman D, Rouleau MF, Bergeron JJM. Direct *in vivo* demonstration by radioautography of specific binding sites for calcitonin in skeletal and renal tissues of the rat. *J Cell Biol* 1980; **85**: 682–694.

Williams CC, Matthews EW, Moseley JM, MacIntyre I. The effects of synthetic human and salmon calcitonins on electrolyte excretion in the rat. *Clin Sci* 1972; **42**: 129–137.

Wimalawansa SJ, De Marco G, Gangula P, Yallampalli C. Nitric oxide donor alleviates ovariectomy-induced bone loss. *Bone* 1996; **18(4)**: 301–304.

Zaidi M, Chambers TJ, Bevis PJR et al. The effects of peptides from the calcitonin genes on bone. *Q J Exp Physiol* 1987; **73**: 471.

5

Physiology of Cartilage

Andrew C Hall

INTRODUCTION

Cartilage is of three varieties; each differs in the composition and proportions of the extracellular fibrous (collagen) and non-fibrous macromolecules (principally proteoglycans), in the distribution and morphology of the cells, and in their anatomical location and functions within the body.

In **hyaline cartilage** (e.g. articular cartilage) the proportions of collagen:proteoglycan are such that cartilage has a glassy, sometimes translucent, blue-white appearance in young age, turning yellow-white and opaque in old age. This cartilage forms the temporary skeleton in the embryo before it is gradually replaced by bone and is also present in the epiphyseal plates found between the diaphysis and epiphysis of growing long bones, and is responsible for the longitudinal growth of bone. In adults, hyaline cartilage is found in the articulating surfaces of movable joints, in the walls of the larger respiratory passages (e.g. nose, larynx, trachea, bronchus) and at the ventral ends of ribs that articulate with the sternum. No fibres are seen either macroscopically or on routine histological examination. The tissue is avascular and populated by the cells, or chondrocytes, that synthesise, export and degrade the components of the extracellular matrix. This comprises much proteoglycan, fibrous collagen, (principally type II, but also small amounts of the important types VI, IX and XI, and others) and other proteins. The tissue is adapted principally to withstand compressive forces, although the surface regions of articular cartilage have some capacity to resist tensile forces associated with joint motion.

Fibrocartilage (white fibrocartilage) is found in the intervertebral discs of the spine, the attachments of some ligaments to bone, and in the pubic symphysis. This cartilage is always associated with dense connective tissue, the border between the two structures often being difficult to distinguish. Indeed, fibrocartilage develops from dense connective tissues by means of differentiation of fibroblastic cells into chondrocytes. Fibrocartilage is usually manufactured by fibroblast-like cells that synthesise a matrix principally of type I collagen in association with relatively little proteoglycan but often with some elastic material. The higher proportion of collagen:proteoglycan is clear since fibres are relatively easily seen (e.g. in intervertebral disc), and the structure is that of an oriented, compact, avascular, fibrous meshwork, containing relatively little water. Although tendon (which is not a fibrocartilage) is adapted principally to withstand tensile forces, it has local fibrocartilaginous regions rather like cartilage where the tendon wraps around bone, giving some capacity to withstand compression.

Elastic cartilage (yellow fibrocartilage) is characterised by elastic fibres as well as collagen and proteoglycan (e.g. auricle of the ear, in the eustachian tubes, epiglottis), and is like rubber, being highly and reversibly deformable. The chondrocytes in elastic cartilage closely resemble those of hyaline cartilage but synthesise elastin in addition to collagens and proteoglycans.

In this chapter the physiology of cartilaginous tissue will be considered with particular reference to articular cartilage, which has been studied most extensively. However, where appropriate, properties of intervertebral disc and tendon are considered because of their interesting comparative characteristics. The reader is referred to recent texts for further information (Maroudas and Kuettner, 1990; Gardner, 1992; Kuettner et al, 1992; Muir, 1995).

CHONDROCYTE FUNCTION

Connective tissues are not inert engineering materials, but living tissues whose capacity for support and resistance to mechanical forces are crucial for the functioning of the musculoskeletal system. By a synchronised balance between anabolism (synthesis) and catabolism (breakdown), the cells of connective tissues continually produce and maintain the appropriate macromolecules, giving the tissue its required mechanical properties. Indeed, it has been said that the cells of connective tissues are the 'functional units of health and disease' (Gardner, 1992). In normal connective tissue, the cells are programmed to synthesise and secrete every form of fibrous and non-fibrous connective tissue macromolecule. However, in practice, differentiated normal connective tissue chondrocytes preferentially produce substantial quantities of a limited repertoire of macromolecules. When there are changes to the physicochemical environment of the cells, as occur during altered loading patterns, different genetic programmes become dominant and the connective tissue cells synthesise an altered pattern of macromolecules. It is this property that allows chondrocytes to respond to altered mechanical forces and produce a mechanically viable matrix.

The mechanical functions of articular cartilage are described in Chapter 16, and these are achieved because cartilage acts like a fibre-reinforced gel. Cartilage is more deformable than bone and so can distribute the load over its surface. Cartilage also resists compression, and with synovial fluid gives a very low friction surface essential for withstanding the tensile and shearing forces associated with joint motion and thereby permits ease of movement. The absence of vulnerable structures such as nerves, blood vessels, lymphatic vessels and epithelia on, or within, cartilage is also essential for its load-bearing properties. Despite the importance of the mechanical properties of the cartilage extracellular matrix, it is the chondrocytes and their response to physico-chemical factors that ultimately determine the characteristics of the tissue. Chondrocytes are remarkable because they can produce unique extracellular matrix components and maintain their orderly interactions within connective tissues relatively remote from nutritional sources or obvious control mechanisms such as cell-to-cell contact.

Although the **macroscopic** appearance of cartilage might be thought of as deceptively simple and homogeneous, it is really quite complex and variable. There is marked heterogeneity throughout the tissue in terms of the matrix macromolecules and the size and shape of chondrocytes. Thus, it is the **avascular nature** of cartilage, the physical properties of the **matrix macromolecules** and the **mechanical forces** occurring routinely that markedly alter the environment of chondrocytes. In this chapter we will initially consider the physical environment of chondrocytes, which is rather unusual compared to that of most other cell types, and then the cellular aspects of cartilage, and give examples of how changes to the chondrocytes' environment can influence matrix metabolism.

It is becoming evident that the study of the fundamental properties of the cellular aspects of connective tissue is an important prerequisite for understanding the normal functioning of the tissue and ultimately providing a rational framework for the treatment of disease processes. Unfortunately, there has been rather slow progress in this field, possibly because laboratories working on connective tissue approach the problem from the perspective either of joint biomechanics or of the biochemistry of the extracellular matrix, rather than cellular biology and physiology.

In the past, the role of chondrocytes has often been marginalised, which is surprising because they are the only living agents that can synthesise or breakdown the matrix, and initiate repair if it is damaged. In addition, in skeletally mature healthy animals and humans, it appears that there is very little, if any, chondrocyte division, and thus the chondrocytes in adult cartilage are those that are present for life. Chondrocytes that are lost, for example through mechanical damage, are probably not replaced, leaving the remaining cells with a greater burden to maintain normal matrix turnover.

Connective tissues are, however, not easy to study because the cells are heterogeneous and surrounded by a complex extracellular matrix which plays an important, but poorly understood, role in mediating the cellular response. Although it is possible to investigate some cellular responses *in situ*, for example using confocal laser scanning microscopy of fluorescently labelled cells, these approaches are in their infancy. Even experiments on cartilage explants require careful interpretation because the apparently simple act of cutting cartilage from bone can alter the forces within the collagen architecture of the tissue and may change chondrocyte behaviour, particularly when the matrix is compromised mechanically as occurs in the disease (osteoarthrosis[1]) processes.

There has, therefore, been considerable interest using isolated chondrocytes as experimental systems with the ultimate aim of understanding cartilage function, and this chapter attempts to clarify some of the properties of the chondrocyte's environment and how they may influence chondrocyte metabolism, and hopefully to stimulate interest in these areas. Although one must be aware of the problems associated with the use of chondrocytes isolated from the matrix, there is no doubt that often this information cannot be obtained in any other way. Thus, studies on isolated chondrocytes are an essential part of cartilage research but it is appreciated that ultimately the aim is to understand the behaviour of the cells in the intact tissue.

PRINCIPAL COMPONENTS OF ARTICULAR CARTILAGE

The mechanical resilience of cartilage arises from the four main constituents of the extracellular matrix and their properties (*Figure 5.1*).

Proteoglycans

The proteoglycans of articular cartilage are proteins that have one or more glycosaminoglycan (GAG) chains attached, usually chondroitin sulphate (CS) or keratan sulphate (KS), and that are covalently bound to the core protein. **Aggrecan** (the large species of proteoglycan), which comprises monomers of GAG, represents the bulk of the proteoglycans, interacts non-covalently with hyaluronan and link proteins to form huge multimolecular aggregates (hence the name), typically of $M_r = 5 \times 10^7$ to 5×10^8 Da, trapped within the collagen meshwork. Most of the aggrecan mass is carbohydrate which is usually in the ratio 4:1 (CS:KS) in articular cartilage, although this varies within the tissue and with age. These molecules are highly hydrated and play a key role in cartilage function by giving the tissue the capacity to resist compression.

---

[1]Osteoarthrosis is the European and preferred term; osteoarthritis is the American term. The suffix -*itis* is possibly misleading because it implies that the primary event is inflammatory, which is not the case for this disease, but is for rheumatoid arthritis.

The smaller leucine-rich proteoglycans **decorin, biglycan** and **fibromodulin** (core protein size about 40 kDa) are found in most connective tissues and can account for 20–25% of cartilage proteoglycans. Decorin and biglycan covalently link one or two CS or dermatan sulphate (DS) chains respectively, and fibromodulin bears KS chains (Hardingham and Fosang, 1992). Associated with the proteoglycans are proteins, collectively known as the 'ground substance'.

The turnover of proteoglycans is relatively rapid and, as we consider later, changes to proteoglycan composition are the primary response to variations to the loading pattern and physical environment because they control the capacity of cartilage to withstand mechanical stresses. Turnover rates depend on the cartilage source and the species studied; for example, in human adult femoral head, values vary over 300–800 days, whereas in adult rabbit articular cartilage a value of more than 100 days has been obtained; turnover rates vary between different types of proteoglycans, for example that of KS is less than with CS.

Another essential component of the matrix, although present in relatively small amounts, is **hyaluronan**, a non-sulphated glycosaminoglycan. Chondrocytes have surface receptors for these molecules (CD44), which belong to a large family of hyaluronan-binding proteins termed **hyaloadherins**. Hyaluronan therefore provides a gel to which chondrocytes are able to attach, as well as providing the central component of the proteoglycan aggregates (see *Figure 5.1*).

Collagen

The collagens (principally type II comprising more than 95% of the total) form a three-dimensional fibrillar network of rope-like molecular aggregates which maintains the tissue volume, shape and tensile strength. The type II (and type X) collagen molecules are homotrimers (i.e. they are composed of three identical polypeptide α chains up to several micrometres long and 8–500 nm thick), each possessing the characteristic repeating tripeptide sequence (gly–x–y) which forms a left-handed helix. The three chains are twisted together into a right-handed helix. The other collagens are heterotrimers, being composed of three distinct peptide chains. The minor collagens of connective tissues play essential roles; for example, type IX, a non-fibril-forming highly glycosylated collagen covalently linked to the surface of type II

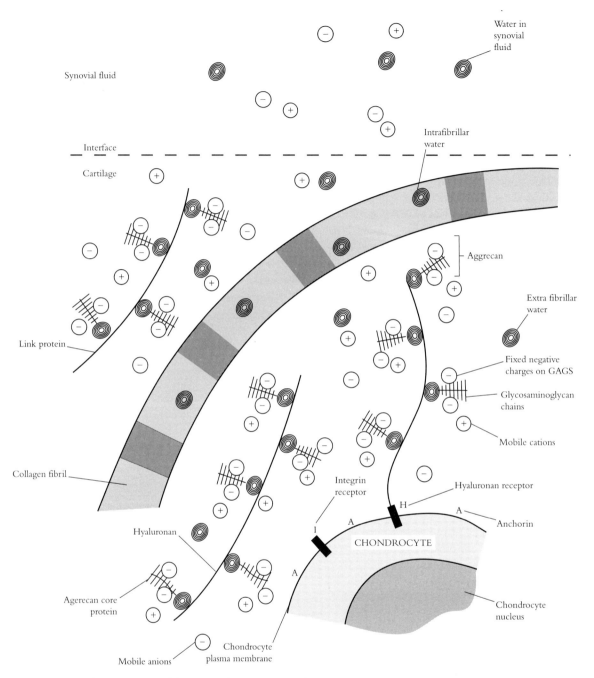

Figure 5.1 A schematic view of the principal components of cartilage and the chondrocyte's environment. The collagen fibrils immobilise the glycosaminoglycan (GAG) chains which bear a high density of fixed negative charges resulting in a marked increase/decrease in the concentration of mobile cations/anions respectively. The GAG chains are linked to the aggrecan core protein, which is attached via link protein to hyaluronan (hyaluronic acid). **A** indicates anchorin CII, a 34-kDa protein found on the chondrocyte plasma membrane which binds to a collagen type II fibre to which type VI collagen is anchored via its globular domain. (This molecule differs from **ankyrin** an intracellular protein of several cell types, which anchors the cytoskeleton to the plasma membrane). Also shown are the **hyaluronan** (CD44) and **integrin** receptors of chondrocytes, which may bind directly to type VI collagen or via intermediate matrix macromolecules, and which may be important for mechanotransduction (not shown). For clarity, divalent anions and cations and the chondron are not shown (see text for details).

collagen fibrils, appears to be important for cross-linking the collagen molecules.

The classification of proteoglycans and collagens is complex because type IX collagen is regarded as both a collagen and a proteoglycan because it bears one CS chain. It should be noted here that, in contrast to the proteoglycans, there is very little collagen turnover in adult human articular cartilage. Studies on the racemisation[2] of aspartic acid residues of collagen from young and aged healthy human femoral head cartilage (Maroudas et al, 1992) indicate very slow turnover, and therefore it is perhaps more accurate to view the repair of the collagen network as being more relevant than its bulk turnover.

Interstitial fluid

The interstitial fluid has an unusual composition because the proteoglycans are highly negatively charged with acidic (sulphate, SO_4^{2-}; and carboxyl, COO^-) groups and therefore attract cations from the synovial fluid, increasing the osmotic pressure in the matrix. Water is imbibed and the tissue inflates, but this is limited by the increasing tension that develops within the collagen network. The proteoglycans account for 3–10% of the tissue on a wet weight basis and are restricted to about 20% of their maximum molecular domain present in dilute solutions, thereby imparting significant compressibility to the tissue. The fibrillar component, or collagens (accounting for 15–30% of the tissue on a wet weight basis), forms a complex 'basketweave' which gives the tissue tensile strength and essentially immobilises the proteoglycans preventing their swelling and thereby limiting tissue hydration. The interstitial fluid, which on a wet weight basis accounts for 65–80% of the tissue, forms the aqueous environment in which chondrocytes live, and supplies nutrients, substrates and precursors for matrix biosynthesis, and also permits the removal of metabolic byproducts.

[2]Amino acids in natural proteins exist as the L-configuration optical isomers but will convert to the biologically uncommon D-isomer by a spontaneous process termed racemisation, which is dependent on time, temperature and, to a lesser extent, pH. Aspartic acid is one of the fastest of the racemising amino acids so that D-aspartic acid can be detected in proteins that are not renewed or that have a slow turnover.

Chondrocytes

The **chondrocytes** are present at a very low density (1–5% of volume in adult tissue, with approximately 10 000 chondrocytes per mm^3 in human femoral head) and, because they do not play direct mechanical role, they are often ignored (Stockwell, 1979). Nevertheless chondrocytes continuously synthesise and degrade the matrix, and there is important physical feedback from the chondrocyte environment which determines matrix metabolism and ultimately the mechanical characteristics of the tissue.

These effects are either (a) on the ionic/osmotic composition of the interstitial fluid; (b) via cell–matrix interactions; and (c) by virtue of their control of the permeability properties of the matrix, which determine the rates of permeation of substances from the synovial fluid through the matrix and hence to the chondrocytes. Obviously there is no epithelium between the cartilage and synovial fluid, or between the bone surface and the cartilage, because its presence would significantly compromise the load-bearing properties of the tissue. Cartilage must also be avascular, which has consequences for nutrient diffusion through the matrix to the chondrocytes and removal of metabolic byproducts.

ORGANISATION OF MATRIX AND CHONDROCYTES

Benninghoff's observations on the fine structure of cartilage using polarised light (see Stockwell, 1991) formed the basis on which most classical views on the organisation of the cartilage matrix have been based. He described **arcades** of collagen bundles originating in the calcified zone (zone V), binding the non-calcified cartilage and extending in arches towards the articular surface before curving down again (*Figure 5.2*). Thus, in sequence from above down, the collagen bundles were suggested to be tangential, radial and perpendicular. Scanning electron microscopy shows some of the collagen fibres emerging from the calcified cartilage and passing through the tide-line (or tide-mark[3]) but there are other fibres that lie parallel to the irregular surface of the calcified cartilage or are arranged at random.

[3]The tide-mark represents the interface plane between hyaline articular cartilage and the zone of calcified cartilage, and marks the normal mineralisation front.

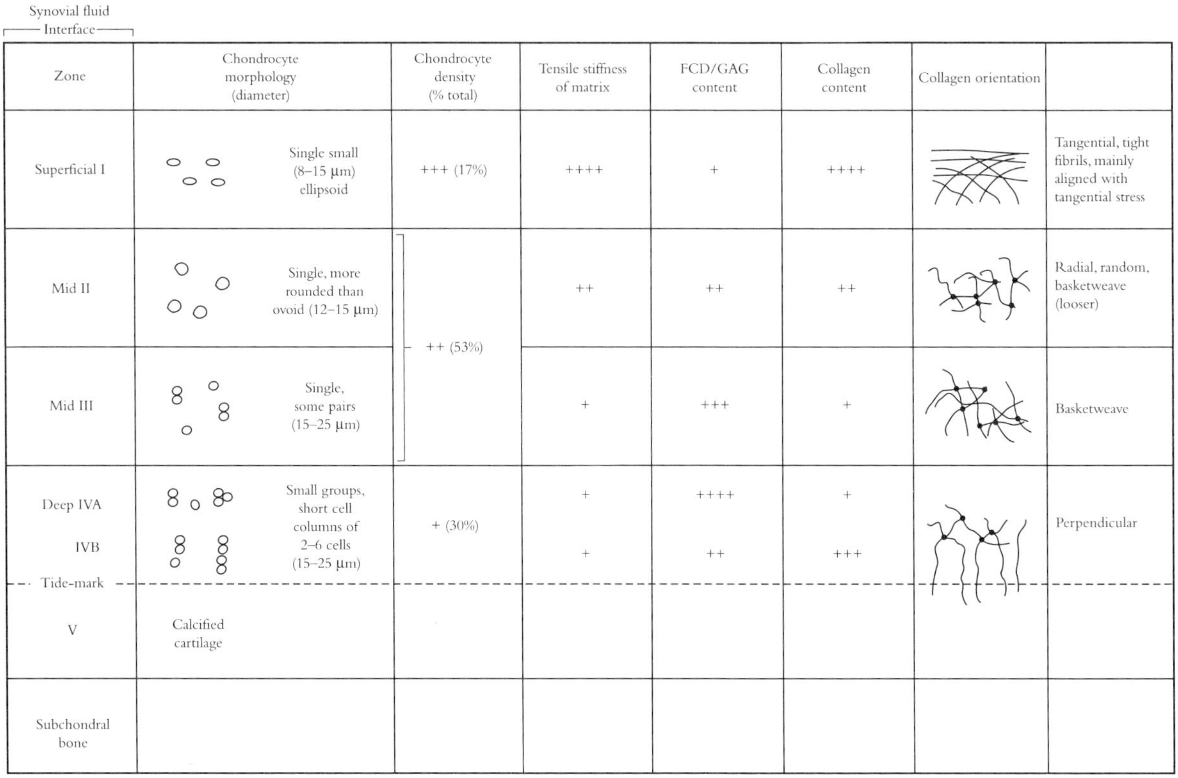

Synovial fluid
Interface

Zone	Chondrocyte morphology (diameter)	Chondrocyte density (% total)	Tensile stiffness of matrix	FCD/GAG content	Collagen content	Collagen orientation	
Superficial I	Single small (8–15 μm) ellipsoid	+++ (17%)	++++	+	++++		Tangential, tight fibrils, mainly aligned with tangential stress
Mid II	Single, more rounded than ovoid (12–15 μm)	++ (53%)	++	++	++		Radial, random, basketweave (looser)
Mid III	Single, some pairs (15–25 μm)		+	+++	+		Basketweave
Deep IVA	Small groups, short cell columns of 2–6 cells (15–25 μm)	+ (30%)	+	++++	+		Perpendicular
IVB			+	++	+++		
Tide-mark							
V	Calcified cartilage						
Subchondral bone							

Figure 5.2   The various zones of articular cartilage and some of their characteristics. This is a simplified picture of a perpendicular section of articular cartilage and underlying bone showing some of the heterogeneity that exists in the chondrocytes and extracellular matrix. The terminology associated with the different zones is convenient, although highly simplistic. The diagram does not represent articular cartilage from a specific species, but these features are reasonable representations of dog, primate and human tissue.

These models did not adequately take account of the theoretical concepts of the tissue organisation required to resist compressive load in the mid-zone, which required oblique fibrils or a random mesh. There is now evidence for extensive fibril interweaving and interlinking which traps the hydrated proteoglycans, and it has been suggested that type IX collagen (which is part collagen, part proteoglycan, because a high proportion of these molecules have a single CS chain attached to them) may play a key role in this process. This macromolecule is a *fibril-associated collagen with interrupted triple helices* collagen (FACIT collagen) which is covalently attached to type II collagen and is thought to give lateral strength and flexibility to the fibrillar network.

Thus, the mechanical properties of collagen depend on covalent cross-linking within and between α chains. The associations between the collagen fibrils give rise to a 'chicken-wire' arrangement, which is thought to account for the mechanism of reversible deformation under load, and possibly also, when it is damaged, to the pattern of development of fibrillation in osteoarthrosis.

It is interesting to consider the alignment of the collagen fibrils and the chondrocytes with respect to the mechanical forces to which the tissue is subjected. Thus, during joint movement, the surface regions will experience mainly shearing/tangential forces and deformation of the surface under joint load, whereas in the deeper regions the compressive component will dominate. During static loading (e.g. when standing), all areas will experience compressive load.

Within cartilage and other connective tissues there are marked topographical variations in the amount and types of GAG present. This has an important effect on the physical properties of the matrix and, as we will consider later, on the chondrocyte's environment.

The distribution of GAGs within tissue is usually

described and quantified using the fixed charge density (FCD). At physiological pH, the FCD is due entirely to the presence of the negative charges on the GAGs, because if all the GAGs are removed chemically/enzymically the collagen fibres that remain carry no detectable charge.

The measurement of FCD is based on a range of methods (e.g. radiotracers, chemical analysis, nuclear magnetic resonance). The radiotracer cation method is non–destructive, very rapid and simple, and can be used to measure the FCD in specimens of any size or shape, or weighing between 1 mg and 1 g. Cartilage is equilibrated in a dilute electrolyte solution (15 mmol l^{-1} NaCl to which ^{22}Na has been added as a radioactive tracer) at physiological pH (7.4), so that free electrolyte is virtually excluded from the tissue because of the Donnan equilibrium (see below). The only ions left in cartilage under these conditions should be those balancing the fixed, negatively charged groups in the cartilage. Thus, by measuring the concentration of ^{22}Na in the tissue after equilibration, and by determining the collagen and water content to calculate the extrafibrillar water content, a value can be obtained for the total concentration of fixed negatively charged groups. The FCD is decreased when the pH is reduced below about 5 (i.e. outside the physiological range) because the protons displace ^{22}Na from the negative groups on the GAGs. For human femoral head cartilage with a collagen content of 15–20% and water content of 70–75%, the FCD ranges over 0.1–0.2 mEq per g wet cartilage.

The profile of FCD and hence of GAGs throughout articular cartilages shows that the surface always has the lowest levels, increasing towards the middle zones, and usually decreasing again at the deepest zones (see *Figure 5.2*). Measurements have shown that the synthesis of aggrecan in surface zones is less than that in the deeper regions, but the catabolism of proteoglycans is more rapid in the surface region. Recent work (Schumacher et al, 1994) has shown a proteoglycan synthesised exclusively by surface chondrocytes (superficial zone protein, SZP) which contains both CS and KS. The proteoglycan content is significantly less in the surface than in the deep zones and, because of the properties of these molecules, this changes the water content throughout the tissue giving a complex hydration profile.

In the intervertebral disc, the FCD and water content are thought to be highest in the nucleus and lowest in the outer annulus. The FCD and hydration are lower in older than younger discs, and the older discs have flatter hydration profiles. In contrast to cartilage, in the disc the collagen fibre network is rather loose, hence the disc tissue can swell and the water content increases in proportion to the FCD, being highest in the nucleus.

For experiments where it is essential to maintain disc hydration close to *in vivo* levels, this is achieved by placing disc samples in dialysis bags, which are sealed and placed in a concentrated polyethylene glycol (PEG) solution. Water is drawn out from the tissue by endosmosis, and by using a range of PEG solutions a concentration can be used that maintains tissue hydration near to *in vivo* levels. In other experiments, mechanical load can be used to balance the tendency of the disc to swell.

Chondrocyte heterogeneity is related to topography within different regions of tissue (surface versus deep zones), and there is also local heterogeneity, because chondrocytes can exist singly or in small groups (of about six cells), which is superimposed on this zonal variation (*Figure 5.2*) It might therefore be expected that there would be differences in the nutritional and metabolic properties of chondrocytes whether they are arranged singly or in groups; however, the significance of this microheterogeneity is to a large extent unknown.

Chondrocytes in the superficial zone are small, sparsely distributed and are flattened, oblate spheroids or discoidal (10 × 2–3 μm) in morphology, occurring singly or occasionally as pairs. In deeper regions, the cells are more rounded or egg-shaped (*Figure 5.2*) and 15–25 μm in diameter, occurring as radially oriented groups of cells or as short cell columns near the 'tide-mark'. The differences in shape are fascinating, because there is evidence for a relationship between cell shape, metabolism and differentiation (Zanetti and Solursh, 1992).

Chondrocytes are larger in embryonic than in infantile cartilage, in younger than older tissue, and in growing than mature tissue. In non-articular cartilage (e.g. bronchus), chondrocytes are relatively uniform in structure and size. When chondrocytes of chondrosarcoma tumours are excluded, the largest cells of non-articular cartilage are those of the hypertrophic zones of the epiphyseal growth plate. The increase in cell volume associated with hypertrophy is quite remarkable (over tenfold) and is thought to underlie and regulate the growth of the long bones; however, the physiological events that drive the process of controlled cell swelling are poorly understood (Hunziker and Schenk, 1989; Cancedda et al, 1995).

In a single mammalian species, when articular cartilage from large joints is compared with that from small joints, there is a wide range in cellularity (i.e. cell density) which decreases almost inversely in proportion to cartilage thickness (in mm, x), as $y = 28\,000\,x^{-0.88}$. Cell density is also inversely proportional to the size of a joint irrespective of animal size, and thus articular cartilage in the small joints of large animals is no less cellular than that in the large joints of small animals.

Clearly the chondrocytes within thicker cartilage are more susceptible to nutritional deprivation and this probably is the major determinant of cell density. Diffusion distances can be large; for example, femoral head cartilage can be 2 mm thick, and in the intervertebral disc chondrocytes can be as much as 6–8 mm from the nearest blood supply. In thicker cartilage this reduction in cell density appears to cease at varying distances from the joint surface and it reaches a 'basal' level.

The number of cells that derive nutrients from each unit area (e.g. 1 mm^2) of load-bearing articular cartilage is thought to be uniform and the quantity of cartilage covering each unit of load-bearing bone is determined by factors such as the mechanical load to which the surface is routinely subjected. It has been suggested that the survival of chondrocytes in heavily loaded areas may require thicker cartilage, because this will spread larger loads on to a greater area of bone. It has been proposed that this relatively constant cell number is a consequence of a limit to the total number of cells that can be supported by nutritional diffusion (and possibly removal of metabolic byproducts by diffusion) located at the boundary of the tissue with the synovial fluid.

It is worth noting that the overall cellularity of cartilage changes greatly with the stage of development. Thus, in the embryonic limb before bone is formed, the proportionate volume of cells to extracellular matrix is approximately 1 : 3. As the limb grows, the relative volume of the matrix increases such that, in adult articular cartilage, the chondrocytes of zone I tend to be single, and the proportion of cells to matrix relatively high (about 1 : 50). In zones II and III the chondrocytes are often paired, occupying a larger volume, but the proportion of matrix is much greater.

It has been recognised from the very early studies on the structure of hyaline cartilage that the chondrocyte is surrounded by a specialised territorial matrix with properties distinctly different from the bulk of the intercellular (or interterritorial) matrix which makes up more than 90% of the volume of the tissue. Benninghoff (Poole, 1992) identified a unit he termed the 'chondron', which consists of one, or sometimes several, chondrocytes, its pericellular (or 'lacunar') space and a 'pericellular rim', and proposed that the chondron was the primary functional and metabolic unit responsible for cartilage homoeostasis. Although for many years his ideas received little attention, there has been a revival of interest (particularly through the studies of Poole and co-workers), partly because chondrons can now be extracted, apparently intact, from adult articular cartilage by gentle mechanical disruption of the tissue and filtration.

Chondrocytes within their chondrons are surrounded by a specialised microenvironment which, it has been suggested, might serve to protect the chondrocyte by dampening the mechanical, physicochemical and osmotic changes that occur during dynamic loading (Poole, 1992). The immediate extracellular vicinity of the chondrocyte membrane is called the 'pericellular' or 'lacunar matrix', and is characterised by a richness of proteoglycans and possibly hyaluronic acid, and a relative absence of organised fibrillar collagen. Contiguous with this pericellular matrix lies the territorial or capsular matrix, which is composed of a basket-like network of cross-linked fibrillar collagen encapsulating the individual cells. Several constituents are present in this space, including types VI, II and IX collagen, with the latter localised mainly in the outer margins of the chondron capsule. Type VI collagen is thought to be particularly important here and could possibly play a dual role: (a) in binding to the collagens, proteoglycans and glycoproteins in the pericellular environment to give structural and functional integrity to the chondron; and (b) because several types of chondrocyte plasma membrane surface receptors exist, interactions between this collagen and the chondrocyte could provide anchorage and signalling pathways between the pericellular matrix and the cell nucleus (Poole et al, 1992).

The chondrocyte establishes contacts with the capsular matrix through numerous cytoplasmic processes rich in microfilaments, as well as through anchorin CII (see *Figure 5.1*). The fine pericellular collagen fibrils converge and diverge at the superficial ('articular') pole of the capsule, and here (the 'cupola') there is an ultrastructural 'pericellular channel' open to the articular substance between the interior of the chondron and the bulk matrix. The presence of membrane-bound matrix vesicles immediately beyond this pericellular channel has been taken to indicate that a flow of materials (possibly water) through such channels during compressive deformation of cartilage may be a mechanism by which chondrocytes sense aspects of mechanical load and thereby regulate matrix metabolism. The formation of chondrons is thought to be intrinsic and specific to chondrocytes because of the appearance of chondron-like structures around chondrocytes when they have been cultured for several weeks in alginate beads.

There is considerable activity and cell division in growing cartilage of embryonic limbs and this contrasts markedly with the inert behaviour of adult hyaline articular cartilages. Young embryonic cartilage is highly cellular ($2–3 \times 10^6$ cells per mm^3) and this decreases throughout the growth period despite the occurrence of cell division, with the process continuing until completion of maturation. Human newborn femoral condylar articular cartilage contains about 10^5 chrondrocytes per mm^3, whereas in the young adult there are only $10–15 \times 10^3$ cells per mm^3. The change in cell density is due to: (a) matrix deposition, which is responsible for the bulk of the cellularity change during development; (b) cell death (leading to increased intercellular distance); and (c) interstitial mitosis, tending to reduce intercellular spacing.

It is very rare to see cell division in mature articular cartilage. However, even in aged articular cartilage, the chondrocytes do not lose their capacity for cell growth and division. In osteoarthrotic cartilage, chondrocyte clumping (or 'cloning') is observed, but it is not clear whether this is due to increased cell division or to the accumulation of cells in certain areas as a result of mechanical breakdown and 'splitting' of the cartilage. It has been observed that the degradation or removal of matrix, for example by the intra-articular injection of papain (a protein-digesting enzyme extracted from the fruit and leaves of the papaya tree, *Carica papaya*) into adult cartilage, provokes marked cell multiplication.

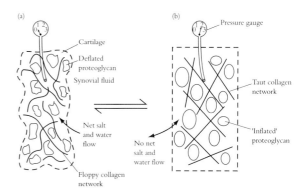

Figure 5.3 A simple model to illustrate some of the consequences of impermeant charged GAGs on the physico-chemical environment of chondrocytes. (a) Initially, the proteoglycans are shown as deflated balloons entrapped by the floppy collagen fibrils with the tissue suspended in a saline solution representing synovial fluid. The negative charges on the GAGs of the matrix attract cations, increasing the osmotic pressure within the cartilage and drawing in water, thereby 'inflating' the proteoglycans, as shown in (b). Anions are also attracted into the matrix, although to a lesser extent than cations, so as to balance charge. The raised osmolyte content increases the GAG hydration/swelling pressure and the tension within the collagen network, increasing the hydrostatic pressure in the matrix to approximately 2 atmospheres above normal pressure. At a given load, an equilibrium is reached (i.e. when there is no net water flux), when the restraining force within the collagen network balances the driving force for water imbibition. Changing the load on the tissue will vary the point at which equilibrium occurs. It has been noted that the earliest detectable change in osteoarthrosis is tissue swelling in the mid-zone (Stockwell, 1991). This is possibly because of damage to the collagen network, which will mean that the GAGs can swell more than normal, lowering the interstitial osmotic pressure. In addition, the ability of the tissue to resist a given load will be less, and the chondrocytes will be exposed to greater variations in osmotic pressure during normal joint activity.

THE DONNAN EQUILIBRIUM AND TISSUE SWELLING

The high negative charge density of the GAGs, and the fact that they are immobilised within cartilage, markedly influences the distribution of ions and hence the osmotic pressure between the synovial fluid and the interstitial fluid that surrounds the chondrocytes. This can be illustrated with a simple model, as in *Figure 5.3*, which shows the loose collagen meshwork enclosing deflated proteoglycans suspended in a saline solution. Salt and water will pass into the matrix until a thermodynamic equilibrium (the Donnan, or Gibbs–Donnan equilibrium) is reached.

The Donnan rule states that, in the presence of an impermeant anion (i.e. GAG), the products of the concentrations of the diffusible ions on both sides or compartments (i.e. interstitial fluid and synovial fluid) of the membrane are equal at equilibrium. However, because of the impermeable GAGs in the tissue, sodium (Na^+) and chloride (Cl^-) ions will redistribute such that the Na^+ concentration in the tissue will be greater than for Cl^- because some of the Na^+ in the tissue is associated with Cl^- and some with the negatively charged GAGs. Clearly, the number of osmotically active particles and hence the total osmotic pressure is greater in the tissue, and thus water tends to be imbibed by the tissue. There will, therefore, be contributions from the mobile co- and counter-ions, non-ionic solutes, and the colloid osmotic pressure of the proteoglycans (and to a very small extent by the collagen fibrils) to the interstitial osmotic pressure; the contribution from the mobile ions is far more significant because their large numbers greatly exceed the number of protein molecules.

In the absence of any restraint on the relative volumes of the two compartments, the movements of cations, and to a lesser extent anions and associated water movement into the tissue, will continue unless a pressure is exerted that equals the difference of osmotic pressure between tissue and synovial fluid. This is achieved by the tension generated within the basketweave network of collagen fibrils and by the external load on the joint. The tension in the collagen fibrils increases progressively until it balances the pressure driving water movement into the tissue (*Figure 5.3*); the resulting hydrostatic pressure within the unloaded cartilage matrix, and that to which the chondrocytes experience *in situ*, is about 2 atmospheres (atm) above normal pressure.

Because the Donnan distribution is a thermodynamic equilibrium for all passively distributed ions, the Donnan factor in a system is identical for all such univalent ions. If it is known for one ion, the activity of which in the solution of the two compartments has been determined, the activity of another ion need be known in only one compartment (e.g. in the synovial fluid) to calculate its activity in the other (in the interstitial fluid) by the Donnan factor. For multivalent ions, with a valency of n, the factor corresponds to the nth root of the concentration ratio. However, there are some other considerations that must be taken into account; for example, there is thought to be binding of Ca^{2+} to the intrafibrillar component, for reasons that are not yet understood.

When cartilage is not subjected to an external load, the difference in the osmotic pressure between the inside of the tissue and the outside medium (the so-called swelling pressure) is balanced by the hydrostatic pressure (about 2 atm) owing to the elastic forces in the collagen network,

so that they are equal. The application of a local external compressive load changes this equilibrium such that the sum of the applied hydrostatic pressure and the elastic forces exceeds the swelling pressure. This results in fluid flow away from the loaded region under the effect of a net difference in pressure. As fluid is squeezed out of the matrix, the swelling pressure rises, because the concentration of the GAGs increases, whereas the elastic forces decrease. Thus, as the load on articular cartilage is increased and water is lost, the proteoglycan–water gel of the matrix develops a higher swelling pressure which tends to resist further changes in this direction until eventually a new steady state is reached.

The water content of the tissue is therefore influenced by the osmotic pressure of the proteoglycans, the tension in the collagen network, and the external load on the tissue. The effects of normal loading on cartilage water can be quite complex and depend on various factors such as the applied pressure, cartilage permeability, osmotic pressure, the length of the fluid flow paths within cartilage and also the size of the high and low pressure zone through which the fluid can escape.

In terms of swelling, because the collagen network of normal human joints, mature hip and knee cartilage is very stiff, the cartilage has little tendency to swell above its normal water content when excised from the underlying bone or when the osmotic pressure gradients between it and the equilibrating solution are altered. Indeed, normal adult human femoral head cartilage swells by only about 3% when placed in distilled water. Thus, the value of the water content determined after exposure of the tissue to solution is near to the value 'as excised' and thus close to the value *in vivo* when the cartilage is in an unloaded state. This means that near the normal hydration value the stresses in the collagen network are high and must rise very steeply with an increase in tissue hydration (i.e. the collagen network is very nearly inextensible, does not resist compression, but counteracts and limits expansion). However, in young bovine knee cartilage there is significant swelling by up to 15–25% following excision of the cartilage from the underlying bone as the collagen fibrils linking cartilage to bone are severed and the restraining forces removed.

More marked is the case of intervertebral disc tissue studied either whole or in sections, which will swell considerably (by up to two times its volume) when excised from the spine and placed in physiological saline. This is because the collagen fibre network is much looser in the disc and its tension is not sufficiently high to oppose the swelling pressure of the proteoglycans. *In vivo*, the disc is always loaded even when the body is in the supine position, and the swelling pressure of the proteoglycans is thus resisted not only by the tension in the collagen fibre network, which particularly in the nucleus is very weak, but also by body-weight and muscle and ligament forces. The swelling of isolated disc explants can be accompanied by the leaching of proteoglycans, and therefore, if accurate measurements are to be made *in vitro*, it is crucial to prevent tissue swelling.

The importance of GAGs in the maintenance of cartilage hydration and hence mechanical stability is nicely shown by studies on the 'floppy ear syndrome' of rabbits (*Figure 5.4*). The injection into the ears of active or inactive crude papain proteinase within a few hours causes a marked degradation of cartilage GAGs, leading to loss of tissue water and a dramatic reversible loss in the mechanical properties of the ear. The fact that active or inactive enzyme causes the ears to droop suggests that the effect is not directly on the tissue but is cell-mediated. It is thought that the effects are due to increased permeability of the lysosomal membrane of chondrocytes, which

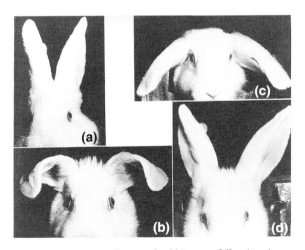

Figure 5.4 The collapse of rabbit ears following intravenous injection of crude papain proteinase. (a) Appearance before papain was injected; (b) after 4 hours, during which there was degradation of GAGs, loss of cartilage water and subsequent failure of the mechanical properties of the tissue; (c) partial recovery after 24 hours; and (d) after 5 days. The ear-collapsing effect was observed with both active and inactive papain, and was markedly prolonged by cortisone, which delayed the recovery of the cartilage matrix. From Thomas (1956), with permission.

releases activated hydrolytic enzymes which then act on the adjacent cartilage. It is remarkable how quickly the chondrocytes resynthesise and repack the GAGs within the fibrillar network to restore the mechanical properties of the tissue to normal.

THE IONIC AND OSMOTIC ENVIRONMENT OF CHONDROCYTES

As described in the previous section, the fixed negative charges of the GAGs markedly alter the ionic composition of the interstitial fluid compared with that of most extracellular fluids (e.g. synovial fluid, plasma) (Hall et al, 1996). This gives rise to a Donnan equilibrium such that cations (e.g. Na^+, K^+, Mg^{2+}, Ca^{2+}, H^+) are attracted into the matrix, whereas anions (e.g. Cl^- SO_4^{2-}, HCO_3^-) are repelled, resulting in marked differences in the ionic and osmotic properties of the interstitial fluid that bathes the chondrocytes (summarised in *Table 5.1*). Thus, cations have partition coefficients[4] that are higher than unity and depend on the size and charge of the solute and on the properties of the matrix, in particular its charge and excluded volume which increase and decrease respectively with the GAG content. Conversely, anions have partition coefficients less than unity and which decrease further with raised GAG content. The monovalent ions are free to move within the fluid, and have the same mobility as in aqueous solution.

Water is freely mobile within cartilage and behaves as if 99% is in a single compartment, with about 1% as 'bound' water. Evidence in support of the high water mobility is that the partition coefficients of small solutes (e.g. some amino acids, urea, oxygen, glucose), which are uncharged at neutral pH, are close to unity whether in the intrafibrillar or extrafibrillar water space. The diffusion coefficients of small uncharged and ionic solutes are about half those expected in aqueous solution, and this is due to steric factors associated with the presence of the 'immobile' constituents of the matrix.

It is important to note that because the GAG distribution is not homogenous throughout cartilage, being lowest in the surface zone and highest in the middle to

---

[4]The 'partition coefficient is the maximum concentration of the unbound solute in the matrix relative to its concentration in the external contacting fluid (e.g. synovial fluid or plasma).

Table 5.1   Estimates of the free ion concentrations and other environmental factors surrounding chondrocytes in articular cartilage.

	Tissue culture medium	*Surface zone*	*Deep zone*
FCD[a] (mEq $l^{-1}H_2O$)	0	120–160	200–250
Na^+ (mmol l^{-1})	140	240–270	300–350
K^+ (mmol l^{-1})	5	7–9	9–12
Ca^{2+} (mmol l^{-1})	2	6–9	14–20
Cl^- (mmol l^{-1})	140	60–90	50–100
Osmolarity (mOsm)	280	310–370	370–480
pH	7.4	7.1–7.3	About 6.9–7.0
Oxygen tension as % of blood	Depends on culture conditions	6%	1%

[a]FCD = Fixed charge density.

Values are mainly from human femoral head cartilage (see Maroudas and Evans, 1974; Maroudas, 1980; Urban and Hall, 1992; Hall et al, 1996).

deep zones (see *Figure 5.2*), the actual ionic or osmotic environment experienced by a given chondrocyte will depend mainly on the local GAG concentration.

The situation for Ca^{2+} (and other divalent cations) is interesting because they have partition coefficients that are much higher (about threefold) than those of monovalent ions. This is due in part to the higher valency in accordance with the Donnan equilibrium equation, and there is also the suggestion of Ca^{2+} binding to collagen, although this does not affect the partition coefficient. However, if the actual ratio of the mean activity coefficient[5] of Ca^{2+} in cartilage to that in the external solution is estimated from the partition data, a ratio of about 0.3 is obtained.

The fact that cartilage is rather selective towards Ca^{2+} also implies a low activity coefficient, and thus there are strong interactions between Ca^{2+} and the negatively charged groups on the GAGs in cartilage compared with its behaviour free in solution. One result of this low activity coefficient is that cartilage can tolerate a much higher concentration of Ca^{2+} in the presence of normal phosphate levels than would be possible in aqueous solution without precipitation of calcium orthophosphate.

It is interesting to speculate that proteoglycans may control calcification by allowing the concentration of Ca^{2+} within the cartilage matrix to rise (and reducing phosphate levels because of the negatively charged GAGs) without precipitation. However, if the proteoglycan concentration fell, this might result in a local

decrease in Ca^{2+} concentration and a rise in phosphate levels and, if suitable nucleation sites were present in these areas, the energy barrier for calcification within the matrix might therefore be reduced, resulting in focal crystallisation. This might induce a mechanical instability within the matrix, or if the crystals were released into the synovial fluid, could form an abrasive slurry weakening the superficial surface of cartilage with joint motion; there is, however, little evidence at present to suggest that failure of joint lubrication is a causative factor in the initiation of cartilage degeneration. This does not, however, exclude the possibility of superficial cartilage wear at the molecular level during normal joint usage, which usually could be repaired. However, once a surface defect has been initiated, such crystals might act as focal points for high mechanical stresses, accelerating tissue damage.

Divalent anions are excluded from the matrix more than monovalent ones. The partition coefficient for divalents (e.g. SO_4^{2-}, HPO_4^{2-}) is about 0.5, whereas that for monovalent anions (Cl^-, HCO_3^-) is about 0.6, both decreasing as the GAG concentration increases. Clearly, the ionic environment of chondrocytes is strongly dependent on the local GAG concentration. Although the influence of ionic environment on chondrocyte metabolism is considered in detail below, one could envisage a simple feedback loop such that a reduction in local GAG concentration would alter the ionic environment of the cells and hence intracellular composition, in such a way as to stimulate matrix synthesis, thereby restoring the GAG content to normal.

In the past, partition coefficients have usually been calculated with respect to total matrix water, but it is obvious that for some substances these values will be very different depending on whether intrafibrillar or extra-

[5]The activity coefficient is the ratio of the ideal or thermodynamic concentration of a substance to its true concentration. This is often a more useful term than concentration, because it reflects what is actually experienced by the cells within the tissue.

fibrillar water is being considered. Intrafibrillar space has no overall charge at physiological pH, whereas the extrafibrillar space has a strong negative charge; it is particularly important to note this difference when calculating the partition coefficients of small ionic solutes. Again, larger solutes are excluded only partially from the extrafibrillar compartment because of the 'excluded volume' properties of the proteoglycans, whereas they are excluded completely from the intrafibrillar compartment into which they simply cannot fit.

Compression of cartilage changes the concentrations of mobile ions and molecules significantly on the basis of extrafibrillar water; thus there is a twofold increase in tissue $[Na^+]$[6] and a fivefold increase in $[Ca^{2+}]$. Changes in tissue osmolarity[7], whether produced by alterations to the GAG content or during loading of the tissue, will change the movement of water across the chondrocyte plasma membrane, which is highly permeable to water. Thus, increasing tissue osmotic pressure, such as would occur when GAGs are concentrated and water expressed during static loading, would tend to draw water by endosmosis from chondrocytes (i.e. the cells would shrink), so that a new equilibrium at a reduced cell volume was achieved. There is evidence that chondrocytes are osmotically sensitive despite the rigidity of the cartilage matrix, and this is another method by which the cells could 'sense' and modulate, by altered synthesis or degradation of matrix macromolecules, the mechanical properties of cartilage.

The avascular nature of articular and other cartilages has important consequences for the availability of metabolic substrates and the loss of harmful byproducts (e.g. acids). Perhaps because of the low oxygen tension (PO_2) within cartilage (*Table 5.1*), estimated to be even lower in the nucleus of the intervertebral disc at 0.3%, the energy for chondrocyte metabolism (which is needed for a range of processes from the regulation of intracellular composition to synthesis of matrix macromolecules) comes mostly from glycolysis. This is, of course, metabolically ineffi-cient because complete oxidation of 1 mol of glucose (via Krebs' cycle) gives rise to 36 mol adenosine 5'-triphosphate (ATP), whereas glycolysis produces only 2 mol ATP. However, cartilage metabolism appears to be optimal under anaerobic conditions, and is favoured even in an aerobic environment; it has been suggested that the chondrocyte phenotype may be more stable at a low PO_2, although oxygen is still required in some poorly understood way for various aspects of chondrocyte metabolism.

Clearly, glucose diffusion from the synovial fluid or serum through the matrix to chondrocytes must be adequate to meet cellular demand, and it has been suggested that this limits cartilage thickness. There is very little contribution (probably less than 10%) from the blood within the subchondral bone, although this may be more important when the joint is immobile. The efficient diffusion of lactate away from chondrocytes back to the synovial fluid or serum, and of oxygen from the synovium to the cells, is important because otherwise chondrocytes would be surrounded by raised acidity. This can be deleterious to matrix synthesis (see below) and because proteinases secreted by chondrocytes may be activated as the local pH is reduced.

There is a rapid rise in the concentration of metabolic byproducts with distance from the blood or synovium. For example, in articular cartilage the lactate concentration rises from about $1 \, \mu mol \, g^{-1}$ wet weight of cartilage at the surface, to about $6 \, \mu mol \, g^{-1}$ at a depth of about 1 mm. At the centre of the intervertebral disc (i.e. the nucleus), lactic acid concentrations can be up to ten times greater than those in plasma. This combined with the proton-attracting capacity of the GAGs, can reduce the pH to about 6.9; values below 6.5 have been reported for degenerate discs. During static loading there will be an increase in the proteoglycan concentration, which will raise the $[H^+]$ further and lower the pH even more. There are, therefore, likely to be complex pH profiles within the tissue, depending on GAG distribution, the metabolic gradients near chondrocytes and the loading pattern.

[6]Square brackets are taken to represent the concentration in millimoles per litre. The subscripts i and o indicate intracellular (i.e. inside the chondrocyte) or extracellular (i.e. outside the chondrocyte) concentrations respectively.

[7]Osmotic pressure is given as either the osmolarity (mOsm per litre water, i.e. with water added to the 1-litre mark) or osmolality (mOsm per kg water, i.e. with 1 kg water added); for concentrated solutions the latter term is preferred because it is independent of the volume occupied by salts, etc., and is unaffected by temperature.

SELECTIVE PERMEABILITY OF THE CARTILAGE MATRIX

The proteoglycans not only influence ion distributions, and the partitions of a range of electrolytes and

58

non-electrolytes, they also perform an important selectivity barrier or 'sieve' function. The concentration and properties of proteoglycans determine the extent and nature of the molecules that can penetrate the matrix from the synovial fluid, and hence gain access to the chondrocytes. The accessibility of factors in the synovial fluid to the cartilage matrix, and the subsequent movement of substances through the matrix (e.g. water as fluid flow), is controlled in part by the gaps or 'pores' between the GAG chains which have a diameter ranging over 30–40 Å, and their domains interpenetrate the matrix.

The size, shape and charge of the permeating substance also strongly influence the rate of solute transport. Large molecules have a lower diffusion coefficient in water than smaller ones, but in cartilage they are retarded further as a result of **friction** between the solute and the matrix macromolecules. The controlling factor is the GAG concentration and charge density: a twofold increase in GAG concentration can decrease the partition coefficient of, for example, serum albumin by about tenfold (*Figure 5.5*). Reductions to GAG content not only alter the distribution of pore sizes but also increase the number of large pores. Small molecules and ions (e.g. urea, amino acids, cations, anions) can permeate the matrix freely (although note the Donnan effect); large molecules such as immunoglobulins or serum albumin are virtually excluded from normal cartilage, with concentrations 100-fold lower than those in the serum.

The permeation of all these ions and molecules through the matrix is tortuous; it is the molecular size, not the molecular weight, that is the important determinant. The concentrations of the potent cytokines or growth factors (e.g. insulin-like growth factor 1) are only one-tenth of those in the serum, and thus chondrocytes in healthy intact cartilage are exposed to much lower concentrations of these agents than many other cell types. However, when the cartilage becomes damaged (e.g. in osteoarthrosis where damage to the collagen fibrils results in tissue swelling, or when proteoglycan loss occurs), the properties of the selectivity barrier will change markedly; molecules (e.g. growth factors) previously excluded will penetrate, and concentrations of partially excluded factors will rise.

The permeation rate is determined by: (a) the thickness, as this determines the concentration gradient across the tissue; (b) the partition coefficient of the solute between the cartilage and the surrounding fluid; (c) the diffusion coefficient of the solute through the cartilage;

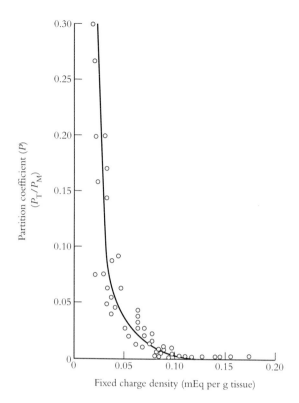

Figure 5.5 Changes to the partition coefficient (*P*) of serum albumin with the fixed charge density (FCD) of human articular cartilage. Note the marked increase in partition coefficient (concentration in tissue, P_T/concentration in medium, P_M) as the FCD was changed in samples of normal and fibrillated human articular cartilage, or in normal tissue by reducing the FCD by chemical treatment. From Maroudas (1980), with permission.

and (d) the surface area available for diffusion. It is interesting to note that the permeability is reduced at the superficial zone of articular cartilage, partly because the collagen network is very dense and also because hydration in this region is low as a result of the reduced GAG content.

The permeability properties of the matrix will dampen any kinetic responses because diffusion through the matrix is slow and a change in the concentration of substances in the synovial fluid could take hours to reach the chondrocytes in the deep zones of articular cartilage or intervertebral disc. There are other consequences; for example, matrix permeability will affect the turnover of matrix macromolecules themselves, because the passage of degradative enzymes and newly synthesised molecules from chondrocytes is restricted.

It has been suggested that cartilage obtains some of its nutrition from the action of a 'physiological pump' by which the compression of cartilage under load leads to fluid expression, whereas the subsequent relaxation is accompanied by the reabsorption of fresh fluid. Although cartilage pumping does appear to assist the transport of large solutes (e.g. serum albumin, M_r 69 kDa), pump-aided transport of small solutes (e.g. amino acids, urea, glucose) is far less significant, and free diffusion is the dominant mechanism for permeation. It should be noted that free diffusion of substrates from the joint cavity into the loaded area will be significantly reduced during the loading part of the cycle, because the cartilage under load is not in immediate contact with the solute-rich synovial fluid. Joint **loading** is important for mass transfer of fluid through the matrix, whereas joint **motion** is a key factor for minimising the 'stagnant fluid' film at the articular cartilage surface by 'stirring' the synovial fluid. These selectivity properties of the matrix are complex but very important and, apart from a few notable exceptions (see Maroudas, 1980), have not received the attention they deserve.

CULTURE OF CHONDROCYTES: ADVANTAGES AND DISADVANTAGES

It will be clear from the previous sections that the physical nature of the extracellular matrix is complex. Indeed, the selective permeability and binding or exclusion properties of the matrix prevent a wide range of experiments on the physiology and cell biology of chondrocytes. The precise extracellular conditions to which chondrocytes are exposed are often not known and therefore methods have been developed for the removal of chondrocytes from their matrix, and subsequent culturing under a range of experimental conditions. As there has been an enormous amount of work performed using cultured chondrocytes, it is important at the outset to point out some of the advantages and disadvantages of these procedures.

First, it must be appreciated that the apparently simple act of cutting cartilage from the bone can often alter the tensions in the collagen network, and can change the mechanical environment of the cells. Second, the isolation of chondrocytes by enzymic digestion (for example, with collagenase) of cartilage explants releases the cells from the pressures that exist within the matrix, and there is also a loss of cell–matrix interactions which may be an important determinant of the sensitivity to pressure or load (see below). Third, cell isolation exposes chondrocytes to a different ionic and osmotic environment (see *Table 5.1*) and, although it is possible to mimic some of the characteristics of the *in situ* environment of the cells (e.g. raising the osmolarity of the medium used for cell isolation with NaCl), it must be remembered that this might alter their behaviour in culture. However, some changes are very difficult to control, for example the gradients of pH, lactate and Po_2 within the tissue, and the high cation, low anion ratios characteristic of tissues with high GAG content, although for the latter point the use of pressure-dialysed solutions is helpful for comparative studies.

Although there are many studies using cultured chondrocytes, the results of which are often related back to chondrocyte behaviour in cartilage, it is important to remember the possible effects of culture conditions on chondrocyte behaviour. Studies using monolayer culture have given valuable information about chondrocyte metabolism, but are limited by the possibility of phenotypic instability of chondrocytes, especially when the cells are cultured and passaged at low density. Thus the de-differentiation of chondrocytes into fibroblasts, which occurs under these proliferative conditions associated with changes to the synthesis of matrix macromolecules, has been viewed as a problem with these approaches.

Chondrocytes normally produce predominantly type II collagen (frequently taken as a marker for the maintenance of the chondrocyte phenotype), high molecular weight GAGs (aggrecan) and a few small proteoglycans, whereas fibroblasts synthesise mainly type I collagen, little aggrecan and large amounts of small non-aggregating proteoglycans. Alkaline phosphatase activity (an enzyme required in the mineralisation process), which is negligible or low in chondrocytes, is high in fibroblasts and has also been taken as an index of the stability of the chondrocyte phenotype.

These changes in phenotype occur after the cells come in contact with a surface (e.g. a plastic Petri culture dish), possibly as a result of a morphological change involving cell shape or the cytoskeleton (Stein and Bronner, 1992). Substrates that enhance the adhesion and spreading of chondrocytes (e.g. fibronectin) increase the rate at which the differentiated phenotype (i.e. chondrocytes) is lost. Conversely, agents that disrupt the actin component of the cytoskeleton (e.g. cytochalasin D) stimulate chondrogenesis by maintaining the rounded morphology. Loss of chondrocyte phenotype can be prevented by various manoeuvres (e.g. seeding at high densities so that the growth factors normally produced by chondrocytes maintain phenotype) or by the addition of growth factors present in serum, which are thought to prevent the shape change.

A recent publication on the long-term culture of human articular chondrocytes undergoing proliferation has shown that they replicate much more slowly than either human fibroblasts or chondrocytes from other species. About 35 population doublings occurred before the cells became senescent and ceased to divide; however, they retained type II collagen expression, albeit at a low level, despite the fact that their morphology had become fibroblastic (Kolettas et al, 1995). Additionally, type I collagen synthesis, which is often taken as indicating loss of chondrocyte phenotype, is expressed even by chondrocytes in fresh human articular cartilage explants, suggesting that the production of type I collagen does not by itself indicate a loss of phenotype.

Currently the most popular method is the culture of chondrocytes within an artificial matrix such as that formed by agarose or alginate. Chondrocytes thus treated are largely immobilised and separated from surrounding interactions so that the development of their matrix can be examined microscopically at different stages of culture and under various conditions. Because fibroblasts and other anchorage-dependent cells fail to grow within agarose, this method allows for the selection of anchorage-independent cells from a mixed population such as those derived from chondrosarcoma tissue.

The normal phenotype of chondrocytes is thought to be stabilised under these conditions, and these methods have been used to show that chondrocytes isolated from different depths of articular cartilage and cultured in agarose under identical environmental conditions maintain metabolic differences and for months show the characteristics of the tissue zones from which they were derived (Aydelotte et al, 1992). For example, the quantitative differences in the synthesis of KS by subpopulations of cultured chondrocytes are consistent with regional differences in concentration within intact articular cartilage. De-differentiated chondrocytes can be induced to re-express the normal collagen type II phenotype when cultured in agarose gels. Chondrocytes, which have been cultured in alginate to which Ca^{2+} is added as an essential co-factor for the stability of the gel, can be released with a Ca^{2+}-chelating agent (ethylene-bis(oxy-ethylenenitrilo)-tetraacetic acid; (EGTA)) which causes the disruption of the gel and chondrocyte release.

Thus, although there are changes to the chondrocyte's environment under culture conditions, there is no doubt that these studies are crucial for understanding cartilage function. It is important, nevertheless, that the limitations of using cultured chondrocytes are remembered, and that data are compared wherever possible with intact cartilage in which the chondrocytes are less perturbed and maintenance of morphology and topography is assured.

TENDON – A CONNECTIVE TISSUE EXPOSED TO TENSIONAL AND COMPRESSIVE FORCES

Mechanical forces on articular joints are very complex, and the relationship between chondrocyte metabolism and its mechanical environment is often difficult to interpret. It is therefore of interest to consider related tissues in order to gain a better understanding of the possible relationships between connective tissue cells and their mechanical environment, and vice versa.

Tendon, which plays a crucial role in transmitting tensional forces associated with joint movement, is a good example to illustrate this. In some tendons, the tissue can be divided into regions that experience mainly **tension** or mainly **compression**; the latter region in bovine flexor tendon is found where the tissue wraps around the sesamoid bones and is subjected to compressive and frictional forces, in addition to tensile forces. The properties of the region exposed to compressive forces are sharply localised and are markedly different (*Table 5.2*), and extend to about a one-third of tissue depth. In the region exposed primarily to compressive forces, the tissue possesses a 'cartilage-like' matrix and its properties are sensitive to the prevailing mechanical load. For example, dislocation of the rabbit flexor digitorum profundus tendon *in vivo*, so as to remove the tendon from load, produces a marked loss of GAG from the region normally exposed to compression (up to 60% loss of GAG within 8 days), whereas little change was observed in other areas (Vogel and Koob, 1989).

Immobilisation also produced a significant reduction in the tensile strength of rabbit tendons. The loss of the

Table 5.2 Characteristics of different regions of tendon showing some of the major differences between the composition and ultrastructure of regions exposed to either tensile forces or a combination of compressive and tensile forces.

Tissue property	Region exposed to:	
	Tension	*Tension and compression*
Collagen	**Clear orientation**; parallel arrays along length of tendon in direction of tensile force	**Basketweave**; cartilage-like matrix collagen bundles, thinner, often at right angles to tendon axis
GAG content	Very low, mostly small, proteoglycans (10^5Da), e.g. decorin (possibly regulate collagen fibril growth)	High – large (10^6Da) 'fibrocartilage-like' proteoglycans; levels of CS, KS, aggrecan, biglycan up to tenfold higher; give tissue compressive strength. Some small proteoglycans
Cells	'Tenocytes' – fibroblast-like cells elongated/flattened parallel to collagen fibrils, low density	Cells tend to be rounded and 'chondrocytic'
Water content (wet)	About 55%	About 75% (cartilage also approx. 75%)
Collagen content (by hydroxyproline assay)	About 80% (principally type I, no type II)	About 69% (principally type II; some type I present)
General microstructure	Little association between GAGs and collagen	Large globular proteoglycans (CS, KS) in interfibrillar space, like cartilage

Note the 'cartilage-like' properties of the region exposed to tension and compression, even though the proteoglycan content is much lower than that of cartilage (Vogel and Koob, 1989).

cartilaginous character of this region (loss of 'basketweave' collagen structure, changes to cellular behaviour, etc.) was reversible when the tendon was replaced and normal mechanical loading restored. Further experiments removing the GAGs from the fibrocartilaginous region by enzyme treatment abolished the difference between tensional and pressure-bearing regions, and removed cartilage-like properties from load-bearing regions. Interestingly, in foetal bovine tendon, where the compressive forces are very weak, the molecular weight of the proteoglycans is relatively small, and increases only when the animal begins to walk, when the compressive forces increase. In the Achilles tendons of rabbits, exercise increased collagen fibril diameter whereas it remained unchanged in untrained rabbits. Thus, there is evidence that mechanical forces (compression and tension) play a major role in determining the nature of the macromolecules produced by the cells, and hence the mechanical characteristics of the tissue.

It is thought that compressive loads *in vivo* are important for the maintenance of the cartilage phenotype, and cell shape may be a determinant; however, load does not simply upregulate or downregulate overall cell metabolism: the effects are considerably more subtle. The 'sensor'

on (or possibly in) the cells for detecting the changes in loading pattern and thereby initiating a response to remodel the extracellular matrix is poorly understood. Possible mediators include an ion channel in the cell membrane sensitive to membrane stretch (stretch-activated channel), changes to cell morphology, movement of soluble factors (e.g. flow of nutrients, changes in oxygen tension) and genetic programming. Because the cells in culture appear not only to synthesise region-specific macromolecules, but also have some inherent capacity to respond to changes in loading pattern, it seems likely that both genetic and mechanical factors are involved.

IMPORTANCE OF MECHANICAL LOAD IN MAINTAINING THE HEALTH OF ARTICULAR CARTILAGE

It has been known for a long time that load is essential for the health of cartilage *in vivo* (reviewed in Helminen et al, 1987; see also Urban, 1994). It is worth emphasising that the forces to which articular cartilage are routinely exposed are very large; *Figure 5.6* shows the changes in hydrostatic pressure (one major component of load) during *in vivo* activity where high pressures can be generated very quickly.

Within limits, chondrocytes respond to mechanical stress and remodel the tissue so that in future it is better able to withstand these forces. In this context, Wolff's law (Helminen et al, 1987) is often cited, which, although was initially established to apply to bone, is relevant for

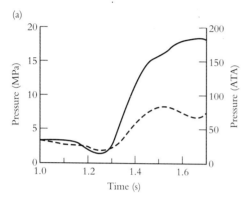

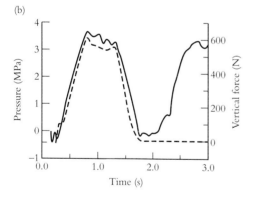

Figure 5.6 Changes in hydrostatic pressure measured in an instrumented hip prosthesis of a 74-year-old woman. (a) As the woman rose from a chair there was a rapid increase in pressure to about 8 MPa (80 ATA (atmospheres absolute); 1 ATA = 0.1 MPa) at 6 months (broken line), and to about 18 MPa (180 ATA) 12 months (solid line) after surgery. The rate of pressure rise was estimated to be over 100 MPa s^{-1}. (b) During level walking, pressures cycled between atmospheric pressure and 3–4 MPa(30–40 ATA) at a frequency of about 1 Hz (solid line); the vertical force (in newtons) between foot and floor is also shown (broken line). From Hodge et al (1986), with permission.

load-bearing cartilage. In simple terms, this law states that 'form follows function', thereby suggesting that, within limits, chondrocytes have the capacity to remodel cartilage to withstand the prevailing level of mechanical stress. Thus, in normal joints, load-bearing areas are thicker, have a higher proteoglycan concentration, and are mechanically stronger than non-load-bearing regions of the same joint. Additionally, the chondrocytes are larger and have a greater volume of intracellular organelles.

The chondrocytes and cartilage are affected if the loading pattern across the joint is altered. Thus, after prolonged exercise, chondrocytes of young rabbits were larger and more metabolically active, and, in beagles, cartilage thickness, proteoglycan content and the stiffness of the extracellular matrix all increased. In experiments where animals had one limb immobilised, an increase in proteoglycan content occurred in the contralateral limb exposed to load. In the immobilised joint, there was a marked loss of proteoglycans, which was gradually restored when the joint was remobilised. This loss of proteoglycans was due to the lack of loading rather than reduced movement, because passive motion did not maintain cartilage health.

The clear conclusion from a wide range of studies is that the routine application of mechanical load is necessary for the cartilage matrix to maintain its resilience. It should be noted that the most marked changes in the matrix are to the proteoglycan content (which controls tissue compressibility), whereas no significant changes are found in collagen content. If loading patterns are excessive, this can damage cartilage that was previously healthy and there is evidence that this is due in part to changes in chondrocyte activity. For example, the mechanically induced joint instability caused by section of the canine anterior cruciate ligament affects chondrocyte behaviour and matrix structure within days and can eventually result in the loss of cartilage. Thus, it has been suggested that the mechanical breakdown of cartilage (as occurs in osteoarthrosis) can be initiated by normal load on an abnormal joint, or abnormal load on a normal joint (Gardner, 1992).

Despite the clear link between these *in vivo* studies showing that load can markedly influence chondrocyte behaviour in terms of proteoglycan turnover, it is very difficult to design *in vivo* experiments that investigate the response of chondrocytes in detail. The joint is too complex and experiments rely on animal models where differences in loading pattern, growth and circulating agents cannot be controlled properly. Therefore, most studies have focused on the effects of load on *in vitro* models, particularly cartilage explants and cultured chondrocytes.

In vitro experiments have usually studied the effects of mechanical load on the metabolism of cartilage plugs taken from defined regions of a joint maintained in a standard tissue culture medium for up to several days. An important conclusion from this work is that the stimulus required for the cartilage to respond to the mechanical load is present in the isolated explant. The chondrocyte response is strongly dependent on the loading pattern such that static loading leads to a proportionate **fall** in synthesis rates, whereas dynamic (cyclic, oscillatory) loading can **stimulate** synthesis, although the response depends on the frequency of the applied stress (*Figure 5.7*). It is likely that the dynamic components of load are superimposed on a slowly evolving, time-averaged, static component, and separating out the possible events experimentally is clearly essential before the results obtained are meaningful.

The metabolic response to load is not simply an increase or decrease in proteoglycan synthesis, as there appear to be differences in matrix macromolecules produced by chondrocytes and in the agents that influence cartilage breakdown (e.g. degradative enzymes). The overall effects of load on proteinases and their inhibitors is very important (although beyond the scope of this chapter; Tyler et al, 1992; Alexander and Werb, 1991), because it has been shown that the loss of proteoglycans after immobilisation occurs too quickly to be accounted for by the suppression of synthesis alone. The response to mechanical loads *in vitro* are rapid (from minutes to hours) and, although there is little information about intracellular events, the extracellular signals appear to arise from changes to the physical environment of chondrocytes.

EFFECT OF LOAD ON CHONDROCYTE ENVIRONMENT

Chondrocytes are continually exposed to mechanical loads which, *in vivo*, depend not only on body-weight but also on muscle tension, and will therefore vary with posture and activity. The effects of load are complex and will alter the physical environment of the chondrocytes in many ways, any or all of which might be the stimulus for the chondrocyte's response (*Table 5.3*).

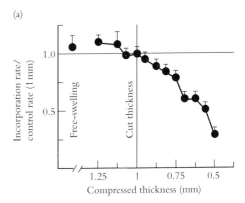

(a)

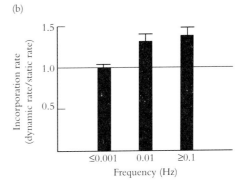

(b)

Figure 5.7 Differential effects of static and dynamic loading on bovine articular cartilage matrix synthesis. (a) Static compression (for 12 hours) of cartilage inhibits proteoglycan synthesis. Incorporation of the radiotracer $^{35}SO_4$ into proteoglycans (over 12 hours) was expressed relative to discs maintained at 1 mm (the thickness 'as cut'). Note the increase in free-swelling thickness following removal of cartilage from the joint ('cut thickness'), which arises from the so-called 'stress–relaxation' phenomenon. (b) The increase in proteoglycan synthesis with dynamic load. Cartilage disks were radiolabelled over the last 8 hours of 23-hour dynamic compression protocols. The discs were statically compressed to 1 mm and a superimposed dynamic/oscillatory strain of 1–2% was applied at frequencies of 0.0001–0.1 Hz, with control discs being maintained at 1 mm thickness by static compression. Data are expressed as dynamic/static synthesis rates. From Sah et al (1992), with permission; see this reference in Kuettner et al (1992) for further details.

When load is applied, the first events are cell and tissue deformation and a rapid rise in hydrostatic pressure. If the load is removed immediately, the cartilage returns to its original state and the pressure quickly falls. However, if the load is maintained, because cartilage is an osmotic system (see *Figure 5.3*) this will disturb the equilibrium

Table 5.3 Time course of the effects of loading on chondrocytes and their environment (Grodzinsky, 1983).

1. Tissue and chondrocytes deform (possible cell stretch, shape change, cell–matrix interaction; milliseconds

2. Hydrostatic pressure increases (milliseconds for dynamic load, minutes to hours for static load)

3. Fluid expressed, solute transport influenced (seconds to hours)
   (a) high local fluid flows/streaming potentials (seconds to hours)
   (b) proteoglycan concentration and fixed charge density increases (minutes to hours)
   (c) matrix cation concentration and osmolarity increase (minutes to hours)
   (d) cell volume decreases, changes to cell composition (minutes to hours)

and fluid will be lost, eventually reaching a new osmotic steady state. This loss of fluid will increase the proteoglycan concentration and thus raise the cation concentration and conversely reduce the anion concentration. This will continue until either the osmotic balance is restored or the load is removed and fluid re-imbibed. The extent of the changes to the ionic and osmotic composition of the interstitial fluid will therefore depend on the loading pattern applied. The degree of cartilage deformation will depend mainly on the **magnitude** of the load, whereas the extent of fluid loss will depend mainly on the **duration** of the load. During normal walking, 1–5% of the fluid of articular cartilage is moved in or out of the cartilage, whereas about 20% of the fluid of the intervertebral disc is lost and regained during a diurnal cycle of activity and rest. It is clear that the chondrocyte environment is influenced strongly by the nature of the load to which the tissue is subjected.

As noted earlier, the extracellular matrix is not uniform in composition and structure, and thus the degree of deformation produced by a given load will not be homogeneous throughout the tissue. It is likely that the surface is more compliant because of the relatively low proteoglycan : collagen ratio, whereas the mid-deep zones are more resilient because of the higher ratio. The effects of load on cartilage will not only depend on the loading pattern, but will also vary with the structure and composition of the matrix. In particular, the extent of deformation will depend on the integrity of the collagen network and the GAG content, and will be greater in degenerate (osteoarthrotic) cartilage where the mechan-

ical resilience of the matrix is compromised. Because the rate and amount of fluid loss are controlled to a large extent by the proteoglycan concentration, diseased cartilage will lose fluid faster and to a greater extent than normal cartilage. The chondrocytes in diseased cartilage will therefore experience much wider variations in osmotic and ionic environment, deformation, etc., compared to cells in healthy tissue.

It is interesting to note that there is a striking difference in water content between aged and osteoarthrotic cartilage. With ageing, cartilage becomes 'drier', in marked contrast to osteoarthrotic cartilage where there is a significant increase in tissue hydration (which, when expressed as ratio of tissue water weight : dry weight, can be up to 60% greater). Some workers have interpreted this as indicating that osteoarthrotic degeneration does not follow naturally from the tissue changes during ageing. However, the factors leading to the cellular and matrix changes in osteoarthrosis could still be a consequence of these and other, as yet unknown, age-related changes.

EXTRACELLULAR SIGNALS INDUCED BY MECHANICAL FORCES

There are several changes occurring in the matrix during loading (*Table 5.3*) that alter the extracellular environment of the chondrocytes, and some of these have been suggested as signals that link the loading pattern on the joint to chondrocyte matrix biosynthesis. They are: (a) a shape change of chondrocytes arising from tissue deformation, possibly involving a cell–matrix interaction; (b) the rise in hydrostatic pressure; (c) fluid flow, which causes streaming potentials as ions move past the fixed negative charges on the GAGs; and (d) loss of fluid, producing changes in the extracellular ionic composition. In the following sections, the role of these factors is considered with reference to some recent publications, to which the reader can refer for more detailed information.

Deformation

Changes to the shape of a range of cell types has been shown to initiate a variety of cellular responses, including the activation (and inactivation) of various ion channels, alterations in the activity of the membrane transport proteins (e.g. the Na^+/H^+ exchanger which regulates intracellular pH), modulation of adenylate cyclase activity (which controls intracellular levels of adenosine $3',5'$-cyclic monophosphate (cAMP), and alterations to the activity of enzymes associated with second-messenger pathways (e.g. phosphatidylinositol turnover; see Watson, 1991). It has been proposed that cell shape is a dynamic balance between counterbalancing forces (contraction and resistance) within cells, giving rise to the phenomenon of **tensegrity** (Stein and Bronner, 1992; Schwartz and Ingber, 1994).

Recent work suggests that, in adherent endothelial cells, the extracellular matrix receptor integrin β_1 acts as a mechanoreceptor and transmits signals to the tensionally integrated cytoskeleton. Unfortunately studies in chondrocytes are still at a very early stage and it is not known to what extent (if any) these processes are involved in mediating the signals from the matrix to chondrocyte (Hall et al, 1996). Indeed, it is still an open question whether chondrocyte deformation under load is possible, given the resilience of the extracellular matrix. It has been reported that chondrocytes possess a monocilium (Wilsman, 1978). The function of the monocilium is unknown but it has been suggested that it operates as a mechanoreceptor transmitting information from the extracellular matrix to the chondrocyte.

A role for the extracellular matrix in mediating the response to load has been suggested by recent experiments on chondrocytes maintained in alginate culture synthesising a mechanically functional cartilage matrix (Buschmann et al, 1995). It was shown that the chondrocyte response to static compression was controlled to a significant extent by cell–matrix interactions and extracellular physicochemical effects (e.g. increase in $[Na^+]_O$, decreased pH). For dynamic compression, fluid flow and streaming potentials (see below), in addition to cell–matrix interactions, were thought to be important determinants of the synthetic response by chondrocytes.

Hydrostatic pressure

This component dominates during high-frequency dynamic loading, as there is elastic-like tissue deformation with very little expression or imbibition of fluid. Studies have shown that short applications of hydrostatic pressure *per se* (i.e. without a gas phase present), within the physiological range (up to about 18 MPa; see *Figure 5.6*), can stimulate matrix synthesis (Hall et al, 1991). However, when the same pressure levels are maintained for longer periods, the stimulatory effect is considerably reduced, suggesting at least two processes. Our knowledge of the nature of the signals involved is rudimentary at present, and although for the dynamic response several possible mediators have been proposed (chondrocyte cytoskeleton/shape change, second-messenger pathways, e.g. cAMP, inositol trisphosphate, Ca^{2+}), a clear explanation has not yet been obtained.

There have been suggestions, although relatively few supporting experiments, that changes to the activity of ion channels in the plasma membrane might account for the effects of pressure on chondrocyte metabolism. An interesting study on cultured human articular chondrocytes has shown marked changes to the electrophysiological properties following cyclical pressure-induced strain (Wright et al, 1996). Evidence was presented which suggested that membrane deformation resulted in the stimulation of 'stretch-activated' ion channels, leading to chondrocyte hyperpolarisation, and that this correlated with a rise in GAG synthesis. It was thought possible that cell surface integrins may act as 'mechanosensors' linking the changes in the physico-chemical environment that occur during loading, to the stretch-activated ion channels, and hence control matrix synthesis.

Fluid flow or streaming potentials and currents

Electrical fields (streaming potentials) are generated by the fluid flow convecting mobile counter-ions past the ionised charged groups on the immobilised GAGs (Grodzinsky, 1983). Streaming potentials are proportional to both the fluid velocity (estimated to be about $1\,\mu m\,s^{-1}$) and FCD. Experiments have shown a greater stimulation of chondrocyte biosynthesis at the periphery of cartilage explants where fluid flow is greater, compared with that in the central region where fluid flow is less. In addition, the response of chondrocytes to dynamic compression was greater when the cells had been cultured for some time and had synthesised more matrix, resulting in a smaller change in shape when they were loaded. Thus, it was suggested that cell deformation was not a very important signal under these conditions, but that the larger streaming currents arising from the increased GAG content around the cells were (Buschmann et al, 1995). Although it is not yet clear how streaming potentials exert their effects on cell metabolism, this is thought to be an important mechanism by which chondrocytes detect changes to their environment.

Changes to the ionic and osmotic environment of chondrocytes

It has been established *in vitro* that fluid expression either by osmotic load, or directional mechanical load, decreases matrix synthesis rates proportionally, and that this results directly from changes to tissue hydration. Osmotic load is given either by using PEG, which cannot permeate the matrix but which draws water out of the tissue, or sucrose, which penetrates the matrix (but not the chondrocytes) increasing the osmotic pressure around the cells, causing them to shrink. As fluid leaves the tissue, the GAG concentration will rise, increasing the concentration of cations (e.g. Na^+, K^+, H^+) and the osmotic pressure, which will change intracellular composition thereby modulating matrix synthesis.

If cartilage plugs are subjected to mechanical load, or equilibrated in a solution of PEG at high osmolarity, fluid is lost in proportion to the applied mechanical or osmotic stress. In the first case, the plugs deform anisotropically (i.e. not unidirectionally) and hydrostatic pressure increases, and in the second case there is no increase in hydrostatic pressure, the stress is isotropic and the shape of the cartilage plugs and chondrocytes at equilibrium is very different from those that had been loaded. If, however, synthesis rates are plotted as a function of fluid loss, there is no significant difference between the two curves (Schneiderman et al, 1986). Fluid loss increases extracellular osmolarity and, at equivalent degress of fluid loss, the change in extracellular osmolarity is very similar. This suggests that, although mechanical load and osmotic load might be considered to be different physiological stimuli, the common effect on chondrocyte matrix synthesis arises from changes to cell volume resulting from loss of water.

In view of the changing osmotic environment of chondrocytes, it is interesting to compare the effects of osmolarity on matrix synthesis rates by cartilage explants and isolated chondrocytes (*Figure 5.8*). Clearly, because of the Donnan effect of the GAGs in cartilage, the extracellular osmolarity of chondrocytes in cartilage explants is always higher than that of isolated cells at the same medium osmolarity. If the osmolarity is increased, general

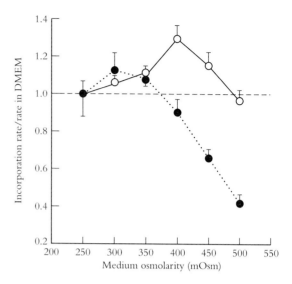

Figure 5.8 Effects of extracellular osmolarity using NaCl addition on matrix synthesis by bovine articular cartilage explants (●) or isolated bovine articular chondrocytes (○). The synthesis rates (measured as the rate of incorporation of the radiotracer $^{35}SO_4$ into proteoglycans) were normalised to the rate in tissue culture medium (Dulbecco's Modified Eagles medium, DMEM; about 280 mOsm), although the synthesis rate of isolated cells was about ten times less per cell compared with cells *in situ*. Optimal synthesis rates for cartilage explants were found at a medium osmolarity of about 300 mOsm. This corresponds to an interstitial osmolarity (i.e. that which the chondrocytes experience *in situ*) of about 380 mOsm. For isolated chondrocytes, optimal rates were at about 400 mOsm. Modified from Urban et al (1993); see this reference for further details.

protein synthesis and that of proteoglycans are affected. For isolated cells, normalised synthesis rates peak at around 400 mOsm and then decrease with raised osmolarity. Synthesis rates for articular cartilage explants show a similar pattern, but the peak rate is at a lower osmolarity (about 300 mOsm). If the curves are plotted as a function of extracellular osmolarity, rather than medium osmolarity, the curves superimpose. This suggests that it is cell volume *per se* that is involved in the response of chondrocytes to extracellular osmolarity, rather than other factors (e.g. cell–matrix interactions).

Changes to the ionic environment of either *in situ* or isolated chondrocytes (to simulate some of the effects of mechanical load) can also affect matrix synthesis markedly. Variations in pH, either indirectly by tissue loading (Gray et al, 1988) or directly by changes to medium pH, can have complex effects (*Figure 5.9*), and there is evidence

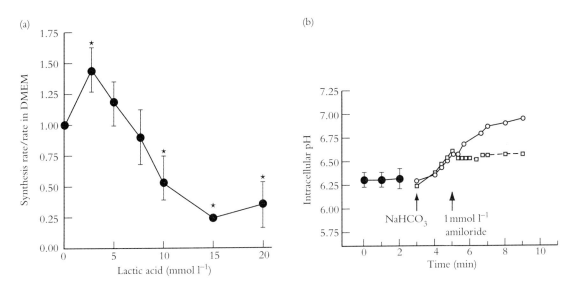

Figure 5.9 Effects of acidity on (a) matrix synthesis rates and (b) regulation of intracellular pH (pH$_i$) in isolated bovine articular chondrocytes. In (a), synthesis rates (measured as the incorporation of $^{35}SO_4$ into proteoglycans) have been normalised to those in standard tissue culture medium (DMEM) at pH 7.4 in the absence of lactate. Note the initial stimulation of synthesis at a lactate concentration of 2.5 mmol l^{-1} (corresponding to a decrease in pH of about 0.1 units), whereas with increasing acidity there was marked inhibition such that at [lactate]$_0$ of 20 mmol l^{-1} (pH approx. 6.2) synthesis had been reduced to about 30% of the control value. In separate experiments, synthesis was measured in medium containing 10 mmol l^{-1} lactic acid with the pH reset to 7.4. The results were no different from control values, showing that it was the acidity associated with the lactate (rather than the lactate ion itself) that influenced synthesis. In (b), chondrocytes were isolated from cartilage explants using collagenase and were then incubated with a membrane-permeant pH-sensitive fluorescent dye (BCECF-AM) which becomes trapped inside the cells. The chondrocytes were then washed free of extracellular dye, suspended in Na$^+$ and HCO$_3^-$-free medium (using N-methyl-D-glucamine chloride, 150 mmol l^{-1}) and the cells acidified to about pH 6.0. Note that pH remained constant at about 6.25 (●—●). However, when this solution was replaced by 150 mmol l^{-1} NaHCO$_3$ (open symbols: ○—○, control; □—□, before amiloride) there was a rapid recovery in pH$_i$ which was determined by the transport of H$^+$ across the plasma membrane out of the cell, thereby increasing the pH$_i$. When amiloride (a potassium-sparing diuretic which inhibits the Na$^+$/H$^+$ exchanger) was added, the recovery of pH$_i$ was prevented (□- - -□, after amiloride). A role for HCO$_3$-dependent pathways was ruled out because of the lack of effect of inhibitors of these systems on restoration of pH$_i$ after acid load. The absence of recovery of pH$_i$ in Na$^+$-free solutions, and the inhibitory effect of amiloride, showed that the Na$^+$/H$^+$ exchanger played the major role in pH$_i$ regulation in these cells. This system uses the inwardly directed Na$^+$ gradient to expel intracellular protons. Figure courtesy of Dr R.J. Wilkins reproduced with permission; see Wilkins and Hall (1995) and Hall et al (1996) for further details.

that it is the changes to intracellular pH (pH$_i$) that initiate the chondrocyte's response. Alterations to the extracellular K$^+$ concentration (and hence [K$^+$]$_i$) can also influence synthesis rates, but interestingly variation in extracellular [Ca^{2+}] over the physiological range has little effect. Measurements of [Ca^{2+}]$_i$ under these conditions show little change, and it is likely that this is achieved principally by means of the powerful outwardly directed Ca^{2+} pump present in these cells which prevents a rise in [Ca^{2+}]$_i$.

In summary, it is likely that chondrocytes 'sense' and respond to a range of signals resulting from physiological loading. There is, however, a considerable amount of research required before an understanding of these processes in normal and diseased cartilage is obtained.

CHONDROCYTE PHYSIOLOGY AND CARTILAGE DEFECTS

There is evidence to show that the biosynthetic response of chondrocytes following altered mechanical loading is mediated by changes to the physiology of the cells. The role of chondrocytes in the initiation and progression of osteoarthrosis is unclear at present, because the disease process is very complex and can be highly localised, with focal lesions surrounded by viable tissue. The initiation and progression of the disease within an individual joint, and possibly also the distribution of the disease between joints, may be determined by a balance between local and systemic factors (Dieppe and Kirwan, 1994). There are situations in which it is likely that chondrocytes are not involved directly, where, for example, excessive mechanical loads can cause micro-damage, initiating a sequence of lesions in the extracellular matrix before any changes to chondrocyte activity or cartilage composition are detected.

The focal defects observed in osteoarthrosis of knee and hip cartilage at positions of peak loading suggest that in some cases mechanical factors are an important determinant by their effects on cellular function (Kuettner et al, 1992). It used to be thought that cartilage loss in osteoarthrosis was the result of normal 'wear and tear', but there is evidence that cartilage breakdown is part of a disease process in which abnormal chondrocyte function is central to the progression, and possibly also to the initiation, of the disease (Stockwell, 1991; Gardner, 1992). The increase in mid-zone tissue hydration in osteoarthrosis is reported to be the earliest detectable change and, because no change in the collagen content occurs, this must result from a weakening of the fibrillar network. Clearly this will alter the biochemical properties of the joint and the microenvironment (ionic and osmotic environment, cell–matrix interactions) of the chondrocytes during normal activity.

It is worth remembering that these pathological changes differ markedly from those that occur during ageing, where the cartilage in some joints becomes 'drier'. In view of the effects of the physicochemical environment on chondrocyte metabolism, it is possible that changes to the physiology of a susceptible group of cells may start a sequence of events that results in the production of a mechanically compromised matrix. The increased permeability of the damaged matrix could significantly reduce the selectivity of the matrix to various potent factors in the synovial fluid, exposing the defective chondrocytes to much higher concentrations than normal, and an increased P_{O_2}.

Finally, if it was known how mechanical factors influenced chondrocyte physiology to alter the synthesis and degradation of the matrix, and how this was perturbed in osteoarthrosis, this might open up new targets for pharmacological intervention to limit, or even stimulate, the repair of the damaged extracellular matrix.

ACKNOWLEDGEMENTS

The author thanks the Wellcome Trust and the Arthritis and Rheumatism Council for support. He also thanks Dr J.P.G. Urban, who initially stimulated his interest in cartilage research, and Dr M.O. Wright and Dr R.J. Wilkins who gave useful comments on the manuscript.

REFERENCES

Alexander CM, Werb Z. Extracellular matrix degradation. In: Hay ED (ed.) *Cell Biology of Extracellular Matrix*, 2nd edn. New York: Plenum Press, 1991: 255–302.

Aydelotte MB, Schumacher BL, Kuettner KE. Heterogeneity of articular chondrocytes. In: Kuettner KE, Schleyerbach R, Peyron JG, Hascall VC (eds). *Articular Cartilage and Osteoarthritis*. New York: Raven Press, 1992: 237–249.

Buschmann MD, Gluzband YA, Grodzinsky AJ, Hunziker EB. Mechanical compression modulates matrix biosynthesis in chondrocyte/agarose culture. *J Cell Sci* 1995; **108**: 1497–1508.

Cancedda R, Cancedda FD, Castagnola P. Chondrocyte differentiation. *Int Rev Cytol* 1995; **159**: 265–358.

Dieppe P, Kirwan J. The localization of osteoarthritis. *Br J Rheumatol* 1994; **33**: 201–204.

Gardner DL. *The Pathological Basis of Connective Tissue Disease*. London: Edward Arnold, 1992.

Gray ML, Pizzanelli AM, Grodzinsky AJ, Lee RC. Mechanical and physicochemical determinants of the chondrocyte biosynthetic response. *J Orthop Res* 1988; **6**: 777–792.

Grodzinsky AJ. Electromechanical and physicochemical properties of connective tissue. *CRC Critical Reviews in Bioengineering* 1983; **9**: 133–199.

Hall AC, Urban JPG, Gehl KA. The effects of hydrostatic pressure on matrix synthesis in articular cartilage. *J Orthop Res* 1991; **9**: 1–10.

Hall AC, Horwitz ER, Wilkins RJ. The cellular physiology of articular cartilage. *Exp Physiol* 1996; **81**: 535–545.

Hardingham TE, Fosang AJ. Proteoglycans: many forms and many functions. *FASEB J* 1992; **6**: 861–870.

Helminen HJ, Kiviranta I, Säämänen A-M, Tammi M, Paukkonen K, Jurvelin J (eds). *Joint Loading*. Bristol: Wright, 1987.

Hodge WA, Fijan RS, Carlson KL, Burgess RG, Harris WH, Mann RW. Contact pressures in the human hip joint measured *in vivo*. *Proc Nat Acad Sci USA* 1986; **83**: 2879–2883.

Hunziker EB, Schenk RK. Physiological mechanisms adopted by chondrocytes in regulating longditudinal bone growth in rats. *J Physiol (Lond)* 1989; **414**: 55–71.

Kolettas E, Buluwela L, Bayliss MT, Muir H. Expression of cartilage-specific molecules is retained on long-term culture of human articular chondrocytes. *J Cell Sci* 1995; **108**, 1991–1999.

Kuettner KE, Schleyerbach R, Peyron JG, Hascall VC (eds). *Articular Cartilage and Osteoarthritis*. New York: Raven Press, 1992.

Maroudas A. Physical chemistry of articular cartilage and the intervertebral disc. In: Sokoloff L (ed.) *The Joints and Synovial Fluid*. New York: Academic Press 1980: 240–291.

Maroudas A, Evans H. A study of ionic equilibria in cartilage. *Connect Tissue Res* 1974; **1**, 69–77.

Maroudas A, Kuettner KE (eds). *Methods in Cartilage Research*. London: Academic Press, 1990.

Maroudas A, Palla G, Gilav E. Racemization of aspartic acid in human articular cartilage. *Connect Tissue Res* 1992; **28**, 161–169.

Muir H. The chondrocyte, architect of cartilage. *BioEssays* 1995; **17(12)**: 1039–1048.

Poole CA. Chondrons – the chondrocyte and its pericellular microenvironment. In: Kuettner KE, Schleyerbach R, Peyron JG, Hascall VC (eds). *Articular Cartilage and Osteoarthritis*. New York: Raven Press, 1992: 201–210.

Poole CA, Ayad S, Gilbert, RT. Chondrons from articular cartilage. *J Cell Sci* 1992; **103**: 1101–1110.

Schneiderman R, Keret D, Maroudas A. Effect of mechanical and osmotic pressure on the rate of glycosaminoglycan synthesis in human femoral head cartilage. An *in vitro* study. *J Orthop Res* 1986; **4**, 393–408.

Schumacher BL, Block JA, Schmid TM, Aydelotte MB, Kuettner, KE. A novel proteoglycan synthesized and secreted by chondrocytes of the superficial zone of articular cartilage. *Arch Biochem Biophys* 1994; **311(1)**: 144–152.

Schwartz MA, Ingber DE. Integrating with integrins. *Mol Biol Cell* 1994; **5**, 389–393.

Stein WD, Bronner F (eds). *Cell Shape – Determinants, Regulation and Regulatory Role*. London: Academic Press, 1992.

Stockwell RA. *The Biology of Cartilage Cells*. Cambridge: Cambridge University Press, 1979.

Stockwell RA. Cartilage failure in osteoarthritis: relevance of normal structure and function. A review. *Clin Anat* 1991; **4**, 161–191.

Thomas L. Reversible collapse of rabbit ears after intravenous papain, and prevention of recovery by cortisone. *J Exp Med* 1956; **104**, 245–252.

Tyler JA, Bolis S, Dingle JT, Middleton JFS. Mediators of matrix metabolism. In: Kuettner KE, Schleyerbach, Peyron JG, Hascall VC (eds). *Articular Cartilage and Osteoarthritis*. New York: Raven Press, 1992: 237–249.

Urban JPG. The chondrocyte: a cell under pressure. *Br J Rheumatol* 1994; **33**, 901–908.

Urban JPG, Hall AC. Physical modifiers of cartilage metabolism. In: Kuettner KE, Schleyerbach R, Peyron JG, Hascall VC (eds) *Articular Cartilage and Osteoarthritis*. New York: Raven Press, 1992: 393–406.

Urban JPG, Hall AC, Gehl KA. Regulation of matrix synthesis rates by the ionic and osmotic environment of articular chondrocytes. *J Cell Physiol* 1993; **154**: 262–270.

Vogel KG, Koob TJ. Structural specialization in tendons under compression. *Int Rev Cytol* 1989; **115**, 267–293.

Watson PA. Function follows form: generation of intracellular signals by cell deformation. *FASEB J* 1991; **5**: 2013–2019.

Wilkins RJ, Hall AC. Control of matrix synthesis in isolated bovine chondrocytes by extracellular and intracellular pH. *J Cell Physiol* 1995; **164**, 474–481.

Wilsman NJ. Cilia of adult canine articular chondrocytes. *J Ultrastructural Research* 1978; **64**, 270–281.

Wright MO, Jobanputra P, Barington C, Salter DM, Nuki G. Effects of intermittent pressure-induced strain on electrophysiology of cultured human chondrocytes: evidence for the presence of stretch-activated membrane ion channels. *Clin Sci* 1996; **90(1)**: 61–71.

Zanetti NC, Solursh M. Effect of cell shape on cartilage differentiation. In: Stein WD, Bronner F (eds) *Cell Shape – Determinants, Regulation and Regulatory Role*. London: Academic Press, 1992: 291–327.

6

Peripheral Nerves

Michael A Glasby and Christopher L-H Huang

INTRODUCTION

The detailed anatomy of nerve cells is beyond the scope of this book. It is of little direct concern to surgeons. The make-up of peripheral nerves is, however, of paramount importance in the assessment and treatment of nerve injuries. A simple appreciation of the components of, for example, the facial nerve will explain the difference in the clinical findings with injury in the cerebellopontine angle compared with injury in the preparotid region.

Certain aspects of the anatomy of nerves are frequently confused and these will be considered as a priority in this chapter. For a full appreciation of the structure of nerve cells and the topographical anatomy of peripheral nerves, the reader should consult a text such as *Gray's Anatomy*.

The nerve cell

Figure 6.1 is a diagrammatic representation of the nerve cell. Although these cells are large, they are in a considerable minority within the nervous system compared with the glial cells. Recent studies of the latter have indicated that, far from merely supporting neurones, the Schwann cells have a role in the regeneration of nerve cells in the periphery, and substances elaborated by oligodendrocytes

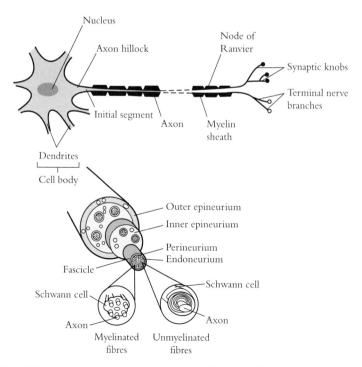

Figure 6.1 Diagrammatic representation of a typical nerve cell, nerve fibre and nerve trunk.

in the central nervous system (CNS) actively inhibit regeneration. This has led to the important concept that nerve cell regeneration is determined by the **environment** provided by the supporting cells.

The cell body of a neurone is the site of metabolic activity and its integrity is essential for cell function and for regeneration. It is thus axiomatic that only nerve fibres connected to a cell body are capable of regeneration in whatever environment. The precise shape and the arrangement of processes depends on the function which the cell has to perform. Classical examples are the motor neurone with a cell body with multiple short dendrites lying in the anterior funiculus of the spinal cord and a single long axon reaching muscles in the periphery. The typical pseudounipolar sensory cell has its cell body in the dorsal root ganglion, a single very long peripheral dendrite and an axon lying mainly within the spinal cord. It should be noted that the terms **axon** and **dendrite** have specific functional meanings. An axon carries the nerve impulse away from the cell body whereas a dendrite carries it towards the cell body. Thus, in, for example, the median nerve at the wrist, the motor fibres will be axons and the sensory fibres dendrites.

The term **nerve fibre**, when applied to a myelinated nerve, comprises the axon or dendrite, its myelin sheath which is laid down by and contains Schwann cells and, surrounding both of these, a Schwann cell **basement membrane** sheath or **endoneurial tube**. The term basement membrane sheath is much to be preferred but the term 'endoneurial tube' is hallowed by usage although anatomically inaccurate.

Unmyelinated nerve fibres are made up differently. A single Schwann cell has several axons or dendrites embedded in it and, of course, does not lay down myelin. This arrangement is often called a **Remak bundle**. When considering nerve repair, unmyelinated fibres are rarely implicated but it should never be forgotten that they make up a substantial proportion of most peripheral nerves.

The arrangement of the nerve fibres in relation to nonneural elements within a nerve trunk is of great importance in nerve repair. The terminology is often confused, even by experienced surgeons, and this has led to much misunderstanding of the processes of nerve degeneration and regeneration. There are three non-neural elements which, along with blood vessels, are to be found in peripheral nerves. By far the most important of these is the **perineurium**. This is a **cellular** layer which sur-

rounds groups of nerve fibres separating them into **fascicles** or **funiculi**. Individual funiculi may serve specific functions (i.e. be wholly sensory or motor) and may be directed to particular sites (e.g. within a particular nerve specific funiculi may be directed to flexor or extensor muscles uniquely). Within a nerve trunk there is often extensive branching of the funiculi with exchange of fibres between them. This is a particular problem which faces the surgeon wishing to repair a nerve trunk especially as the branching is not constant in different individuals.

In most nerves the **perineurium** is made up of a single layer of cells although in nerves which have been repaired and have regenerated across the repair site the perineurium may develop several layers of cells. Between individual perineurial cells there are **tight junctions**, which indicate a function of these cells in defining an enclosed environment. Although study has proved difficult, it seems likely that the environment enclosed within the perineurium may be chemically different from that outside, which is part of the body's extracellular fluid space. It seems likely that the environment enclosed within the perineurium (**endoneurial space**) is particularly appropriate both for nerve conduction and for nerve regeneration, and a better understanding of its composition is one of the prizes for researchers in this field. In a regenerated nerve, although the perineurium becomes multilaminate, tight junctions are found only at the innermost layer of cells.

Understanding the nature of the **perineurium** makes defining the other non-neural structures in a nerve trunk easy. Anything outside the perineurium which is not a nerve fibre or a blood vessel is **epineurium**. For the most part, epineurium is collagen and is mechanically the strongest supporting structure in nerve. The collagen fibres are the same as those which form connective tissue elsewhere in the body and are secreted by fibroblasts derived from **mesoderm**.

Within the perineurial space (i.e. inside funiculi) is the endoneurial space, and the collagen contained within it is termed **endoneurium**. The individual endoneurial collagen fibres have a different chemical structure and are thinner than those of epineurium. At least two subpopulations have been seen, with smaller fibres lying closer to the nerve fibres themselves. There is evidence to suggest that they have a different embryological origin and are derived from **ectoderm** like the nerve cells. Some authors have suggested transformations between

Table 6.1 Classification of nerve fibre types.

Nerve fibre type	Aα	Aβ	Aγ	Aδ	B	C
Fibre diameter (μm)	12–20	5–12	3–6	2–5	< 3	0.4–1.2
Conduction velocity (m s^{-1})	70–110	30–65	20–30	15–30	3–15	0.5–2
Function	Motor to skeletal muscle proprioception	Touch pressure	Fusimotor to muscle spindles	Mechanical pain, temperature, touch	Autonomic, preganglionic	Chemical pain

Schwann cells, perineurial cells and ectodermally derived fibroblasts, with the latter producing endoneurial collagen. This transformation is triggered by regenerating nerve cells or by factors which they elaborate. Endoneurial collagen appears to be 'friendly' to developing or regenerating nerve cells when it is separated from 'hostile' epineurial collagen by the protective perineurial cell layer.

Nerve fibre types

Nerve fibres may be classified by their structural and their functional characteristics. This is important in both the diagnosis and assessment of nerve injuries because it allows comparisons to be made. For a myelinated nerve the following relationship exists:

$$v \propto d$$

For a non-myelinated nerve fibre the relationship is:

$$v \propto \sqrt{d}$$

where v is the conduction velocity (m s^{-1}) and d is fibre diameter (μm).

Table 6.1 shows the relationship between nerve conduction velocities, fibre size and function. All of the nerve fibres except group C are myelinated.

Most authorities today add to the confusion by preferring a classification which uses Lloyd's nomenclature for sensory fibres innervating muscle spindles and Golgi tendon organs, while they use Erlanger and Gasser's classification for everything else. This makes sense inasmuch as the precise descriptions are more fitting with this arrangement.

In diagnosing nerve injuries two questions must be asked. These are:

- What is the exact site of injury?
- What functional nerve fibre types does the nerve contain **at this site**?

Only if these facts are known can the true nature of the functional loss and the prospects of recovery after repair be assessed. In reality, the questions are more often considered from their answers. The surgeon assesses the functional loss and, from a knowledge of the make-up of the nerve, identifies the site of injury. Even where all of these things are seemingly obvious (i.e. there is a precise gash at the wrist and we know where the median nerve lies and what it contains here), the exercise of answering the above questions acts as an internal correlation and complete appraisal of the findings.

All nerve fibres below the cranial nerves fall into four major groups. At the level of the cranial nerves a further three groups are added to make a total of seven functional groups. These groups and their subgroups are summarized in *Figure 6.2* and represent, along with spinal levels and the topography of nerve trunks, the three most important ingredients for the study and treatment of nerve injuries.

PHYSIOLOGY OF PERIPHERAL NERVES

The term 'neurophysiology' is often used in clinical circles specifically to refer to electrophysiological methods used in the diagnosis of nerve injuries and in assessment of progress after nerve repair. This very specific aspect of peripheral nerve surgery will be dealt with later. The paragraphs that follow immediately are an

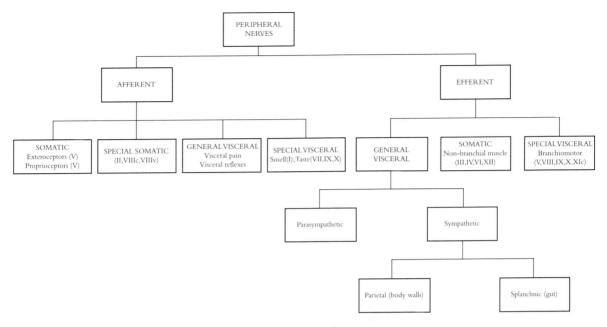

Figure 6.2 Classification of nerve fibre types.

introduction to the biophysics of excitable tissues and provide the scientific basis on which the applied principles of clinical neurophysiology are based.

The nerve cell

A neurone, or nerve cell, consists of several recognisable parts (see *Figure 6.1*). There is a cell body, or perikaryon, containing a nucleus, endoplasmic reticulum, mitochondria and other organelles. The biochemical processes that take place in the cell body are ultimately responsible for maintaining the extensive structure of the nerve cell. Thus, the cell body is rich in ribosomes, which are associated with protein synthesis. The nerve cell functions as a unit of information processing, and communication must therefore take place between component cells of the nervous system.

Each cell receives incoming (afferent) information from functional points of contact (synapses) with other cells or from sensory stimuli acting upon particular specialisations in the form of receptor cells. The structural process which conveys impulses towards the cell body is known as a dendrite. The incoming information has to be processed, and is then conveyed to distant effector sites (e.g. muscles) away from the cell body by its axon. The axon is typically terminated by branchings into synaptic

terminals, motor endplates or vascular capillaries in the case of neurosecretory cells.

In addition to the rapid conduction of electrical activity, the axon is responsible for protein transport processes. There is a process of rapid axonal transport (40 cm day^{-1}) and a process of a slow transport (1–3 mm day^{-1}). This latter mechanism may translocate structural elements such as microtubular proteins and this may be an important factor that limits axonal regeneration after nerve fibre transection.

The nerve cell surface membrane

The most important structure in the generation and conduction of nerve impulses is the cell membrane. This is also the surface across which the cell makes its chemical transactions with the environment; it is about 5–10 nm thick and consists of two monolayer phospholipid leaflets in which proteins are embedded. It separates the cell interior from the extracellular fluid. The lipid component of the cell membrane in mammals contains substantial quantities of phosphatidylcholine, phosphatidylethanolamine and cholesterol.

These substances are made up of both polar (hydrophilic) head-groups and non-polar (hydrophobic) tails. Typically, two hydrophobic tails are linked to a glycerol

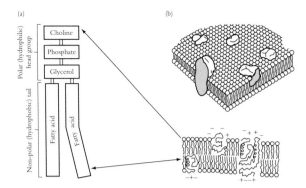

Figure 6.3 (a) Basic structure of the phospholipid phosphatidylcholine, showing linkage of two hydrophobic tails by a hydrophilic glycerol moiety, conjugated to choline through phosphate. (b) The fluid mosaic hypothesis for the structure of membranes, which suggests that the greater part of the surface area consists of a lipid bilayer matrix forming two leaflets containing integral and peripheral membrane proteins scattered through the phospholipid. From Singer and Nicolson (1972), with permission.

head-group conjugated with a phosphatidylcholine moiety (*Figure 6.3a*). The polar head-groups face and are stabilised by association with the aqueous phase whereas the non-polar tails are oriented towards the centre of the membrane. The membrane is thus assembled as a bilaminar leaflet which forms a barrier to permeation by polar molecules. The lipid bilayer acts as an insulator which prevents charged particles from crossing the membrane, and so any charge becomes deposited and remains on the membrane surface. The result is a stored charge which can be remobilised on removal of the voltage that caused its accumulation. The amount of charge stored (Q) depends both on the imposed voltage (V) and on the properties of the material of which the membrane is composed and its geometry. These latter properties can be described by a constant, termed the capacitance (C) of the membrane. Thus:

$$C = Q/V$$

The result of any charge separation across a biological membrane is the genesis of a membrane potential. This refers to the voltage within the cell, V_i, relative to that outside the cell, V_o, and is typically expressed in millivolts (mV). In the quiescent state, the inside of a cell is normally negative with respect to the extracellular fluid. An increase in this negativity is referred to as a hyperpo-larisation; a shift in the potential towards more positive values is called a depolarisation.

The lipid bilayer forms a largely fluid matrix in which discrete macromolecular components composed typically of protein and glycoprotein are embedded (*Figure 6.3*). The latter mediate the specific physiological processes that are associated with cell membranes. These macromolecules are anchored within the membrane matrix by the non-polar amino acid residues which they contain. There, they tend to associate with the non-polar tail groups of the lipid in the membrane interior. Folding of the protein exposes the polar head-groups to the aqueous environment that faces the membrane surface. At least some of the proteins are tethered to specific regions within the plane of the membrane by intracellular cytoskeletal elements.

Transmembrane or integral proteins span the entire membrane thickness. Their central hydrophobic regions are composed largely of α helices that make contact with the lipid tails of the phospholipids. Transmembrane proteins mediate membrane processes which involve communication between both sides of the membrane. They include ionic pumps, ion channels and hormone receptors. Other peripheral membrane proteins are only partially inserted into the membrane.

Membranes mediate important exchanges of solutes and water between the cell and its environment. Of these, active transport processes utilise metabolic energy to transport ions or metabolites against electrochemical gradients. In contrast, passive transport mechanisms simply facilitate translocation down a concentration gradient, and/or an electrical gradient if the particles concerned are charged. Passive transport may take a number of routes. Lipid-soluble molecules including oxygen and carbon dioxide cross the membrane readily by simple diffusion owing to their capacity to dissolve in the lipid bilayer. Such a capacity is not shared by hydrophilic molecules such as glucose and amino acids whose membrane permeation requires their combination with carrier proteins which must then transport the bound substance to the opposite side of the membrane before its release into the cytosol. Such transfer would take place at a rate limited by the number of available carrier sites and, consequently, it would reach a saturating maximum value at high substrate concentrations.

Finally, specific charged species may traverse the membrane through particular 'pores' or channels. These confer a small ionic permeability on the membrane (around 10^{-10} times that of the membrane H_2O and 10^{-5} times that of glucose), which is nevertheless essential for the excitable phenomena shown by nerve cell membranes.

Ionic gradients across cell membranes

The active transport processes contribute to the maintenance of ionic concentration differences between the intracellular and extracellular fluids. Thus, concentration differences in Na^+ and K^+ on either side of the membrane are set up by a metabolically driven Na^+/K^+ pump. This integral membrane protein contains extracellular K^+ and intracellular Na^+ binding sites. Its operation cycle transports three Na^+ ions out of the cell for each inward transport of two K^+ ions. This generates large inward Na^+ and outward K^+ concentration gradients across the cell membrane. Consequently, each operation of the pump requires energy, which it derives from being coupled to the hydrolysis of a molecule of adenosine $5'$-triphosphate (ATP).

The Na^+/K^+-ATPase system is of fundamental importance to cellular function and survival of all cells. The function of the pump also results in the extrusion of a quantity of water osmotically equivalent to the Na^+ expelled. This prevents the cellular accumulation of water that would have otherwise resulted from the osmotic effect of intracellular proteins and which would tend to cause cell disruption and lysis. The Na^+ gradients additionally form a chemical energy reservoir that is necessary to drive the secondary active transport mechanisms for other substances such as amino acids and monosaccharides into cells against their concentration gradients. These processes are central to renal function and gastrointestinal absorption. Similar processes are also important in the secondary active transport of Ca^{2+} out of cells through Na^+/Ca^{2+} exchange. Finally, the gradients of Na^+/K^+, and secondarily of Ca^{2+} provide an electrochemical energy reservoir essential for electrical conduction in excitable membranes.

The resting potential

The consequence of Na^+/K^+ pump activity in eukaryotic cells is a high internal K^+ concentration; $[K^+]_i$, and a low internal Na^+ concentration $[Na^+]_i$ (*Table 6.2*). The concentration difference between intracellular and extracellular fluids leads to a number of physical consequences. Any ion that can permeate the membrane will diffuse through it down its concentration gradient as the latter provides a chemical potential for such a flux. In addition, the voltage across the membrane will influence movement of the charged ion. Thus the overall movement of the ion is determined by both chemical and electrical forces.

The concentrations of the ion on either side of the membrane will tend towards values where the sum of the chemical and electrical energies is minimised, whereupon the system attains electrochemical equilibrium. This can be exemplified for a membrane which separates two compartments with different K^+ concentrations. A membrane that was impermeable to all ions would generate no voltage drop between the compartments. However, if the membrane were exclusively permeable to K^+, this ion would flow from its region of higher concentration to one of lower concentration. This would result in a transfer of positive charge and consequently the development of a voltage across the membrane. Such a voltage, however, would oppose further movement of charge and lead to a state of equilibrium in which the membrane potential precisely balanced the chemical potential (see *Figure 6.4a*).

Table 6.2 Intracellular and extracellular concentrations of major ions.

Ionic species	External concentration (mmol l^{-1})	Internal concentration (mmol l^{-1})	Ratio (internal : external)
Na^+	145	12	0.08
K^+	4	140	35
Ca^{2+}	1.5	<0.0001	0
Cl^-	125	4	0.03

(a)

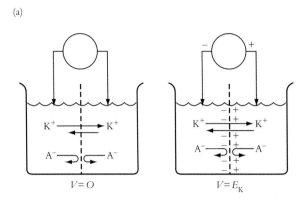

(b)

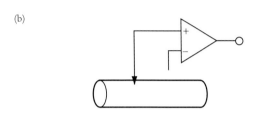

(c)

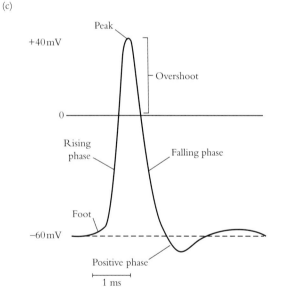

Figure 6.4 (a) A membrane uniquely permeable to K$^+$ will allow selective permeation of K$^+$ from the compartment of higher to that of lower [K$^+$]. This results in an associated transfer of charge. The process is complete when the resulting voltage equals the Nernst, or equilibrium, potential for K$^+$. (b) Intracellular recording of the difference between intracellular and extracellular potentials with glass microelectrodes. (c) Components of the action potential. From Glasby and Huang (1995), with permission.

The Nernst equation relates this equilibrium (Nernst) potential (*E*) to the concentrations on either side of the membrane of the particular ion in question. For K$^+$ ions, this potential, E_K, is related to the concentrations, [K$^+$]$_o$ and [K$^+$]$_i$, on either side of the membrane by:

$$E_K = \frac{RT}{zF} \ln\left(\frac{[K^+]_o}{[K^+]_i}\right) mV$$

The symbols *R, T* and *F* denote the gas constant, the absolute temperature and Faraday's constant respectively. The valency, *z*, for K$^+$ is unity. For any ion, X, at physiological temperatures, one may also use the approximate form:

$$E_X = \left(\frac{58}{z}\right) \log_{10}\left(\frac{[X]_o}{[X]_i}\right) mV$$

These principles enable a prediction of the equilibrium potentials towards which the concentration differences of any given ion would drive even a quiescent biological membrane. For example, for the K$^+$ ion, [K$^+$]$_o$ = 4 mM and [K$^+$]$_i$ = 140 mM, and this gives an equilibrium potential of E_K = −90 mV. Thus a membrane exclusively permeable to K$^+$ would show a membrane potential that tended to an equilibrium value at E_K = −90 mV. At this voltage there would then be no net driving force on K$^+$ transfer and therefore no net movement of that ion across the membrane. In contrast, for Na$^+$, the corresponding substitutions are [Na$^+$]$_o$ = 145 mM and [Na$^+$]$_i$ = 12 mM. This gives E_{Na} = +62 mV. Thus a membrane exclusively permeable to Na$^+$ would have a membrane potential E_{Na} = +62 mV at equilibrium.

Biological potentials observed *in vivo* generally fall between these limits. Thus the resting potential in a quiescent nerve cell is around −70 mV. Membrane potentials in excitable cells can be recorded using microelectrodes made by drawing glass capillary tubes to fine (0.1 μm) tips which are then filled with electrolyte, typically KCl. After the electrode impales an excitable cell, the cell membrane seals around the pipette. One then typically observes a resting potential of between −70 and −90 mV (inside relative to outside) in a quiescent cell that shows the normal physiological intracellular and extracellular electrolyte concentrations.

Thus neither Na$^+$ nor K$^+$ is in equilibrium, although the resting potential is closer to E_K than to E_{Na}. Furthermore, variations in the external concentration of sodium, [Na$^+$]$_o$, produce relatively little effect on the resting potential, whereas the resting potential varies roughly linearly as the logarithm of the external concentration of potassium, $[K^+]_o$. These findings suggest that the resting potential results largely from the electrochemical gradients of K^+ across the cell membrane (reflecting relatively high membrane permeability to K^+) and only a small contribution is made by the oppositely directed electrochemical gradients of Na^+.

This situation can be described in more formal terms by considering the permeability of the membrane in terms of its conductance to the ion in question. If the membrane obeys Ohm's law, then the current (I_{Na} or I_K) carried by a given ion will depend on the conductance (g_{Na} or g_K) of the membrane to that ion, and on the net driving force for the movement of the ion across the membrane. The latter would be the difference between the membrane potential, V, and the equilibrium potential of the ion, E_{Na} or E_K, at which this driving force is zero. Thus:

$$I_K = g_K(V - E_K)$$

and

$$I_{Na} = g_{Na}(V - E_{Na})$$

When the potential across the membrane is not changing, the total current due to the sodium and potassium currents is zero, thus:

$$I_K + I_{Na} = g_K(V - E_K) + g_{Na}(V - E_{Na}) = 0$$

and so the resting potential:

$$V = \frac{(g_K E_K) + (g_{Na} E_{Na})}{g_K + g_{Na}}$$

Thus if the K^+ conductance greatly exceeds the Na^+ conductance, the membrane potential will tend towards the equilibrium potential for K^+. This explains the closeness of the resting potential to the equilibrium potential for K^+. It also explains the marked dependence of the resting potential on varying conditions of intracellular and extracellular K^+ concentrations and its relative independence of Na^+ concentration.

Initiation of the action potential

A range of stimuli can initiate propagated electrical activity when applied to a quiescent nerve fibre or some other excitable cell. Intracellular recording indicates that the electrical stimulation of an axon elicits in a momentary overshoot of the membrane potential from its -70 mV resting level to a positive reading of $+40$ mV, before a recovery within around 1.5 ms, an event called the action potential (*Figure 6.4b,c*).

The properties of the action potential are often followed in clinical practice by extracellular recording (see Nerve conduction studies below). At its simplest, this approach measures the potential between pairs of external surface electrodes (*Figure 6.5*). The resulting recording is a biphasic rather than a monophasic wave as each electrode senses the external voltage change in succession. Variants of such a recording scheme have clinical applications in the recording of electrical activity in the heart (the electrocardiogram) and muscle (electromyogram), as well as in nerve (*Figure 6.5a,b*).

The all-or-none law states that a single axon shows a distinct threshold for firing. Once this threshold is attained, a full-sized action potential of fixed size that is not graded with the size of stimulus results. The action potential is associated with an overall increase in membrane conductivity. Its amplitude varies with the logarithm of the external Na^+ concentration. Hodgkin and Huxley's sodium hypothesis suggested that, whereas the resting potential results largely from a high membrane conductance to K^+, the action potential is the consequence of a momentary but marked increase in Na^+ conductance.

The current view of action potential generation suggests that the membrane conductance to Na^+ and K^+ ions is controlled by the opening and closing of specific ionic channels in response to an initiating change in membrane potential triggered by current spread from an adjacent activated region of nerve. The Na^+ channel opens in response to depolarisation. This results in an increase in g_{Na}, which in turn causes further depolarisation and therefore a further opening of more Na^+ channels. This results in a regenerative increase in Na^+ conductance, which in turn drives the membrane potential towards $+40$ mV, close to the equilibrium potential for sodium, E_{Na}. However, within around 0.5 ms (at 18°C) the Na^+ channels then become inactivated as a result of the depolarising voltage.

The K^+ conductance also increases with depolarisation but with a slower time course. However, the increased g_K eventually drives the membrane potential back towards the Nernst potential for potassium, E_K. This restores the membrane to the resting potential, and may even cause a brief after-hyperpolarization. Total membrane conductance thus increases through an action potential, owing to activation, in turn, of Na^+ and K^+ channels (*Figure 6.6*).

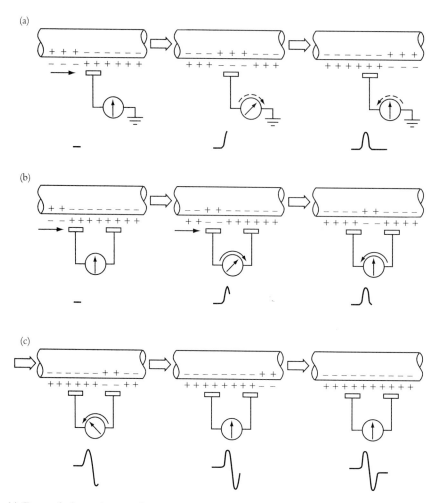

Figure 6.5 (a) External electrode recording: unipolar recording. (b) Bipolar recording of propagated activity, giving (c) biphasic records. From Glasby and Huang (1995), with permission.

A refractory period in which membrane excitability is diminished follows the action potential. It reflects the time required for the Na$^+$ channels to recover from inactivation. The absolute refractory period refers to the interval over which a further stimulus, however large, cannot elicit a fresh action potential. In the relative refractory period that follows, an all-or-none response can be elicited, but this requires a larger stimulus than normal. The refractory period is important in ensuring that the direction of conduction of the action potential remains constant.

The properties of the contributions made by ionic current to the action potential can be studied by applying voltage steps to the membrane and measuring the currents. Individual Na$^+$ and K$^+$ currents can be examined using such a voltage clamp technique. Thus I_{Na} is abolished by replacing extracellular Na$^+$ with the impermeant cation substitute (choline$^+$) to isolate the I_K contribution. Subtraction of this latter trace from that of the total current yields I_{Na}. Subsequent work has also achieved a separation of I_{Na} and I_K through blocking I_{Na} using the puffer fish venom, tetrodotoxin, or blocking I_K by externally applied tetraethylammonium ions, or internally applied Cs$^+$. The corresponding conductances can then be deduced from the currents as functions of time, t, and test voltage, V.

$$g_{Na} = \frac{I_{Na}}{(V - E_{Na})} \quad \text{and} \quad g_K = \frac{I_K}{(V - E_K)}$$

The properties of the conductances, g_{Na} and g_K, that were

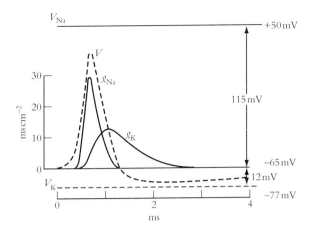

Figure 6.6 Reconstruction of the time course of the propagated action potential with the underlying changes in g_{Na} and g_K. From Hodgkin and Huxley (1952), with permission.

deduced in such studies were appropriate to roles in regenerative activity in nerve membrane. Thus the sodium conductance is turned on rapidly early in response to a depolarising step.

Both the extent and the rate of its activation increase with greater degrees of depolarisation. Furthermore, the Na^+ current is spontaneously inactivated with prolonged depolarisation. The K^+ current is also activated, and also to an increasing extent, with increasing depolarisation. However, this takes place over a considerably slower time course than with the Na^+ current. Additionally, in squid giant axon the activation is sustained with prolonged depolarisation and is not followed by inactivation.

Propagation of electrical activity

The electrical change described above must next pass down the nerve if the initial perturbation is to be signalled at a locus remote from the triggering site. The action potential results in an inversion of polarity in the active region of membrane, with the result that the membrane inside becomes relatively positive to the outside. This results in an electrical gradient between the active and inactive regions of both the inner and outer surfaces of membrane, which produces a local circuit of current flow between the active and inactive regions (*Figure 6.7a,b*). Quiescent regions of nerve become depolarised and, when they reach threshold, a fresh action potential is produced and the process is repeated.

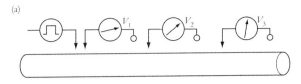

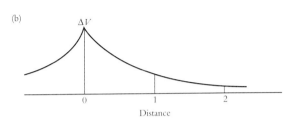

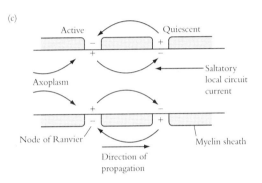

Figure 6.7 (a) Attenuation of a voltage change as induced at a distance $x = 0$ by a current I, along the length (b) of an unmyelinated nerve. (c) Saltatory conduction of local circuit currents in a myelinated nerve. From Glasby and Huang (1995), with permission.

A number of factors influence conduction velocity. First, changes in the size of the action potential or its rate of rise affect the electrical signal that initiates the conduction process. These changes could be the result of alterations in temperature and external Na^+ concentrations, and of pharmacological interventions that influence Na^+ channel function such as local anaesthesia.

Second, factors that increase the extent of current spread would result in a discharge of more remote regions of the membrane and therefore enhance conduction. The same would be true of a reduction in the leakage current across the intervening regions of membrane that would otherwise diminish the relative capacitative current flow. Thus, any reduction of resistance (r_o) to external current flow, or of the resistance (r_i) of the intracellular conducting pathway, would cause a decrease in the extent to which the voltage change imposed at any point would attenuate along the length of a nerve, and so would enhance conduction. Accordingly intracellular resistance diminishes, and conduction velocity increases, with any increase in fibre diameter and, conversely, a decline in membrane resistance (r_m) would increase the leak current shunting through the membrane and so decrease conduction velocity.

Third, factors that influence the effectiveness with which local circuit currents cause activation should also modify conduction velocity. These include the number of Na^+ channels available for activation. The membrane capacitance determines the amount of charge required for the membrane potential to reach the threshold for Na^+ channel activation. In an unmyelinated axon, the capacitance of the cell membrane is close to 1.0 $\mu F\ cm^{-2}$. In myelinated nerve fibres, the wrapping of the axon in an insulating sheath both sharply increases the leakage resistance, r_m, and decreases the membrane capacitance. Current flow in such a situation is confined to nodal regions (of Ranvier), which are not insulated, and so conduction appears to jump from node to node (saltatory conduction; *Figure 6.7c*).

In myelinated nerves, the internodal length increases with fibre diameter. Thus, conduction velocity increases in proportion to fibre diameter. In contrast, conduction velocity in unmyelinated axons is proportional to the square root of fibre diameter. These functions intersect at diameters of around 1 μm. Below this diameter, non-myelinated fibres, and above this diameter myelinated fibres, show the higher conduction velocity. It has been observed empirically that nerve fibres with a diameter below 1 μm are unmyelinated and those above 1 μm are myelinated.

Molecular basis of excitability

The ionic channels that produce the action potential are members of a particular class of membrane protein and have structural features in common with other voltage-sensitive channels. All of these show a four-subunit structure with the ion pore running through the centre of the subunits. The subunits of both the Na^+ and Ca^{2+} channels are organised from a single amino acid chain but K^+ channels are assembled from four separate chains into a nevertheless similar overall structure. In contrast, ligand-gated channels open or close in response to the binding of specific chemicals or transmitters. These

typically show a five-subunit structure. The channels through gap junctions show a six-subunit structure.

Cloning and sequencing of the gene that encodes the voltage-operated Na^+ channel suggests that the channel is a protein of 2000 amino acid residues, which forms four homologous repeats. Each of the latter repeats is made up of six membrane-spanning hydrophobic regions. One of these, the S4 segment, has an unusual sequence which includes five positively charged residues, each of which occurs at every third successive position in the helix. It is probable that this region of the protein acts as the 'voltage sensor' that enables the channel's molecular configuration to be responsive to the membrane voltage.

The function of ion channels requires changes in configuration to take place in response to an applied voltage. This would be accompanied by a rearrangement of charged functional groups within the membrane and resulting changes in the overall electrical field. These movements of charge would produce small electric currents even in the absence of the ions that would normally traverse the channel. Such 'gating currents' have been observed experimentally and their study offers a means of examining the configurational changes that precede and accompany activation in the channels.

The experimental studies of membrane conductance described above give an indication of the ensemble behaviour of a large number of channels. It has been possible to record the currents associated with the molecular openings of individual channels using the patch clamp technique. This involves pressing a fire-polished glass micropipette against the cell membrane to form a seal between the glass and the membrane, and following currents from single channels within the patch. Such experiments indicate the existence of discrete open or closed states in the channel (Glasby and Huang, 1995).

DEGENERATION AND REGENERATION IN PERIPHERAL NERVES

The process of degeneration which occurs after injury to a nerve was classically described by Waller and now bears his name. Cajal and other workers enlarged on the anatomical basis of **wallerian degeneration** and, with improving surgical techniques, interest was aroused in the regenerative process which follows nerve repair.

The fundamental concept of wallerian degeneration is that survival of nerve fibres occurs only if they remain connected to the cell body. Hence, if a nerve trunk is transected, those parts distal to the transection undergo the degenerative process. It has long been held that degeneration also proceeds in the proximal segment but only as far as the next proximal node of Ranvier. Recent work has suggested that proximal changes may be more extensive, at least in respect of biochemical changes extending as far as the cell body. However, at present, details are uncertain.

When wallerian degeneration takes place, the earliest peripheral changes are fragmentation of the distal axon and its myelin sheath. In the cell body there is swelling, migration of the nucleus to the periphery, and chromatolysis, giving an increased basophilic appearance to the cell. At the same time there is activation and proliferation of Schwann cells close to the injury site. These are capable of phagocytising the cellular and myelin debris. In this way the Schwann cells come to occupy the now empty endoneurial tubes where they arrange themselves end to end to form the so-called '**bands of von Bungner**'. These bands act to guide the **sprouts** or **neurites** of regenerating or '**pioneering axons**' down the endoneurial tubes. If these sprouts eventually make connections with distal target organs, nerve fibre maturation follows. The axon increases in size and its myelin sheath increases in thickness. However, regenerated axons never reach pre-injury sizes and a study of the frequency histogram of nerve fibre sizes contained within a nerve always shows a leftward shift after nerve repair. Although the mean fibre size of any population of nerve fibres is reduced after regeneration, the smaller fibres have myelin sheaths with a normal thickness for the size of the axon. This relationship is called the **G ratio** (axon diameter ÷ fibre diameter).

Neurites which fail to make distal connections eventually die back and are lost to the regenerative process. The above assumes that the cut ends have been apposed so that there is at least a potential for some proximal and distal endoneurial tubes to be matched up. Where a gap persists, a **neuroma** is formed. This is a knot of randomly distributed neurites in a mass of connective tissue. It can have no functional use on account of its disorderliness and lack of distal connections. For reasons which are not clear, neuromas are often associated with considerable pain, including the **phantom-limb pain** caused by **terminal neuromas** at amputation sites or where a cutaneous nerve has been divided in a surgical incision. It is not known whether the hyperstimulation of pain fibres caused by the neuroma is produced at the neuroma itself or whether it is a central phenomenon. However, it is a major clinical problem. In clinical practice most terminal neuromas are associated with amputation; the **lateral neuroma** or **neuroma-in-continuity** is more often encountered by the peripheral nerve surgeon. This occurs when there has been partial (or sometimes complete) severance of a nerve, which has either gone unrecognised or untreated, or in nerves which have been repaired and where the nerve ends have separated before regeneration across the gap is complete. Thus there is disorganisation at the neuroma site with failure of pioneering axons to gain distal endoneurial tubes. The treatment is complete excision and repair with a graft.

Factors affecting nerve regeneration

A variety of factors naturally influence nerve regeneration. These are mainly chemical and their precise roles are only presently becoming clear. However, the importance to the surgeon of understanding these processes is that they may eventually offer a means of enhancing nerve regeneration. Surgical techniques for nerve repair today are very sophisticated and it is difficult to imagine how there can be any improvement in the mechanics of nerve repair. Future improvements will almost certainly come from chemical manipulation of the environment in which regeneration takes place.

Neurotrophism

Any injured nerve cell survives and regenerates only if it is reached by appropriate **neurotrophic factors**. These are substances which influence survival and growth of nerve cells; they are produced by Schwann cells and other cellular components of the axonal supporting tissue and by the denervated target organs. These chemical signals are transmitted to the cell body of the injured nerve cell by retrograde axonal transport. The first neurotrophic factor to be investigated was nerve growth factor (NGF). *In vitro* studies have shown it to have an enhancing effect on the survival and regeneration of autonomic and some sensory nerve fibres. Other recently described neurotrophic factors include brain-derived neurotrophic factor (BDNF) and ciliary neurotrophic factor (CNTF). New growth factors are being described at a great rate, although so far there is no convincing evidence of their *in vivo* roles. Work in these substances has remained very much the province of *in vitro* scientists. Before they can be of use to the surgeon their *in vivo* function must be established and also a means of maintaining an appropriate concentration at the active site for an adequate time during the regeneration process. These simple practical considerations, unfashionable as science but essential to the surgeon, do not appear to have excited the numerous research workers in this field.

Matrix proteins

The basement membrane of any cell is made up of a **basal lamina** close to the cell membrane and a **reticular lamina** beyond. The basal lamina of Schwann cell basement membrane (and several other tissues such as muscle) carries on its surface certain glycoproteins which are thought to be able to promote neurite activity. Principal among these are **fibronectin** and **laminin**, both of which have been implicated in enhancing neurite growth by a process termed **contact guidance**. This may explain the efficacy of freeze–thawed coaxial skeletal muscle grafts and grafts made of fibronectin mats. At present, however, the evidence is equivocal and remains to be elucidated further.

Neurotropism

Neurotropism is the name given to the well-known biological process of **chemotaxis** when applied to growing or regenerating nerve fibres. There is a clear preference for pioneering axons to grow towards a distal segment of nerve if it is not situated too far away. In the rat, pioneering axons will cross gaps of up to 7 mm to enter a distal stump without forming a neuroma. In the human, sadly, this does not occur and even the smallest gap will often produce a neuroma-in-continuity. The chemotactic influence is probably exerted by factors such as NGF produced by target organs.

CLASSIFICATION OF NERVE INJURIES

To make sense of diagnosis and treatment of nerve injuries it is essential to have a formalised classification of their nature and severity. Several schemes have been suggested; the most widely used is that of Seddon (1975), which is a functional classification relating the anatomical injury to symptomatology. That this is still the most widely used classification is unfortunate because the three groups are inadequate to describe all types of injury and, more importantly, to allow predictions about outcome to be made. A more detailed classification which considers injuries intermediate between those of Seddon's groups is that of Sunderland (1978). Although the inherent conservatism of orthopaedic teaching in the UK still pays homage to Seddon's classification, it is to be hoped that the more useful classification of Sunderland will supersede it before too long.

Seddon's classification of nerve injuries

This classification recognizes three groups.

1. Neurapraxia

($\nu\epsilon\hat{\upsilon}\rho o\nu$ = nerve; $\grave{\alpha}\pi\rho\alpha\xi\acute{\iota}\alpha$ = non-action)
This is a local conduction block in which the nerve fibre remains intact but there is local demyelination. As Seddon originally used the term there was complete motor paralysis, although some sensory function (especially pain) and sympathetic function were preserved. This is because large, thickly myelinated, nerve fibres are much more susceptible to compression damage than thinner fibres. Today the term is used more loosely. Recovery is by repair of the local demyelination by Schwann cell activity, a process which takes several weeks or months.

2. Axonotmesis

($\grave{\alpha}\xi\omega\nu$ = cylinder; $\tau\mu\hat{\eta}\sigma\iota\varsigma$ = a cutting)
The anatomical injury here is severance of the axon (or dendrite) with preservation of the endoneurial tube. This injury is a more severe form of compression (although it often results from traction) than neurapraxia but the cardinal feature is that here **wallerian degeneration** follows. Thus, there must be complete regeneration of the nerve, not simply re-myelination, before recovery can occur. The endoneurial tubes, however, remain intact so there will be no miswiring of the pathway for regeneration and the nerve's axons will regenerate to make contact with their original target organs. As might

be expected, the results are relatively good because of this maintained continuity, especially if the injury is fairly distal. Obviously the distance over which regeneration has to take place is the principal factor determining the outcome. In very proximal injuries the time taken for regeneration may be considerable and there may be irreversible atrophy of target muscles. The poor motor recovery in such cases may therefore be equivalent to more serious injuries situated distally. On the whole, sensory receptors survive longer and the outcome in terms of sensory recovery is better.

3. Neurotmesis

($\nu\epsilon\hat{\nu}\rho o\nu$ = nerve; $\tau\mu\hat{\eta}\sigma\iota\varsigma$ = a cutting)

This injury was defined by Seddon as complete severance of the nerve trunk; all structures are disrupted. In higher animals there is no recovery unless repair is undertaken. Repair would be by direct suture or grafting, depending on the size of the gap. In either case wallerian degeneration and regeneration takes place, but there is the added complication over axonotmesis that the endoneurial tubes have been disrupted so that there is a high probability of mismatch and hence 'miswiring' when regeneration takes place. Pioneering axons reaching their homonymous target organ types (but **not** necessarily the **same** muscles or receptors) will make new connections but those reaching inappropriate end organs die back. There is thus a reduced mass of innervation and considerable miswiring of target organs, leading to the well-known appearances and functional inadequacies associated with nerve repair.

Sunderland's classification

A consideration of the anatomical structures which make up a nerve will indicate that a number of injuries are possible which do not fit into Seddon's classification. These occupy the position between axonotmesis and neurotmesis. The crucial issue is whether the perineurium has been breached, as this represents a major step in severity and poorer prognosis. These problems were considered by Sunderland (1978) who devised the anatomical classification, summarised in *Table 6.3*.

Sunderland's original classification did not contain the 'metabolic block' group. Recent work has shown that this type of injury is ischaemic and is caused by pressure damage to the blood supply of the nerve. It can be either intrinsic, if the damage is to vessels contained within the nerve trunk, or extrinsic, if the compression is outside the nerve trunk. It is thus quite distinct from neurapraxia, which specifically results from compression of the nerve fibres themselves.

Mackinnon and Dellon (1988) have suggested that the situation in which a nerve has been partially or totally severed and has spontaneously 'repaired' itself by forming a **neuroma-in-continuity** (lateral neuroma) should be added to the classification as a group VI. However, because this process is essentially one of disordered 'self-repair' rather than injury, it seems inappropriate in a classification of types of injury.

Table 6.3 Sunderland's classification of nerve injuries.

Tissues	Normal	Injury group					
		Metabolic block*	I	II	III	IV	V
Axon	†	†	†	#	#	#	#
Myelin sheath	†	†	±	±	#	#	#
Endoneurial tube	†	†	†	†	#	#	#
Endoneurium	†	†	†	†	±	#	#
Perineurium	†	†	†	†	†	#	#
Epineurium	†	†	†	†	†	†	#
Blood vessels	†	#	±	±	±	±	#
Seddon group	Normal	—	Neurapraxia	Axonotmesis	—	—	Neurotmesis

*Injury may be intrinsic or extrinsic (see text). †, Intact; # Severed; ±, variable.

Neuropathy

Although beyond the scope of this chapter, diseases of peripheral nerves should not be forgotten. These present formidable diagnostic problems, with some 50% of cases remaining in doubt as to their nature or cause. Diagnostic methods should be aimed at excluding malignancy and nerve injury, in addition to identifying the specific neuropathy. Established causes may be:

- **Chronic**
  - a) Genetic (e.g. acute intermittent porphyria)
  - b) Metabolic (e.g. diabetes mellitus, deficiency of vitamin B_{12})
  - c) Amyloidosis
  - d) Nutritional (alcoholism, thiamine deficiency)
  - e) Iatrogenic (bleomycin, vincristine, phenytoin, nitrofurantoin)
  - f) Neoplastic (Pancoast's tumour)
- **Acute**
  - a) Autoimmune (Guillain–Barré syndrome)

Neuropathies may affect the nerve axon, in which case they are described as **axonal**, or they may affect the myelin sheath, in which case they are described as **demyelinating**.

ASSESSMENT OF NERVE INJURY

Nerve injuries must be assessed before treatment in order to define their site and extent, and after repair to document recovery and subsequent progress. Although nerve injuries are relatively common in any society, individual injuries differ enormously and it becomes very difficult to obtain data based on large populations of identical cases. Because the latter is the ideal in epidemiological research, nerve injury has not fared well in this respect. In addition, many nerve injuries are not followed up for whatever reason, and there has in the past been an unfortunate tendency to leave the repair of injuries to small nerves to inexperienced junior surgeons. Research which does exist has shown, without doubt, that meticulous attention to (micro) surgical technique, and especially the use of the operating microscope, is the single most important determinant of successful outcome.

In the experimental laboratory precise objective studies allow a correlation of clinical findings with electrophy-siological and morphometric findings. In clinical practice the three means of assessment at our disposal are **sensory testing, motor testing** and **electrodiagnosis**.

Before specific assessment can begin, the surgeon must consider the usual factors provided by thorough **history-taking** and **physical examination**. The latter must include a complete neurological examination. The anatomy of the nerve is all-important; it is essential to consider the **autonomous area** (i.e. the topographical field of supply) of any affected nerve or nerve branch along with the dermatomes and myotomes served by the appropriate spinal cord segment. As mentioned above the **nerve fibre types** and hence the functional **modalities** served by the nerve at the site of injury must be taken into account.

These general procedures are part of any neurological examination. Only when they are complete should the more detailed assessment of peripheral nerve function *per se* be undertaken.

Sensory Testing (*Figure 6.8*)

There are only two entirely objective tests of sensory function: the ninhydrin test for sweating (sympathetic innervation), nowadays more efficiently applied by measuring the electrical conductivity of the skin, and the test for denervation whereby the skin of a denervated finger fails to wrinkle when placed for some time in water. All other sensory tests involve some form of subjective input by the patient. Unless the patient is a malingerer, he or she usually tries very hard to be helpful, and this in itself may destroy objectivity in a test. There are some ways in which a degree of compensation can be made. Many nerve injuries involve limbs, and patients are relatively good at discriminating differences between the affected and unaffected limbs. Closing the eyes removes some possible bias but, in the end, all sensory tests must be considered to have a high degree of subjective bias.

All sensory information reaching a patient's CNS is modified along the way. The first point of modification is the **sensory receptor** itself. Sensory nerve fibres are activated by receptors responding to a particular type of stimulus (e.g. light touch, vibration, heat, cold, pressure, stretch and pain), but also respond to the rate at which the receptor adapts. Thus any test must take account of both of these facts. For example, if one wished to assess the density of skin innervation by slowly adapting touch receptors, one would use **Weber's test for two-point**

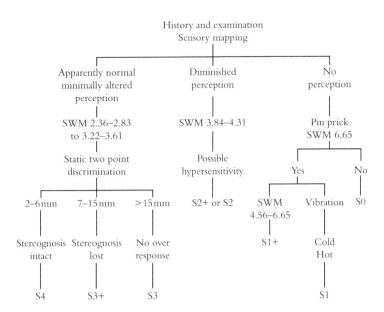

Figure 6.8   A scheme for sensory testing. SWM, Semmes–Weinstein monofilaments (logarithmic scale).

discrimination. To test the related population of rapidly adapting touch receptors, the test for **moving two-point discrimination** would be used. In either case the normal side would be tested first (with the patient's eyes closed), followed by assessment of the affected side.

The following is a list of popular sensory tests, which should by no means be regarded as exhaustive. For a fuller appreciation the reader should consult the classical works of Moberg (1995) and the more recent work by Mackinnon and Dellon (1988).

Hoffmann–Tinel sign

Tinel's sign, first described in 1917, is often regarded as the first good evidence of nerve regeneration. For many surgeons it is, unfortunately, the only sign documented at follow-up clinics. The Tinel sign is based on the fact that the growing point of a regenerating nerve becomes hyperexcitable and the axons can be fired if they receive a sharp tap. Thus the examiner taps along the course of the nerve, beginning at the most distal point. When the point of advancement is reached, the patient experiences 'electric shock-like' sensations – a positive Tinel sign. Unfortunately the sign is not always present and is not easily elicited when the injured nerve lies deeply. The timing of examination is also important. At 4 months after injury it is probably fair to say that a positive Tinel sign at the injury site with no sign distally indicates a failure of

regeneration. A weak sign distal to the repair site **at this time** probably means that recovery is and will remain poor, whereas a strong response distally is more encouraging. It is important not to place too much reliance on this sign: although it is useful as the crudest of discriminators, it is in no manner quantitative.

Pain

Pain sensation usually returns in the same manner as tactile sensation, but sooner. It is often unpleasant and may be a major source of difficulty in managing these patients. Pain is tested for by compressing the nerve against bone or, more often, it is mapped by pin prick. The awareness of an impending painful stimulus often conditions the patient. Where there has been a nerve injury, the increased unpleasantness of painful stimuli leads to an **over-reaction**, which may either precede or succeed the stimulus. The over-reaction is clearly a physical property of the regenerating nerve and in no way a purely psychological phenomenon. It is a useful but non-quantitative sign.

Temperature

Temperature sensation may be tested with hot and cold objects. As might be expected from the anatomical pathways, its recovery occurs at the same rate as that of the pain modality. However, accurate discrimination of temperature represents an advance on the crude sensation of pain because a different population of receptors is involved, and it is thus worth testing for this reason.

Vibration

Vibration sensation is tested over bony prominences using tuning forks of various frequencies (see below). Mackinnon and Dellon (1988) have suggested that a 256-Hz tuning fork is the instrument of choice. It may be used on non-bony areas in the same way as a blunt pin is used for testing tactile discrimination. Dellon suggests that it is a better test immediately after nerve injury as the stimulus it provides is more specific and thus more effective in establishing whether the nerve is transected.

Sudomotor paralysis

When a nerve is divided there is a loss of sweating in its autonomous area. Where overlap occurs, the degree of sweating is reduced in the partially denervated area compared with that in normal skin. The **ninhydrin test**, introduced by Moberg (1995), uses the reaction between ninhydrin and the amino acid components of sweat. This reaction converts the colourless ninhydrin to a purple compound and hence areas of sweating loss can be mapped. Recently a device has appeared that measures the change in electrical conductivity which occurs in skin when sweating occurs. This small battery-operated device is accurate and simple to use, but expensive.

Tactile sensibility

A great deal has been written about testing tactile sensibility. Most clinicians still rely on the wisp of cotton-wool or blunt pin (the distal end of a tie is an excellent substitute). The classical device is a set of **von Frey hairs**, which are short bristles each loaded with a calibrated weight. Von Frey hairs are easy to apply – and very easy to misinterpret. If the hair is properly applied to skin, a specific force should be applied. This works quite well for large differences but is not reliable where small differences need to be discriminated. The cross-sectional area of the filament should be constant for accurate results and the force applied by any given filament will be dependent on both temperature and humidity. Moreover, the possibility of the fibre's buck-

ling upon application may present problems. Different sets of 'hairs' have different types of handles, which affects their application and makes interpretation of measurements very difficult. A more refined set of instruments is the Semmes–Weinstein monofilaments (see *Figure 6.8*). These are similar to von Frey hairs but more uniform and sophisticated. They are calibrated on a logarithmic scale so that the numbers that they each bear are difficult to relate to simple forces. It is arguable whether this degree of sophistication is of great use in the management of most nerve injuries.

Dellon has reported on the development and use of a 'pressure-specifying discriminator', which represents the next generation of testing devices. This computer-driven apparatus is capable of varying the nature of the stimulus (pressure, vibration, two point, etc.). Its use at present is largely experimental and limited to units with a particular interest in sensory testing. However, it may with time lead to the development of less complicated reliable sensory testing devices.

Static and moving two-point discrimination

Weber's test measures the density of innervation for slowly adapting receptors. When a nerve is compressed, changes in sensory threshold occur first and a reduction in two-point discrimination follows as the lesion progresses. **Abnormal two-point discrimination in the sensory system is the equivalent of wasting in the motor system**. It is measured with a pair of dividers or, more conveniently, the useful Disk-Criminator advocated by MacKinnon and Dellon (1988). The threshold distance at which the patient can determine the presence of two specific point-stimuli is recorded for a number of sites. It is one of the most important and useful tests of cutaneous sensibility and should never be omitted from the assessment of a nerve injury. Moberg (1995) held the view that this test correlated particularly well with the ability of the patient to operate a 'precision grip' and as such represented a test which was a good predictor of recovery of hand function.

The moving two-point discrimination test introduced by Moberg addresses the fact that rapidly adapting receptors will be missed by the classical Weber test. The test is performed in exactly the same way as the Weber test, but the two points are moved slowly at constant velocity.

Proprioception

The recovery of proprioception after nerve injury is still a matter of much debate. Reflex proprioceptive activity requires the re-establishment of a specific two-way circuit which, after nerve transection and repair, must be very unlikely indeed. In the hand it is likely that conscious proprioception depends for the most part on tactile sensibility, and this is likely to be the case elsewhere. On this basis both Seddon (1975) and Moberg (1995) have suggested that specific testing of proprioception may be of little use in assessing the outcome of nerve repair.

Stereognosis

This is a modality that returns late – if at all – after nerve repair. There is a considerable central element involved. Testing is by recognition of the geometry of solid objects. The UK heptagonal 50 pence piece has established itself in this role.

Quantification of sensory recovery

No entirely satisfactory system exists. Even with the most refined methods of sensory testing, authorities disagree on how to arrive at some numerical or symbolic result which is a good predictor of outcome or a good means of following recovery. It should be noted that, whereas in the UK it is customary for the surgeon to perform sensory testing in the outpatient department, in the United States and Europe it is becoming common to employ specialist 'therapists' for this task. This undoubtedly saves time and allows for consistency in the assessment, but it nevertheless requires some means of conveying the results of the assessment to the surgeon. Hence the literature from these workers lays much greater emphasis on objectivity (even to the extent of obtaining a single numerical 'score') than is seen in literature from the UK. There are arguments for and against this approach, which are beyond the scope of this chapter.

Almost invariably one returns to the **1954 Medical Research Council Criteria for Sensory Recovery** (*Table 6.4*). There are many problems with this system; it is clearly less than ideal. However, it has stood the test of time if only because there is no clear agreement about what should supersede it.

Table 6.4 1954 Medical Research Council criteria for sensory recovery.

Grade	Description
S_0	Total absence of sensibility **in the autonomous area**
S_1	Recovery of deep cutaneous pain sensibility **specifically within the autonomous area**
S_2	Return of some cutaneous pain and tactile sensibility **within the autonomous area**
S_3	Return of superficial cutaneous pain and tactile sensibility **throughout the autonomous area**, with loss of all previous over-reaction (e.g. hyperesthesia)
S_{3+}	As S_3, with the additional recovery of some two-point discrimination **within the autonomous area**
S_4	Complete recovery

Note the **absolute requirement** to refer all assessment to the **autonomous area** of the nerve under test. In the fingers, for example, there may be considerable overlap from other nerves. This can sometimes be excluded from the test if it is possible to block the overlapping nerve without affecting the one under test. However, this is by no means easy, as an appreciation of the anatomy will usually reveal.

Order of sensory recovery

Experimental and clinical evidence has indicated that after nerve injury and repair there is a reproducible pattern of events in the recovery of sensation. The earliest perception to recover is that of **low-frequency (about 30 Hz) vibration**. This is followed by the recovery of the perception of **moving touch** stimuli, with the perception of **constant touch** following somewhat later. The last perception to recover is that of **high-frequency (around 256 Hz) vibration**. To the surgeon, this sequence of events is a very reassuring indication that things are proceeding normally. The only requirement is two tuning forks and a pair of dividers.

Sensory re-education

There is good evidence that a degree of central plasticity is able to operate so that patients who have had nerve injuries repaired gradually accommodate their permanent sensory losses. The mechanism whereby this accommodation takes place is not understood. There may be a degree of compensation from other systems, especially vision. It will be interesting to see what the future holds in understanding this phenomenon.

Motor testing

Motor testing is used to determine whether specific muscles or muscle groups are capable of contracting and, if so, to assess the power (or more properly the force) of contraction. Animal experiments using isometric myograph testing of reinnervated muscles indicate that, provided there has been no muscle degeneration, reinnervated muscles are capable of generating remarkably normal isometric tensions even though the nerve fibres innervating the muscle are far from normal. As mentioned above, the regenerated fibres will all be of smaller diameter than their predecessors and therefore they will conduct at a slower speed. This does not appear to affect the force with which the muscle contracts, but the twitch curve is prolonged. Presumably the fast fibres are necessary for the rapid initiation of movement and for the reflex control of movement by the muscle spindle/Golgi tendon organ servomechanism. There is no doubt that, although power may recover almost completely after reinnervation, precision of movement does not recover to anything like the same extent.

Besides the reinnervation, the ultimate level of motor recovery will depend on how much irreversible change has occured in the muscle during its denervated period. Physiotherapy is important in preserving muscle survival during the denervated period and there is some evidence to suggest that direct electrical stimulation of the denervated muscle may prevent atrophy and fibrosis during the denervated period. There is also a considerable redistribution of motor units when muscles become reinnervated and an increased randomness in the grouping of fast and slow muscle fibres.

Motor testing is carried out in a variety of ways, and a large number of dynamometers exist for carrying out specific testing tasks. In most cases assessment takes the form of the typical neurological examination in which the patient attempts to move the affected part against resistance supplied by the examiner. Two levels of subjectivism are, therefore, operating. It must be said, however, that the degree of motor recovery which is achieved after all the methods of nerve repair currently available to the surgeon is almost invariably able to be discriminated by this means. This rather pessimistic view reflects the significantly poorer levels of motor recovery than are obtained after sensory nerve repair. The need for early repair, if motor recovery is to be anticipated at all, cannot be emphasised enough. Nuances of recovery

Table 6.5 1954 Medical Research Council criteria for motor recovery.

Grade	Description
M_0	No contraction
M_1	Return of perceptible contraction in the proximal muscles
M_2	Return of perceptible contraction in both proximal and distal muscles
M_3	Return of function in both proximal and distal muscles which is of such a degree that all **important** muscles are sufficiently powerful to act against resistance
M_4	As M_3 with the addition that all synergistic and independent movements are possible
M_5	Complete recovery

requiring high levels of objective discrimination in their assessment are rarely within the purview of the peripheral nerve surgeon. The possible exception to this rule appears to be in the repair of specifically motor (or sensory) nerves rather than mixed nerves. Examples are the facial nerve and the hypoglossal nerve. Where motor recovery is achieved, results are quantified using the **1954 Medical Research Council Criteria for Motor Recovery**. (*Table 6.5*).

Clinical neurophysiology: electrodiagnosis

There is considerable debate even today about the value of electrodiagnosis in assessing the severity of peripheral nerve injury and the effects of repair. The uncertainty is compounded by the relative scarcity of electrodiagnostic services in the UK and the fact that few surgeons have taken the time to gain a thorough understanding of the subject. Although neurophysiology depends considerably on physics, the specialist information needed to understand the more basic tests is by no means beyond the standard of the Primary Fellowship examination. It should be emphasised that the simpler tests are the most useful in the information they yield. Modern electronic technology has led to the development of battery-operated portable meters which give direct read-out recordings of nerve conduction velocities. These are a valuable adjunct to any outpatient department dealing with peripheral nerve injuries, and their use is to be encouraged.

In classical neurophysiology it is customary to stimulate

and record from the same structure, for example nerve or muscle. However, to record large-amplitude compound muscle action potentials (CMAPs) with surface electrodes is much easier than trying to record low-amplitude potentials from nerves (CNAPs). Hence the set-up for surface electrophysiological stimulation and recording using two stimulation sites has evolved. Recording over nerves is, however, necessary for assessing sensory conduction.

Nerve conduction studies

Most peripheral nerves are mixed, although it is often necessary to study the activity of both sensory and motor components separately. The equation:

$$V = \frac{d}{t}$$

where:

V = nerve conduction velocity (m s^{-1})
d = distance (mm) travelled by the impulse
t = latency (ms) i.e. time taken for the impulse to travel distance d)

describes what is needed to obtain the most valuable single variable, the maximum conduction velocity of the fibres in the nerve. For a motor nerve, the recording electrode is a silver or similar plate placed over a superficial muscle supplied by the nerve (e.g. the thenar muscles if the median nerve is being tested). Good electrical contact is made by means of electrolytic electrode jelly between the electrode and carefully cleaned skin. The active recording electrode (cathode) is placed as near as possible over the **motor point**, which is the region at which the nerve enters its muscle, and the indifferent anode is placed a few centimetres away. A ground electrode is placed over inactive muscle nearby. The sites for stimulation are chosen at points where the nerve under test is relatively superficial (e.g. elbow). The active stimulating electrode is the cathode and this is positioned nearest to the recording site. Stimuli consist of short (approximately 0.01–300 ms), square-wave stimuli of either constant current or constant voltage. The former is generally preferred and the apparatus is designed to limit the maximum available voltage to about 200 V. Pulses can be delivered either singly or in trains of between about 0.5 and 50 Hz. When everything is ready, the stimulator is turned on and the current

increased until a clearly defined CMAP just appears. This is the **threshold**. At this point the stimulus amplitude is then increased by a further 50% so that stimulation is now **supramaximal**. This ensures complete activation of the muscle fibres. By convention, **negative** waves are displayed with an **upward** vector on the oscilloscope screen and **positive** voltages are **downward**; also, the latency is measured to the first upward **take-off** from the isoelectric line of the action potential rather than to its peak. If the recording cathode is over the motor-point, this take-off should be very clear. The **latency** is the distance between the **stimulus artefact** and the (usually negative) take-off point. However, with the recording set-up as described, this time would contain a component corresponding to conduction in the motor fibres of the nerve plus components corresponding to the time taken for transmission at the neuromuscular junction and along the muscle membrane. To eliminate these latter two components, which are not usually of interest, stimulation is repeated at a second site nearer to the muscle and the **segment velocity** between the two stimulation sites is calculated as follows:

$$V_{(motor)} = \frac{d_1 - d_2}{t_1 - t_2}$$

where:

$V_{(motor)}$ = **segment velocity** in motor fibres (i.e. between the two stimulation sites)
d_1 = distance between first (proximal) stimulation site and recording cathode
d_2 = distance between second (distal) stimulation site and recording cathode
t_1 = latency between first stimulus artefact and CMAP
t_2 = latency between second stimulus artefact and CMAP

For a sensory nerve, the procedure is much the same; however, because recording cannot take place from muscles the nerve action potential (CNAP), which is of much lower amplitude, must be used. Because of the much-reduced **signal to noise ratio** in this situation, multiple stimuli are applied at each site and the responses averaged by means of a **signal averager**.

With an averaging process, random activity (**noise**) will be lost, whereas constant features of the waveform like the CNAP will be preserved in the averaged trace. To ensure that only sensory nerve fibres are used in the study, a uniquely sensory nerve must be chosen for the stimulation site. In the limbs the digital nerves supply this need. Because there is no component for neuromuscular transmission, it is not necessary to have two stimulation sites and the segment velocity is given by the equation:

$$V_{(sensory)} = \frac{d}{t}$$

where:

$V_{(sensory)}$ = velocity in sensory nerve fibres between stimulating and recording cathodes

d = distance between stimulating and recording cathodes

t = **average** latency between stimulus artefact and CNAP

Although the conduction velocity of nerves is the most useful measurement in nerve conduction studies, the amplitude of the action potential is also an indication of the total amount of electrical activity in the muscle. To reflect this mathematically, the entire CMAP wave can be integrated with respect to time. However, this measurement may be affected by the set-up as it will reflect the quality of the electrical contacts. It is, however, useful for a specific patient and a **given set-up** in that it may be used to differentiate neurapraxia from neurotmesis. In the latter, the CMAP or CNAP will be absent or severely diminished and, with time, will disappear, whereas with neurapraxia an action potential will remain and, although it will be attenuated and deformed, it will return to normal values with time.

When a nerve has been repaired, the regenerated axons never grow to normal diameters and thus the maximum conduction velocity is reduced. Studies such as the above allow this difference to be quantified, and the process of regeneration and maturation with time can be followed by successive velocity measurements.

It is possible also, using a modification of the above, to measure the range of velocities and hence gain an estimate of the distribution of fibre sizes within a nerve. The techniques for achieving this are called **collision studies**. For motor collision studies the set-up would be the same as above except for the fact that two stimulators are used. One is placed proximally on the limb (e.g. elbow), at a distance from the recording electrode, and the other is situated nearer to the recording electrode (e.g. wrist); both stimuli are supramaximal. The apparatus is designed so that the two stimulators can be fired simultaneously or at different times, with the gap between the two impulses able to be 'steplessly' varied by the operator.

When any nerve is stimulated, the impulse will be propagated both **orthodromically** and **antidromically**, although it is only the former which excites the muscle. When the distal stimulator is fired first and the two stimuli are separated by a small time gap, the antidromic impulse from the distal stimulator will collide somewhere between the two stimulating sites with the orthodromic impulse from the proximal stimulator, and the two will cancel each other out. All of the nerve fibres proximal to the distal stimulator will, effectively, be blocked and only the orthodromic impulse from the distal stimulator will reach the muscle.

If the time gap between the stimuli is widened, a point will be reached at which the antidromic impulse from the distal stimulator will have passed the proximal stimulator before the latter fires. The orthodromic impulse from the proximal stimulator will, therefore, be able to excite the muscle and cause a second, recordable, CMAP. However, the excitation thresholds of different nerve fibres differ and in the above situation the larger diameter fibres will become unblocked first.

In practice, the two stimulators are first used independently as described above to obtain a maximal segment velocity. They are then coupled together and the time gap is progressively shortened until the second CMAP disappears; it is then carefully lengthened again until the **second CMAP just reappears**, and this process is continued until the **first and second CMAPs are of equal amplitude**. The latencies of these two points are noted and the difference between them represents the difference in conduction time between the fastest and slowest fibres. If this time is then added on to the original latency used to calculate the maximal segment velocity, a new velocity may be calculated using the new (longer) latency and the same interelectrode distance. This (slower) velocity will represent that of the slowest motor fibres. Hence the range of motor velocities is calculated.

Needle electromyography

More complex electrophysiological studies can be performed on muscles using **needle electrodes**. These may be used both to stimulate the muscle directly and to record from it. Needle electrodes designed for specific tasks may be unipolar, bipolar or multipolar. Their main advantage in peripheral nerve surgery is that they may be used to record activity from a muscle which the patient is activating **voluntarily**. In this way the examiner is testing the entire **upper motor neurone–lower motor neurone** (UMN–LMN) pathway. Modifications of this technique allow testing of **muscle refractory period**, the muscle **strength–duration curve**, individual **motor unit potentials, motor unit density**, the pattern of **motor unit recruitment** and **jitter** (the fluctuation in latency between different motor units due to variability of neuromuscular transmission and a good index of regeneration where jitter progressively decreases with recovery). Details of these measurements are beyond the scope of this book.

Central motor and sensory evoked potentials

Stimulating the brain whilst recording CMAPs or stimulating sensory nerves whilst recording from scalp electrodes are termed respectively central motor and sensory evoked potentials. The brain may be stimulated either electrically (which is quite painful to the scalp) or electromagnetically, which is painless but less focal. Results must be signal-averaged and their interpretation is difficult. However, these techniques may offer valuable information in the future about the relationship of UMN and LMN pathways after nerve repair. A particularly useful technique for the orthopaedic surgeon is intra-operative spinal cord evoked potential monitoring. This is useful to guard against spinal damage when the cord is manipulated during operations. The recording cathode is a fine wire threaded into the vertebral canal rostral to the operating site. It lies on the dura where it records evoked potentials from the dorsal columns. Stimulation is carried out transcutaneously caudal to the operation site. Usually two stimulators are used, one on each leg, so that both sides of the cord are tested. Alternate stimuli are given to each leg and the evoked potentials displayed on the monitor. Injury potentials will be seen if the cord is at risk from rough handling.

SURGICAL METHODS FOR THE REPAIR OF PERIPHERAL NERVES

The milestones in the surgery of peripheral nerves have coincided with world wars in which the number of nerve injuries has greatly increased, and with advances in technology such as the development of synthetic mono-filament sutures and the operating microscope. At present, surgery for peripheral nerves consists of no more than attempting to provide the best possible environment for the natural process of nerve regeneration. Chemical manipulation of this process is a goal still far away. However, over the years, the surgery of peripheral nerves has advanced as we have realised which techniques are useful and which are detrimental. A natural conservatism on the part of surgeons has nevertheless left peripheral nerve surgery in the UK very fragmented. It is particularly unfortunate that the repair of small (e.g. digital) nerves is so often left to inexperienced juniors when one of the few absolute certainties in the field is that attention to technical detail (especially the use of the operating microscope by **trained microsurgeons**) is the surest way to achieve good results. Given the research, both at the laboratory bench and in clinical practice into nerve repair, there is no excuse today for struggling with loupes or even the naked eye, or for using large-diameter needles and sutures to attempt fascicular repair. Yet, all too often, this is the case. No nerve, however minor, should be considered undeserving of the very best expertise and technology available.

Classically, after multiple trauma it has been customary to allow 'things to settle down' and undertake nerve repair at a later date. Recent research has shown beyond doubt that **delayed repair is always inferior** to immediate repair, and the latter should be abandoned only in the most extreme circumstances.

Nerve suture: neurorraphy

Direct suture is the simplest way to repair a nerve. With proper microsurgical technique, individual interrupted sutures are placed in the epineurium of a nerve trunk or in the perineurium of individual fascicles. It is essential that there should be **no tension** between the two stumps; they should be gently coapted[1]. Besides the risk of pulling apart, tension has been shown to be the single largest detrimental factor (apart from incompetent technique) to a successful outcome. It is arguable whether tension exerts its ill effects by strangulation of the intraneural vascular plexus or by a direct stretching of the axons themselves. If repair under tension seems likely, the nerve ends may often be freed a little by dissecting them from anchoring tissues. However, this in itself may reduce the blood supply to the nerve and make the problem worse.

[1]It should be noted that it is impossible to **anastomose** a nerve because nerves do not possess a **stoma**. This is a sloppy (but common) abuse and misuse of a perfectly good word.

A graft may be the only solution and short grafts on the whole do well.

Epineurial versus fascicular repair

Classically, nerves were repaired by epineurial suture. This is still the only method for unifascicular nerves. However, it seems logical that, if a number of individual fascicles can be identified and matched with their counterparts in the other stump, then a small but valuable step to reduce the inevitable miswiring of regeneration will have been made. Matching fascicles can be identified simply by appearance, or use may be made of the fact that individual fascicles are often largely either sensory or motor. Small sterilisable hand-held stimulators can be used to identify motor fascicles by muscle twitching but sensory fascicles can be identified with certainty only if the patient is awake and the nerve in question has been spared from block by local anaesthetic. However, identifying the motor fascicles goes a long way to improving things and allows at least a likely identification of sensory fascicles by 'subtraction'. Fascicular repair should in theory be the goal in every case but its drawback is that it requires a greater level of meticulousness in technique, especially as a greater mass of suture material placed in the nerve may have the effect of increasing scar tissue. It may well be that the surgeon who only occasionally undertakes the microsurgical repair of nerves may achieve a better result with the simpler technique of epineurial repair.

Entubulation

Before the advent of modern microsutures, attempts were made to repair nerves by wrapping the approximated ends in some material which formed a tube, or to insert the ends of the nerve into a tube. Many substances were used. Silicone rubber has enjoyed some fame in the laboratory where it has been used notably in the important experiments of Lundborg (1988) to create chambers at the repair site into which substances could be introduced and from which tissue fluids could be sampled. In clinical practice, however, these tubes remain *in situ*, where, as the nerve matures, compression occurs and is often associated with severe pain. A second operation to remove the tube is highly undesirable and thus permanent tubes appear today to have no clinical use. Biodegradable tubes made of a number of substances have been tried by

a number of authors, but most produce a brisk tissue reaction and would be permeable to any growth factors which might be added to enhance performance. Rigid biodegradable glass tubes used by the present authors have no such reaction and may offer some hope for the future as they degrade only to sodium and phosphate ions, are watertight and their degradation period can be varied by altering their composition. However, these tubes are as yet confined to experimental surgery.

Nerve repair with grafts

Where there is a significant gap, which cannot be closed without tension, some form of graft must be used. There are several possibilities for nerve repair by grafting but the nerve autograft is undoubtedly the best.

Interposed nerve autografts

A nerve autograft is simply a length of nerve taken from another site. Typically, cutaneous nerves are used, most often the sural nerve, but it must be realised that there will always be a sensory deficit. Occasionally, after major injuries, it may be possible to obtain graft material from an irreparable nerve trunk but this is, fortunately, a rare occurrence.

A nerve autograft is not a functioning nerve. It will undergo wallerian degeneration as if it were the distal stump of any transected nerve. In reality, therefore, it is an **oriented matrix of neural supporting tissues**. Important among these for their ability to support nerve regeneration are the endoneurial tubes and Schwann cells which they contain. The option of useful fascicular repair does not exist with the simple nerve autograft and insertion is by epineurial suture.

A theoretical disadvantage of nerve autografts is that, being cutaneous nerves, they will not contain large endoneurial tubes suitable for large motor fibres. However, we know that these largest fibres never regenerate anyway and there is some evidence that endoneurial tubes inflate to accommodate large pioneering axons. A more practical disadvantage is that expendable cutaneous nerves are in relatively short supply.

Vascularised nerve autografts

Usually, nerve autografts are avascular; some degree of vascularisation is established after insertion but a minimum of 72 hours of ischaemia is to be expected. There appears to be some vague evidence that a nerve autograft with an intact blood supply may be preferable although the additional technical difficulties are seldom, if ever, outweighed by the proven neurological advantages. Where the bed for placement of the nerve graft is poorly vascularised, there is a definite theoretical preference for a vascularised nerve graft, but still no clear evidence of its superiority. The reality is that they are used on the strength of an impression; however, the difficulties of quantifying improvement should not be forgotten (Gilbert and Tassin, 1987).

Occasionally a segment of expendable nerve can be moved into position as a graft with its vascular pedicle intact. However, more frequently, a **free vascularised nerve autograft** must be used and microanastomoses of its artery and vein carried out along with its interposition into the nerve gap.

Cable grafts

Where a large nerve trunk has been damaged and the only available graft material is cutaneous nerve, a **cable graft** may be used. This consists of a bundle of segments of equal length of donor nerve, laid in parallel. The individual lengths of donor nerve making up the cable may be glued together with fibrin glue to make them more manageable. The whole is interposed into the nerve gap and held in place with epineurial sutures.

Interfascicular grafts

The natural extension of the cable graft principle is to use the individual lengths of donor nerve to repair individual nerve fascicles; this technique has been pioneered by Millesi (1991). Fascicles should preferably be matched for size and function. The same caveats apply as for fascicular repair, but there is no doubt that in the hands of an expert this is the treatment of choice where a nerve gap exists, and especially where that gap is a long one.

Non-neural autografts

Over the years a number of non-neural autografts have been used, but almost all have met with little success and only one approaches the nerve autograft in effectiveness.

The coaxially aligned freeze–thawed skeletal muscle autograft (FTMG) introduced by the present authors in 1986 has enjoyed more success than most (Glasby, 1990). Skeletal muscle is in plentiful supply and, if taken from a muscle with a parallel arrangement of its fibres, will furnish an oriented matrix of tubular muscle cell basement membrane 'myotubes', which appear to be chemically similar to the endoneurial tubes of nerve although of larger diameter. The muscle sarcoplasm is disrupted by a thermal and a hypo-osmotic shock. The piece of donor muscle, wrapped in sterile foil, is frozen in liquid nitrogen to thermal equilibrium (-196°C) and thawed in sterile distilled water. Shrinkage of up to 50% occurs, so the donor material must be of adequate size. The final graft is then hewn from this piece of treated muscle. It must be emphasised that this treatment is essential for the muscle to function as a graft. A number of surgeons have attempted to 'simplify' the process (despite documentary evidence), by avoiding treatment of the muscle, with disastrous consequences.

After treatment the muscle block is sutured into the nerve gap with the sutures traversing the epineurium of the nerve and the periphery of the muscle block.

Results with short muscle grafts have been encouraging. In the recovery phase there is a very low incidence of hyperaesthesia associated with this technique. In digital nerve repair, the use of small muscle grafts has been shown to be associated with a lower incidence of neuroma formation than direct suture. This is presumably because the latter is more often associated with a degree of tension than was previously imagined.

Unfortunately muscle grafts do not perform well in graft lengths of more than 5 cm. This is presumably because they contain no Schwann cells, and these cannot migrate over the distances involved. The ideal long graft remains to be found.

Nerve allografts

Some authors have experimented with nerve allografts. The results are usually appalling and the logic of subjecting patients with peripheral nerve injuries to immunosuppressive therapy (cyclosporin A) at a dosage similar to that used for cardiac allografts is questionable. There are better alternatives.

Prosthetic grafts

Many entirely prosthetic substances have been tried but as yet none has approached the nerve graft or FTMG in efficacy. An interesting recent addition to the repertoire is the fibronectin mat, which has a theoretical advantage in providing localised matrix protein similar to that in nerves.

Neurotisation

This term was introduced by Narakas (1997) to describe the transfer of the active proximal segments of divided nerves to act as a reinnervating source for the distal segments of injured nerves. It is particularly useful where the injury is one of avulsion of the nerve root from the spinal cord, as in some brachial plexus injuries. The most commonly used 'donor' nerves are the intercostal nerves. One or several of these is divided as distally as possible and dissected free for as much of its length as possible. It may then be passed through the axilla and used to 'neurotise' the distal segments of the plexus in the arm. Similarly the hypoglossal nerve may be (wholly or partially) used to neurotise the facial nerve extracranially after it has been damaged irreparably by, for example, the removal of an acoustic neuroma. In this case primary repair with a nerve graft or short FTMG may not be possible or successful, and late neurotisation may represent the best hope. A major theoretical problem with neurotisation is the inappropriate nature of the upper motor neurone, which drives the reinnervated peripheral nerve. When intercostal nerves are used to reinnervate the brachial plexus, the neurotised fibres in the latter show cyclical firing of their axons in phase with respiration. This is a permanent feature but it is surprising how well patients overcome it.

Spinal root repair

Repairing spinal roots or cranial nerve roots after injury is a very specialised form of nerve repair. The orthopaedic surgeon may encounter this situation in relation to injury to the brachial plexus or cauda equina. These are devastating nerve injuries, and primary repair is very much a goal to be sought. In most cases the injury is one of avulsion. Jamieson and Bonney (1979) were the first to attempt repair and, although their early work in dogs was of limited success, they must be credited with demonstrating the potential for intradural repair.

The central processes (axons) of sensory nerves are unlikely to regenerate because they are entering the hostile CNS environment. However, motor roots have been shown to regenerate centrifugally into the environment of the peripheral nervous system, and sensory nerves peripheral to the dorsal root ganglion behave as any other peripheral nerve. Glasby and Hems (1995) have recently demonstrated the successful reimplantation of ventral nerve roots in both the brachial plexus and cauda equina of sheep using short FTMGs abutted to the anterior funiculus of the spinal cord and attached with fibrin glue. The avulsed roots are trimmed and attached to the distal surface of the FTMG. A small but manageable degree of rotation of the spinal cord is necessary. Carlstedt (1990, 1991) has used nerve autografts channelled to reach the motor neurone pool through the lateral funiculus of the spinal cord in a small number of human patients. The results have been encouraging. There is no doubt that, in the future, operations of this kind, perhaps aided by the use of neurotrophic factors, may open up the possibility of spinal reconstructive surgery.

REFERENCES

Carlstedt T. Experimental studies on surgical treatment of avulsed spinal nerve roots in brachial plexus injury. *J Hand Surg [Br]* 1991; **16B**: 477–482.

Carlstedt T, Risling M, Linda H. Regeneration after spinal nerve root injury. *Restorative Neurol Neurosci* 1990; **1**: 289–295.

Carrick MJ, Fullarton AC, Glasby MA. The tonic vibration reflex as a means of assessing proprioceptive function after nerve repair: a comparison of crush injury and muscle graft repair in the rat. *Neuro-Orthopedics* 1992; **13**: 95–106.

Gattuso JM. Peripheral nerve. In: Glasby MA, Huang CL-H (Eds) *Applied Physiology for Surgery and Critical Care*. Oxford: Butterworth–Heinemann, 1995: 543–548.

Gelberman RH. *Operative Nerve Repair and Reconstruction*. Philadelphia: JB Lippincott, 1991.

Gilbert A, Tassin JL. Obstetrical palsy: a clinical, pathologic and surgical review. In: Terzis JK (ed.) *Microreconstruction of Nerve Injuries*. Philadelphia: WB Saunders, 1987; 529–555.

Glasby MA. Nerve growth in matrices of orientated muscle basement membrane: developing a new method of nerve repair. *Clin Anat* 1990; **3**: 161–182.

Glasby MA. Future possibilities for reconstructive surgery after spinal injuries. *Neuro-Orthopedics* 1995a; **17/18**: 143–149.

Glasby MA. The control of posture and movement. In: Glasby MA, Huang CL-H (eds) *Applied Physiology for Surgery and Critical Care*. Oxford: Butterworth–Heinemann, 1995b.

Glasby MA, Hems TEJ. Basil Kilvington, unknown pioneer of peripheral nerve repair. *J Hand Surg [Br]* 1993; **18B**: 461–464.

Glasby MA, Hems TEJ. Repairing spinal roots after brachial plexus injuries. *Paraplegia* **33**: 359–361.

Glasby MA, Huang CL-H. *Applied Physiology for Surgery and Critical Care*. Oxford: Butterworth–Heinemann, 1995.

Hems TEJ, Glasby MA. Repair of cervical nerve roots proximal to the root ganglia: an experimental study in sheep. *J Bone Joint Surg [Br]* 1992; **74b**: 918–922.

Hems TEJ, Clutton RW, Glasby MA. The repair of avulsed cervical nerve roots; an experimental study in sheep. *J Bone Joint Surg [Br]* 1994; **76B**: 818–823.

Hodgkin, AL, Huxley AF. A quantitative description of membrane current and its application to conduction and excitation in nerve. *J Physiol* 1952; **117**: 500–544.

Huang CL-H. The physiology of excitable cells. In: Glasby MA, Huang CL-H (eds) *Applied Physiology for Surgery and Critical Care*. Oxford: Butterworth–Heinemann, 1995a; 101–1120.

Huang CL-H. Muscle. In: Glasby MA, Huang CL-H (eds) *Applied Physiology for Surgery and Critical Care*. Oxford: Butterworth–Heinemann, 1996b; 119–130.

Jamieson AM, Bonney G. An analysis of the operative findings in brachial plexus traction lesions treated between 1956 and 1978. *J Bone Joint Surg* 1979; **61B**: 516.

Jamieson AM, Eames RA. Reimplantation of avulsed brachial plexus roots: an experimental study in dogs. *Int J Microsurgery* 1980; 75–80.

Kimura J. *Electrodiagnosis in diseases of Nerve and Muscle*. Philadelphia: FA Davis, 1989.

Landon DN. *The Peripheral Nerve*. London: Chapman and Hall, 1976.

Lenman JAR, Ritchie AE. *Clinical Electromyography*. Edinburgh: Churchill Livingstone, 1987.

Lundborg G. *Nerve Injury and Repair*. Edinburgh: Churchill Livingstone, 1988.

Mackinnon SE, Dellon AL. *Surgery of the Peripheral Nerve*. Stuttgart: Georg Thieme, 1988.

Medical Research Council. *Peripheral Nerve Injuries*. London: HMSO, 1954.

Millesi H. Indications and techniques of nerve grafting. In: Gelberman RH (ed.) *Operative Nerve Repair and Reconstruction*. Philadelphia: JB Lippincott, 1991a; 525–544.

Millesi H. Brachial plexus injury in adults: operative repair. In: Gelberman RH (eds.) *Operative Nerve Repair and Reconstruction*. Philadelphia: JB Lippincott, 1991b; 1285–1301.

Millesi H, Meissl G. Consequences of tension at the suture site. In: Gorio A, et al (eds) *Post-traumatic Peripheral Nerve Repair: Experimental Basis and Clinical Implications*. New York: Raven Press, 1995; 277–279.

Moberg E. Methods of examining sensibility. In: Flynn JE (ed.) *Hand Surgery*. Baltimore: Williams and Wilkins, 1995; 435–449.

Narakas, AO. Neurotization in the treatment of brachial plexus injuries. In: Gelberman RH (ed.) *Operative Nerve Repair and Reconstruction*. Philadelphia: JB Lippincott, 1991; 1329–1360.

Seddon HJ. *Surgical Disorders of the Peripheral Nerves*. Edinburgh: Churchill Livingstone, 1975.

Singer SJ, Nicolson GL. The fluid mosaic model of the structure of cell membranes. *Science* 1972; **175**: 720–731.

Sunderland S. *Nerves and Nerve Injuries*. Edinburgh: Churchill Livingstone, 1978.

7

Skeletal Muscle

Christopher L-H Huang

INTRODUCTION

The function of skeletal muscle is to contract and thereby to generate force on its attachments. It is thus responsible both for moving joints and for supporting the skeleton. It comprises 40–50% of the body-weight in an adult male, and a slightly lower proportion of the body-weight in females. This chapter provides an overview of the structure and function of this major component of the musculoskeletal system. More extensive reviews of different aspects of the subject matter are provided in the references.

GROWTH AND DEVELOPMENT OF MUSCLE

Embryology of muscle development

There are basically three stages of development from embryonic mesoderm to definitive muscle fibres (reviews: Kedes & Stockdale, 1989; Adrian & Peachey, 1983). In the sixth embryonic week, the mesoderm differentiates into myoblasts. Most of the myoblasts then fuse or aggregate to form primary myotubes. Some stray out to form satellite cells. The latter are single cells with a potential eventually to differentiate into adult muscle. By the seventh to ninth week, the embryonic primary myotubes become attached to the developing skeleton by tendons. Midway along the primary myotubes, secondary myotubes are formed by a further aggregation of the blast cells. Both the primary and secondary myotubes initially share the same basement membrane.

At the end of about 9 weeks, muscle groups are well defined microscopically and cross-striations in the individual cells may be visible. At around 10 weeks, the

developing nerve fibres come in contact with the myotubes. In response to this development, the muscle fibres differentiate slowly. Tertiary myotubes appear at 16–17 weeks of gestation, and by 18–23 weeks they become mature and gradually migrate to the periphery of the muscle. Initially, the satellite cells are prominent. They are responsible for the regeneration of damaged fibres. Until 39 weeks of intrauterine life, 50% of muscles are expressed as either slow or fast fibres. This differentiation continues in the neonatal period and early infancy. Some embryonic fibres may persist in adult muscle as type IIc fibres.

The chronological events of the developing skeletal muscles can thus be summarised as follows:

6 weeks:	Formation of myoblasts from mesodermal condensation
7 weeks:	Formation of primary myotubes and satellite cells
	Synthesis of the contractile elements actin and myosin
	Appearance of cross-striations
	Attachment to tendons and skeleton
10 weeks:	Nervous system makes contact with developing muscle fibres
	Differentiation of muscle fibres starts
11 weeks:	Hypertrophy and addition of sarcomeres at the ends
16–17 weeks:	Addition of further myotubes and the formation of tertiary myotubes
18–23 weeks:	Independent tertiary myotubes appear
	Appearance of eccentric nuclei
24 weeks:	Number of fibres in each muscle is set
32 weeks:	Differentiation of muscle fibre types
	Production of structural proteins and enzymes
	Participation of metabolic pathways.

This broad outline does not mean that there is no overlap between overall stages. In addition, genetic, hormonal and intrauterine environmental factors exert considerable effects on the stages of development. Before the completion of organogenesis, the teratogenic influences of noxious agents can produce skeletal muscle malformations, but after the stages of organogenesis deformative defects are uncommon.

Growth: size of muscles

Bone grows at the growth plate. In contrast, muscle does not have a growth centre, yet it increases in size to keep up with skeletal development. It is generally accepted that the number of muscle fibres in each muscle is set at around 24 weeks' gestation. Any subsequent changes take place by cell hypertrophy and elongation rather than hyperplasia. This is possibly by an increase in the tendon and by the addition of sarcomeres at the musculotendinous junction during longitudinal growth. Little or no elongation takes place at the middle of the muscle fibres.

From the foetal state to adulthood, division, maturation and decline of the muscle cells are influenced by various hormones, notably the growth hormones, thyroid hormones, insulin and corticosteroids. During postnatal development, there is a surge of luteinising hormone in both sexes. In male neonates, there is considerable release of testosterone, which influences muscle growth. There are also marked changes during the growth spurt at puberty and following cessation of the reproductive age.

Knowledge of muscle growth can contribute to our understanding of the changes that take place in muscle following its immobilisation under different degrees of stretch, or of skeletal lengthening or shortening. When muscles are immobilised in a shortened position, for example with the shortening of the gastrocnemius and soleus muscles in equinus, these muscles will eventually produce more resistance for a given stretch or for given changes of ankle joint angles. Contrasting changes take place following immobilisation under stretch. These include immediate increases in length of the myotubes (increase in length of sarcomere separation of A and I bands) and the eventual addition of new sarcomeres, particularly at the musculotendinous junctions. There is also an increase in muscle protein and in muscle weight, but an unaltered cross-sectional area.

The mechanical end result, even after 2 weeks of such immobilisation, is that achieving a given level of stretch requires the generation of less passive force. These changes in the properties of muscle following imposed changes in length have profound clinical implications in relation to immobilisation, skeletal length changes, tendon transfers or lengthening. The mechanical changes are also influenced by other factors, such as proprioceptive activities, motor innervation, mechanical load, and joint movement and central nervous system influences.

Finally, morphological changes of muscle mass continue to take place between the neonatal period and adulthood. Besides clear sex-related differences, disproportionate growth at various anatomical locations is noticeable even within the same sex. Before puberty, the lower limb grows in proportion to the body-weight and the upper body grows less rapidly. During the adolescent growth spurt, skeletal muscle grows rapidly in relation to weight and height. At this stage, the increased strength of the biceps muscle in boys of the same height as girls could be due to growth influenced by the testosterone surge. The adult human body, as a whole, also shows interesting variations that have been described as falling broadly into three categories of ectomorphic, mesomorphic and endomorphic configurations (*Figure 7.1*).

STRUCTURE OF SKELETAL MUSCLE

Any given skeletal muscle consists of a large number of individual muscle fibres that are organised into bundles or fascicles by connective tissue. Each individual fibre is a cylindrical multinucleate cell of diameter between 50 and 150 μm. The fibres end in connective tissue tendons, which in turn are attached to bone. Muscle contraction therefore results in an approximation of the bony origin and insertion.

Mucsle fibres contain a number of major structural components that reflect their specialised function. The structures that particularly reflect their contractile properties are the bundles of myofibrils that are made up of the contractile proteins that run parallel to the fibre axis. These are long and cylindrical and are between 1 and 2 μm in diameter. There are also extensive, specialised, membrane systems that are involved in regulating cell function. In addition to the surface membrane that surrounds the entire fibre, there are two specialised internal membrane systems. Of these, the transverse

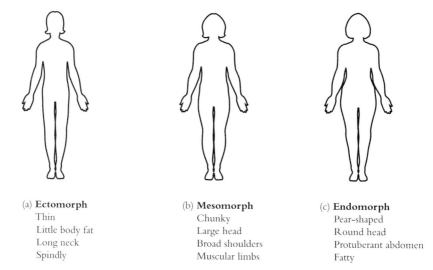

(a) **Ectomorph**
   Thin
   Little body fat
   Long neck
   Spindly

(b) **Mesomorph**
   Chunky
   Large head
   Broad shoulders
   Muscular limbs

(c) **Endomorph**
   Pear-shaped
   Round head
   Protuberant abdomen
   Fatty

Figure 7.1   Mesomorphic, endomorphic and ectomorphic distributions of body tissue.

tubules form a fine system of interconnecting tubes whose lumina are continuous with the extracellular fluid. These tubules form networks at regular intervals along the fibre length that run transversely across the fibre axis. In addition, the sarcoplasmic reticulum forms an intracellular membrane network of tubes and sacs whose lumina are separate from the extracellular space. These act as an intracellular storage site for calcium.

Finally, muscle cells contain organelles that function in energy metabolism, cell repair and protein synthesis, in common with other cells. For example, mitochondria and glycogen granules are involved in the energy metabolism required to support contractile activity. There are also ribosomes, lysosomes and lipid granules. A number of key proteins such as myoglobin and creatinine phosphokinase are found particularly in muscle. Certain proteins such as dystrophin may have an important role in the preservation of cell membrane integrity and have been implicated in the pathogenesis of muscle dystrophy.

MUSCLE FIBRES AND FIBRILS

An isolated muscle fibre examined under a microscope using certain conditions of polarising light or phase contrast shows a characteristic banding structure. This appearance is responsible for the term **striated muscle** that has been used to describe skeletal (as well as cardiac)

muscle. Such patterns were known to nineteenth century microscopists and contribute to our understanding of the contractile mechanism. Thus, the component myofibrils within each muscle fibre also show this banded appearance (*Figure 7.2a*).

The prominent dark A (anisotropic) bands contain thick filaments. The lighter or I (isotropic) bands contain only thin filaments. Both thick and thin filaments are organised into a highly structured configuration within the myofibrils (*Figure 7.2b*). The Z lines occur in the centre of the I bands. They provide attachment sites that ensure an organised arrangement of the thin filaments. The centres of the thick filaments are similarly aligned by cross-connections, which give rise to a dark M line. A sarcomere refers to the repeating anatomical (and functional) unit of a myofibril and extends from Z line to Z line.

Muscle contraction results from the interaction of the proteins of the thick and thin filaments. The thin and the thick filaments thus form the contractile elements of the myofibril and are made up of the proteins actin and myosin. In skeletal and cardiac muscle, the intracellular arrangements of these contractile proteins enhance the generation of force and movement (see Huxley, 1978, for further details).

Myosin

The thick filaments are mainly composed of the protein

(a)

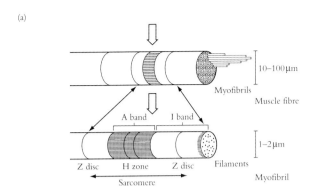

(b)

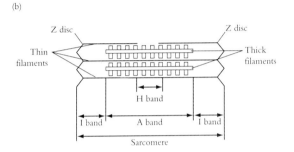

Figure 7.2 (a) Anatomical arrangement of myofibrillar components of skeletal muscle. (b) Arrangement of thick and thin filaments in a muscle sarcomere. Adapted from Lamb et al (1984).

(a)

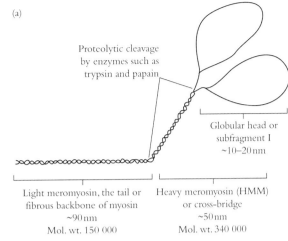

(b)

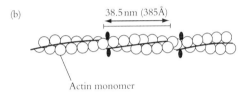

Figure 7.3 (a) Subfragments of myosin showing a fibrous light meromyosin double-stranded backbone and the globular head that contains the actin-binding and ATPase site. (b) Basic actin backbone of the thin filament. The tropomyosin molecule is represented as the line lying in the actin groove. The troponin units are interposed in the actin chain. Adapted from Lamb et al (1984).

myosin. Each myosin molecule consists of a tail of two long light meromyosin strands twisted together; each of these tails in turn is connected to globular heads (*Figure 7.3a*). Each head is made up of a heavy meromyosin molecule that includes two fractions. The S1 fraction contains the globular heads and the S2 fraction contains the necks that connect the heads to the tails. Binding of the myosin head to actin triggers ATPase activity in the S1 fraction. Myosin is assembled into filaments of typically 1.6 μm in length in frog semitendinosus muscle.

Actin

The thin filaments are made up of units of the protein actin in association with the regulatory proteins tropomyosin and troponin (*Figure 7.3b*). Actin occurs not only in muscle but also in a variety of other tissues and cells. Actin forms globular proteins units that become polymerised *in vivo* to form thin filaments that show a unit periodicity of 5 nm. These thin filaments form paired chains that are twisted about each other with a periodicity

of 36.5 nm. Actin can bind strongly with myosin both *in vitro* and *in vivo*. In frog semitendinosus muscle, the thin filaments are typically around 2.05 μm in length.

Tropomyosin and troponin

Tropomyosin is a rod-shaped molecule about 40 nm long with a molecular weight of about 68 kD. It forms α-helical subunits that become packed into the depth of the groove formed by the helical actin chains. One tropomyosin molecule thus spans seven actin units (*Figure 7.3b*). In resting skeletal muscle it prevents the actin from binding to myosin. The latter reaction is permitted only following movement of the tropomyosin molecule deeper into the groove that is formed by the thin filaments. This then stereochemically permits the interaction of the myosin heads with actin. The latter configurational change in the tropomyosin molecule is controlled by troponin, a globular protein of molecular weight 80–90 kDa that consists of three subunits, TnC, TnT and TnI. Troponin is associated with the tropomyosin ribbon through its TnT subunit at the 40-nm intervals in which its own units are intercalated in the actin chain. It is the configurational change triggered by the binding of calcium to the troponin TnC subunit that pulls tropomyosin into the actin grove. The latter then exposes the myosin-binding sites on actin and permits myosin to bind to actin. The latter in turn also activates the ATPase activity of the myosin heads. Troponin also contains a third subunit, TnI, whose function is uncertain.

Other proteins

α-Actinin plays a major role in the structure of the Z line. β-Actinin controls the polymerisation of actin; this determines the length of the thin filament. M line proteins reside in the middle of the A band; they are responsible for the spacing of the thick filaments.

SLIDING FILAMENT THEORY OF MUSCLE CONTRACTION

It is generally accepted that myofilament shortening is produced by the cyclical formation and detachment of bridges between the thick and the thin filaments. Each such cross-bridge cycle generates a force that pulls the thin filaments towards the centre of the sarcomere. In this contractile process, the individual myofilament lengths remain constant and it is the relative sliding of the interdigitated thick and thin filaments that produces the sarcomere shortening. The isometric tension that is generated on stimulation of a single muscle fibre thus varies with the degree of fibre stretch, because the latter in turn determines the degree of myofilament overlap and therefore the opportunities for cross-bridge formation (*Figure 7.4a*). Thus sarcomere lengthening that reduces or abolishes the myofilament overlap reduces the production of force (*Figure 7.4b–e*). Conversely, a greater filament overlap increases the force generation within limits; because the middle of the thick filament lacks myosin heads, the isometric force remains constant at sarcomere lengths below 2.2–2.0 μm as there is then

no further opportunity for cross-bridge formation. Any further shortening will actually diminish the production of force because the thin filaments then collide with one another or the thick filaments collide with the Z lines (*Figure 7.4f*).

The generation of tension by each cross-bridge interaction constitutes a conversion of chemical energy to mechanical energy. The cross-bridges form from the combination of the myosin projections from the thick filament with the actin subunits (*Figure 7.5*). The link between the S1 and S2 segments of heavy meromyosin appears to be flexible. This permits the S1 filament portion to move away from the thick filament and to reach the neighbouring thin filament to make such a contact with an actin unit. This actin–myosin interaction produces the configurational changes that cause the force generation that in turn results in filament sliding and muscle shortening. A reaction with ATP is then required to dissociate this actin–myosin complex, a process that is accompanied by ATP hydrolysis. The dissociation permits a further cross-bridge cycle to begin afresh; otherwise a progressive recruitment of successive crossbridges will result in rigor mortis. The process of cross-bridge formation and release takes place asynchronously among the population of the individual crossbridges; this results in a smooth and sustained production of overall force whose magnitude depends on both the number of interacting sites and the force generated by each site (see Huxley, 1978; Squire, 1990, for detailed reviews).

REGULATION OF FILAMENT INTERACTION BY CALCIUM

Studies have been made both of the ATPase activity of isolated myofibrillar preparations and of the isometric force in 'skinned' muscle fibre preparations from which the surface membrane had been removed. The biological activity in both these preparations depends steeply on the calcium concentration over the range of 10^{-6} to $10^{-4} \, mol \, l^{-1}$. This corresponds to the range of cytosolic calcium levels through which the sarcoplasmic reticulum is able to control the intracellular $[Ca^{2+}]$.

The different muscle types show some variations in the details of such regulation. For example, the regulatory role of calcium is mediated through its binding to the

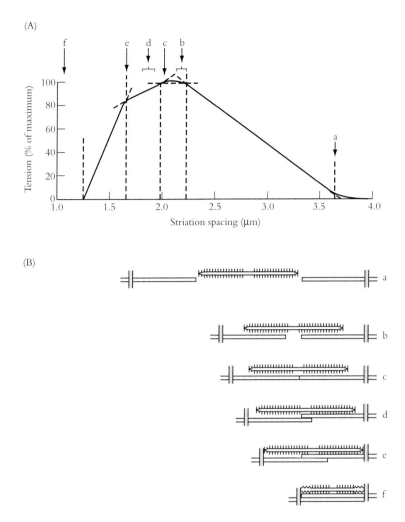

Figure 7.4   The interpretation of the length–tension curve in terms of the corresponding striation spacing in a single muscle fibre. (A) The length–tension relationship in a single amphibian fibre. (B) Anatomical relationships between filaments at different sarcomere lengths. The annotations (a–f) match corresponding markings (a–f) on the length–tension curve. Adapted from Gordon et al (1966).

TnC subunit of troponin in both skeletal and cardiac muscle. Skeletal muscle TnC has four calcium-binding sites; of these, two have a much higher affinity for Ca^{2+} than for Mg^{2+} and are considered to be the critical sites that are involved in the regulation of cross-bridge activation. In contrast, calcium appears first to bind to the protein calmodulin in smooth muscle. The resulting complex in turn activates the phosphorylation of a myosin light chain to produce an ATPase which reacts with actin.

TUBULAR AND SARCOPLASMIC RETICULAR MEMBRANES

The membrane systems in skeletal muscle play a central regulatory role in cellular activation. The structure and electrophysiological function of the surface membrane do not significantly differ from those of the plasma membrane of other excitable cells. However, some of the numerous invaginations of the surface membrane open

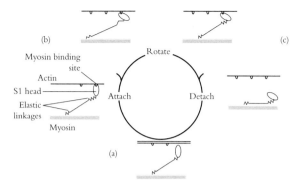

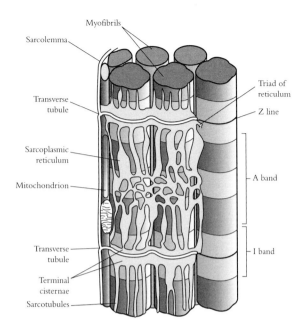

Figure 7.5 Diagrammatic representation of the cross-bridge cycle. (a) Relaxed muscle shows no cross-bridge–actin interaction owing to the low cytosolic Ca^{2+} concentration. Under these conditions the actin-binding sites for myosin are masked by tropomyosin. (b) Excitation–contraction coupling results in troponin activation, tropomyosin displacement with unmasking of the actin-binding site, and myosin binding that is followed by rotation of the myosin head. (c) ATP binding is required to enable detachment of the cross-bridge. Adapted from Lamb et al (1984).

Figure 7.6 The internal membrane systems present in frog sartorius muscle. The transverse tubular system is formed from invaginations of the surface membrane and these form a network that penetrates and surrounds each myofibril. Elements of the transverse tubules come into close proximity with the terminal cisternal regions of the sarcoplasmic reticulum at the triads. Adapted from Peachey (1965).

into a transverse (T) tubular system, which forms an extensive branching membrane network whose lumina remain continuous with the extracellular space (*Figure 7.6*). The transverse tubules thus anastomose repeatedly to form a network that surrounds each individual myofibril. This membrane system presents a total surface area to the extracellular space that is six to ten times greater than that of the sarcolemmal cylinder alone. In mammalian skeletal muscle, such networks occur at the junctions between the A and I bands, whereas in mammalian cardiac muscle and in frog skeletal muscle they appear at the Z line (see Adrian and Peachey, 1983; Huang, 1993, for detailed reviews).

The sarcoplasmic reticulum forms a longitudinal system of tubules and sacs (*Figure 7.6*) that come into close anatomical relationship with the T tubules at localised regions called the terminal cisternae. In these areas, the membranes of the two membrane systems come into close geometrical proximity to give rise to a triad arrangement in which two terminal cisternae sandwich a transverse tubule. Such triadic regions account for around 70% of the transverse tubular membrane surface area in frog muscle. Electronmicrographs of the fine structure of the triads reveal that feet or pillar-like structures appear to project from the sarcoplasmic reticular membranes and extend to the T tubular membranes. It has been suggested that these pillars may form a mechanical link between the

two membrane systems and that this is important in the triggering of calcium release (see below).

ELECTROPHYSIOLOGY OF MUSCLE ACTIVATION

The activation of a motor neurone results in the propagation of an action potential down its axon to its neuromuscular junctions with the individual muscle fibres. The motor neurone, together with the muscle fibres that it innervates, constitutes a functional unit of contraction, the motor unit. Thus, death of the cell body and the subsequent degeneration of the motor axon, as may occur in motor neurone disease or poliomyelitis, results in a flaccid paralysis. The release of chemical transmitter at the neuromuscular junction then triggers an action potential in the muscle fibre membrane that propagates over the surface and into the transverse tubules. Tubular membrane depolarisation leads to the release of intracellularly stored calcium from a sarcoplasmic reticulum membrane system and a consequent increase in the free cytosolic calcium concentration. This activates the contractile proteins and results in force generation with muscle shortening.

A single action potential elicits a single phasic contraction or twitch; this lasts around 50 ms for fast muscles but can extend for up to several hundred milliseconds for slow muscles. However, repetitive stimulation of a muscle, resulting in a train of action potentials that occurs above a critical frequency, produces a sustained and augmented tension generation referred to as tetanus. The stimulation frequency required to produce tetanus varies from 300 per second for rapidly contracting muscles down to about 40 per second for slow muscles.

Many of the electrical properties of muscle membranes are similar to those of nerve cell membranes. Sodium channels are particularly well represented on the surface membrane; they may also occur, but at a lower density, in the tubular membranes. The channels themselves have properties that also closely resemble those found in nerve cell membranes. Familial periodic paralysis results from a genetic abnormality in muscle sodium channel function. Either denervation or motor neurone pathology causes a flaccid paralysis and is accompanied by an early appearance of spontaneous electrical activity and a development of TTX(tetrodotoxin)-resistant sodium channels, as well as enhanced membrane sensitivity to the neurotransmitter acetylcholine.

However, muscle membranes contain at least three kinds of potassium channel, in contrast to the one channel type that appears to predominate in nerve. The first is activated by depolarisation and opens with a time course similar to that found in nerve membranes. The activation of a second channel type takes place over a considerably longer time course of hundreds of milliseconds. Finally, an inward rectification channel whose functional significance is uncertain in skeletal muscle allows potassium to pass more easily into than out of the cell. In cardiac muscle this inward rectifier may be important in minimising leak currents and so may reduce the amount of inward current that is required to sustain the plateau phase of the action potential. Unlike nerve cells, resting skeletal muscle cells show a significant chloride conductance that actually exceeds the resting potassium conductance and may be important in stabilising the membrane potential between episodes of electrical activity. Thus, the condi-

tion myotonia congenita is associated with a deficiency or absence of functioning chloride channels; this condition results in unwanted repetitive action potential firing.

Finally, calcium channels are responsible for the inward currents that give rise to the excitability observed in invertebrate muscles. However, the time course of their activation is too slow to mediate a direct role in electrical properties *in vivo* in amphibian and mammalian skeletal muscle. Nevertheless, they generate the plateau phase of the action potential in mammalian cardiac muscle. Furthermore, recent findings have suggested that normal calcium channel function is required to maintain the motor endplate, and that dystrophic muscle membranes show abnormalities in calcium permeability properties.

The transverse tubular membranes are capable of generating action potentials and thereby conducting the depolarisation that is initiated along the surface membrane into the depths of the muscle fibre. The waveform of the action potential from a skeletal muscle fibre consequently differs from that shown by an axon, in that it shows a long after-depolarisation. This reflects the more prolonged propagation of the depolarising wave into the transverse tubules following its initiation by the action potential depolarisation of the surface membrane. Finally, the presence of the transverse tubular system results in unit cylindrical surface of skeletal muscle showing a fivefold to tenfold higher membrane capacitance compared with axonal membranes. In addition, the transverse tubular lumina give rise to a restricted space in which ions may accumulate or be depleted, and with which diffusion equilibrium with the rest of the extracellular fluid is relatively slow (see Adrian and Peachey, 1983, for a detailed account of skeletal muscle electrophysiology).

EXCITATION–CONTRACTION COUPLING

This refers to the series of events that begins with membrane depolarisation and ends with the actual contractile activation of the myofilaments. Experiments in which local stimuli were applied to different regions along the sarcomere length specifically implicated the transverse tubules in this process. Subsequent studies have demonstrated that the transverse tubules not only passively spread the depolarisation that is initiated by the surface action potential into the depths of the fibre but also themselves propagate action potentials. They thus assume an instrumental role in initiating and synchronising contractile activation through the entire cross-section of the muscle fibre.

The events that actually couple the tubular depolarisation with contractile activation begin with the detection by a voltage sensor of the transverse tubular membrane depolarisation. The sensor is thought to be an integral membrane protein whose molecular configuration varies steeply with changes in membrane potential. Its conformational transitions have been identified and characterised electrically through the small currents or charge movements that it produces by such configurational changes. Pharmacological studies have demonstrated that the molecule involved may be a modified calcium channel. Its marked voltage sensitivity may account for the very steep relationship that has been observed between the membrane potential and either the release of intracellularly stored calcium as measured by experiments that follow absorbance changes in introduced intracellular calcium indicators, or the actual tension generation.

The voltage-sensing process must then be linked to the release of intracellularly stored calcium from the sarcoplasmic reticulum into the cytosol. It is likely that the triad complexes described above constitute the sites at which such transverse tubular depolarisation is transduced into calcium release. In skeletal muscle, the resulting increase in the cytosolic concentration of this activator calcium almost entirely reflects the calcium release from the sarcoplasmic reticular stores that takes place at the terminal cisternae. There is no significant contribution from calcium influx from the extracellular space. However, there is little evidence for direct electrical communication between the component membrane systems of the triads.

On the other hand, electron micrographic studies have demonstrated that the foot processes that join the cisternal and the tubular membranes in the triad complexes occur at regular intervals within the plane of the long axis of the transverse tubules. Recent studies suggest that these foot processes are the cytoplasmic components of a macromolecule that has been characterised through its specific binding for the plant alkaloid ryanodine. The intramembrane portion of this ryanodine receptor resides within the sarcoplasmic reticulum membrane and functions as a calcium channel. A genetic defect in the ryanodine receptor is thought to be responsible for malignant hyperthermia, which is an inheritable condition whose clinical manifestations of muscle spasm and excessive heat generation are typically triggered by halothane anaesthesia.

The foot processes also appear in close geometrical proximity to structures that are embedded within the transverse tubular membrane, which may well be the voltage sensors. Thus both anatomical and electrophysiological studies suggest a possible mechanism for the coupling of changes in the transverse tubular membrane to changes in the sarcoplasmic reticulum which might involve some direct mechanical interaction between the ryanodine receptor and the dihydropyridine-sensitive voltage sensors. This would result in the release of intracellularly stored calcium ions, which ultimately would initiate mechanical activity through their binding to the regulatory protein troponin. This area is reviewed in greater detail in Huang (1993).

The relaxation that follows myofilament activation results from the re-sequestration of the released calcium back from the cytosol into the sarcoplasmic reticulum, a process that takes place by active transport through a membrane Ca–ATPase, a transport protein embedded in regions of the sarcoplasmic reticular membrane that are remote from the terminal cisternae (Martonosi, 1984). This specific ATPase protein, of molecular weight 100 kDa, transports two calcium ions per molecule of ATP hydrolysed. It pumps calcium from the cytosol into the sarcoplasmic reticular lumen and is capable of building up 1000-fold concentration gradients of ionised calcium across the membrane. A number of intraluminal proteins then sequester this transported calcium. One example of such proteins is calsequestrin which has a 1:45 binding ratio for calcium and occurs most abundantly in the terminal cisternal lumina. As a result of this transport process, the cytosolic calcium concentration falls to levels that are below those required for significant troponin binding. This ends the twitch.

BIOMECHANICS OF MUSCLE CONTRACTION

Force generation

The activation of a muscle results in the generation of a force between its attachments. The activation of a single nerve produces a single twitch of the muscle which typically lasts less than 200 ms. Repetitive activation at a low frequency elicits successive twitches with no increase in peak tension. At higher frequencies of stimulation, the muscle may be re-activated before the tension that arose from the previous twitch has returned to baseline; under such conditions, the tension rises above that of a single twitch. As the frequency of activation increases further, the tension summates to reach a maximum level of tetanus.

Length–tension relationship

Tension in a muscle can be developed either passively, by stretching the quiescent muscle, or actively by the initiation of cross-bridge activity following nerve stimulation. Passive tension is generated mainly by the connective tissue and fascia that is present within the muscle. When a muscle is stretched passively there is little initial development of tension, but beyond a certain degree of strain there is a significant non-linear increase in tension.

The isometric force that is generated by a muscle stimulated tetanically at different lengths varies with the length of the muscle. At shorter lengths, most of the tension is due to active contraction. At longer lengths, the contribution made by the active contraction decreases, and the contribution from passive tension becomes more important. The decrease in active tension with increasing length can be explained by the geometric arrangement of the filaments. When the muscle is lengthened beyond a certain limit, the thick filaments fail to overlap the thin filaments, and it is no longer possible for active tension to develop in the muscle.

Force–velocity relationship

The classical experiments by A.V. Hill investigated the relationship between the velocity of muscle contraction and the force generated in the muscle, and demonstrated an inverse relationship between the two. Maximum force is generated at isometric tension and, as the velocity of contraction increases, the force generated by the muscle decreases. Mathematically, this relationship is described by the equation:

$$(F + a)(v + b) = (F_{max} + a)b$$

where F is the muscle force, v is the velocity of contraction, F_{max} is the maximum isometric tension, and a and b are constants (for a review see Hill, 1970).

Joint reaction forces

Calculation of the forces and torques that act on joints as a result of muscular activity is discussed in detail in Section III. However, it is useful to point out at this stage that muscles normally act at a mechanical disadvantage. This is due to the fact that the perpendicular distance from the line of action of the muscle to the joint is, in general, significantly smaller than the distance of the external load to the joint. Therefore, contractile muscle forces are usually significantly larger than those that result from the external load. So are the joint forces: these are determined largely by the magnitude of the muscle force. Although working at a mechanical disadvantage, such an arrangement does amplify the amount of shortening of the muscle to produce a correspondingly larger motion at the position of the external load. Thus, mechanical efficiency is compromised to increase the available velocity and acceleration for movement.

ENERGY SOURCES FOR MUSCLE CONTRACTION

Adenosine 5′-triphosphate (ATP) is the only molecule to provide energy through its hydrolysis that can be used directly to drive cross-bridge cycling. The adenosine moiety in the ATP molecule is attached to three inorganic phosphate bonds. The hydrolytic reaction that dissociates the terminal phosphate releases energy that can drive appropriately coupled biological reactions. The ATP is transformed to adenosine 5′-diphosphate (ADP) in this process. The available pool of ATP in the cell is, by itself, sufficient for only about eight twitches. However, the supply of cellular ATP can be regenerated through the reaction of ADP with phosphocreatine (CP) in the creatine kinase reaction in which the phosphate from CP is transferred to ADP to form ATP (review in Woledge, Curtin and Homsher, 1984).

$$ADP + CP \rightleftharpoons ATP + creatine$$

The creatine kinase reaction ensures that cellular ATP concentrations remain virtually constant during light exercise at the expense of the levels of CP. CP thus provides an immediate back-up energy supply: if all aerobic and anaerobic metabolic pathways are blocked, generation of ATP from CP through the creatine kinase

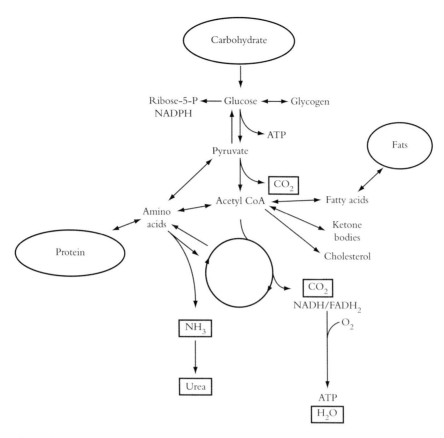

Figure 7.7 Outline of energy metabolism, emphasising major metabolic fuels. The circle in the centre denotes the tricarboxylic acid cycle. Adapted from Reddy and White (1995).

reaction can supply sufficient energy for around 100 twitches. However, at increased intensities of exercise, the ATP requirements cannot be so met, and aerobic or anaerobic mechanisms are used to produce ATP, mainly utilising glucose. Both these forms of metabolism can take place simultaneously.

Aerobic exercise is designed to be performed at an intensity in which oxygen demand can be met by the oxidative energy system. Thus, when oxygen is available, glucose or fatty acid molecules are broken down to pyruvate, which enters the Krebs cycle and produces large quantities of ATP through oxidative phosphorylation. Anaerobic mechanisms are usually required when there is a large increase in energy demand over a relatively short time. However, in the absence of oxygen, glucose molecules are converted to lactic acid with limited conversion of ADP to ATP. When the intensity and duration of the exercise exceeds the oxygen supply required by oxidative phosphorylation, anaerobic respira-

tion results in lactic acid production. However, lactic acid is toxic and produces fatigue.

In addition to carbohydrate, fat and protein also contribute to the energy supply (*Figure 7.7*). Triglyceride is broken down into its three constituent fatty acids, which are exchangeable with the extracellular compartment and are major potential sources of energy in cells. The fatty acids become converted by β-oxidation to acetyl coenzyme A and enter the Krebs cycle. Proteins are accessory sources of energy. Deamination of proteins produces ketoacids, which may be intermediates in, or otherwise enter, the Krebs cycle. The predominance of either aerobic or anaerobic energy metabolism is related to the various types of muscle fibre. Type I fibres have higher concentrations of the aerobic enzymes, type II cells are intermediate, and IIb fibres have higher concentrations of anaerobic enzymes. The role of various forms of exercise in relation to this metabolic background will be discussed below under the heading of Exercise and Training.

MUSCLE FIBRE TYPES

Mammalian muscle fibres can be classified into fast or slow types on the basis of their speeds of contraction, resistance to fatigue and on some of their structural and biochemical properties. For example, rat soleus muscle consists mainly of slow fibre types and has an approximately fivefold slower shortening velocity than does flexor digitorum longus, which is a muscle made up mainly of fast fibres.

A number of common features appear to define the differences between these fibre types. First, the shortening velocity of a muscle fibre is closely related to the rate of its myosin ATPase activity. The latter enzyme activity may vary by as much as a factor of three between fast and slow muscle fibre types. Such differences may reflect differences in the amino acid sequences that are present in their respective myosin light chains. Second, the rate and extent with which calcium is transported by Ca–ATPase into the sarcoplasmic reticulum appears to differ between fast and slow muscle. Third, the different fibre types differ in their glycogen storage capacity and in their balance between aerobic and anaerobic energy metabolism. This results in variations in their ability to withstand fatigue during repetitive activation. Thus slow fibres are capable of maintaining smooth tetanic tensions for long periods whereas fast fibres fatigue under similar conditions.

These structural, biochemical and physiological differences between fibre types are reflected in differences in their histological characteristics. A broad classification on the basis of the histochemical staining of myosin ATPase at various values of pH might recognise type I or slow, fatigue-resistant fibres, or type II or fast, fatiguable fibres. Type I fibres are also called slow oxidative fibres, and are extremely resistant to fatigue. Types IIa and IIb are also known as fast oxidative glycolytic (FOG) and fast glycolytic (FG) fibres respectively. These show increasing contraction velocities and fatiguability compared with Type I (I < IIa < IIb) fibres. Type IIc fibres are relatively common at birth (approximately 10%), but this proportion decreases significantly during the first 12 months of life. Therefore, type IIc fibres are thought by some to be undifferentiated fibres, but they might also represent a transitional state between types I and II. Some characteristics of the different fibre types are summarized in *Table 7.1* (Adrian and Peachey, 1983).

Table 7.1 Muscle fibre types and their basic characteristics.

Type	Characteristic	Staining
I	Slow twitch	ATPase (pH 4.3 and 4.6)
	Low strength	NADH-TR[a]
	Fatigue resistant	
IIa	Fast twitch	Phosphorylase
	High strength	ATPase (pH 9.4)
IIb	Fast twitch	ATPase (pH 4.6 and 9.4)
	High strength	Phosphorylase
IIc	Embryonic fibres	
	Regenerating fibres	

[a]NADH-TR = nicotinamide adenine dinucleotide, reduced-tetrazolium reductase.

FUNCTIONAL SIGNIFICANCE OF FIBRE TYPING

Any given muscle can contain both fibre types, although each individual motor unit is uniformly made up of a single fibre type. The motor units of slow fibres are smaller; their stimulation consequently produces relatively small tension increments. Their motor neurones are also small, and give rise to slowly conducting axons with small diameters. The activation of such motor units accordingly generates finely graded and sustained contractions with little fatigue that are therefore well adapted for maintaining sustained postural movements.

In contrast, motor units of fast fibres are large and so their stimulation produces high tensions and rapid contractions, but the fibres show a greater tendency to fatigue. Such motor units accordingly are adapted for producing phasic movements of short duration in which power and speed are more important than sustained activity. Gradual changes in fibre type from fast fibres to slow fibres can be produced by changing the nerve supply to the muscle, by chronically altering the pattern of its nerve stimulation or even by directly stimulating the muscle fibres involved. Such transformations of slow to fast fibres are associated with increases in capillary density, increases in numbers of their mitochrondria, decreases in the amount of sarcoplasmic reticulum, and changes in troponin and myosin isoenzymes (see, for example, Goldspink, 1980).

In general, postural muscles contain a higher proportion of type I fibres, whereas type II fibres tend to predominate in faster acting muscles. However, this trend is very variable, and differences in the relative proportion of fibre types are observed even when investigating different sites in the same muscle. Trained athletes have a higher proportion of the muscle fibre type relevant to their particular discipline. Sprinters tend to have more type II fibres, and long distance runners more type I. In paraplegics, type I fibres may be missing completely, and there is a considerable reduction in muscle cross-sectional area during prolonged immobilisation. The distribution of fibre types may also be abnormal in the myotonic dystrophies and childhood myopathies. Type IIc fibres are usually absent in the adult, but these are found to be increased in recurrent dislocation of the patella.

EXERCISE AND TRAINING

There are broadly three types of training. First, the primary effect of **strength** training is where the muscle becomes stronger and enlarged. In this type of training, the muscles are subjected to work that they are not strong enough to carry out, but this process induces adaptive changes in the muscle groups involved that results in a long-term increase in contractile strength. Second, aerobic or **endurance** training, such as long distance running, does not involve subjecting the muscle to high resistance or force. Thirdly, **anaerobic** or power training involves the imposition of high-intensity exercise lasting for a few seconds to minutes that calls upon metabolic support using anaerobic pathways.

Training for strength and size

Strength training involves high force, low repetition exercise. In an untrained person, the stimulation of motor nerves can recruit around 60% of the available motor units in the muscle. Strength exercise may achieve a recruitment and synchronisation of up to 90% of the available motor units. In this form of training, shortening of the muscle against resistance is repeated for a few minutes or until fatigue sets in. Sequential use of separate groups of muscles allows recovery of the immediately used muscle group and allows repetition.

Muscle strength is increased as the muscle cross-sectional area also proportionately enlarges. The fibre size increases along with the amount of contractile

protein. There are also adaptations amongst the fibre types; for example, type II fibres show more hypertrophy than type I fibres. The fibres also develop increased amounts of phosphogens without noticeable changes in the size and number of mitochondria and the level of oxidative enzymes following strength exercises. The relative progressive increase in resistance increases the strength and muscle volume (see, for example, Pette, 1980).

Anabolic steroids have seen inappropriate use in attempts to enhance performance and muscular development. They lead to increases of body-weight, in muscle protein synthesis and in aggressive behaviour. They competitively block the catabolic effects of cortisol but slow cortisol metabolism in the liver with a consequent increase in its circulating levels. This may contribute to a prevention of, or enhanced recovery from, injury. However, they produce significant unwanted side-effects that include the following: liver damage leading to development of tumours; feminising of men and virilisation of women mediated by inhibition of the secretion of gonadotrophin-releasing hormones from the hypothalamus, thereby reducing the plasma levels of follicle-stimulating hormone and of luteinising hormone; cardiovascular effects resulting from decreases in plasma levels of high density lipoprotein including stroke; cardiomyopathy, myocardial infarction; negative effects on the reproductive system (oligospermia, azoospermia, testicular atrophy); renal dysfunction; premature epiphyseal closure; and spontaneous rupture of the tendons (resulting from an inhibitory effect on collagen biosynthesis). The American Academy of Orthopedic Surgeons concluded in 1996, on the basis of such evidence, that 'these agents can cause serious harmful physiological, pathological and psychological effects'.

Training for endurance

Aerobic exercise training attempts to enhance the supply of metabolic energy to the muscle rather than developing muscular strength; there is an improvement in muscle metabolic function and overall cardiovascular performance. Endurance training imposes an increase in metabolic demand and promotes an improvement in the muscle blood supply by opening new capillaries. The cardiovascular system also adjusts to adapt to the demand. The left ventricle enlarges, stroke volume increases and, to pump increased amounts of blood to the tissues, the heart rate increases.

Unlike strength training, endurance training promotes adjustments in the oxidative metabolism of muscle cells. This is reflected in an increase in the size and number of mitochondria. The mitochondrial enzyme activities are also increased, leading to an enhanced formation of pyruvic acid from glycogen and of acetyl coenzyme A from fat. The non-carbohydrate energy supply from fatty acids is also increased in endurance exercise, particularly if this is extended over hours.

Glycogen stores in muscles and liver provide the primary source of muscle energy metabolism during exercise of moderate intensity. Accordingly, this storage capacity can be improved with a fat-free carbohydrate diet for several days before competition. The storage can be further enhanced by a programme of depleting the storage of glycogen by exercise followed by carbohydrate loading for a period before the endurance performance. In endurance training, type IIa fibres become more prominent.

Training for power (anaerobic exercise)

This form of high-intensity, short duration, exercise results in a depletion of the available intracellular phosphates and a triggering of anaerobic pathways to replenish ATP. This results in the formation of lactic acid, which can limit the activities. It results in an increase in the cellular levels of glycolytic enzymes such as phosphofructokinase and succinate dehydrogenase, particularly in the fast-twitch muscle fibres.

MUSCLE INJURY AND REGENERATION

Damage to skeletal muscles can result from physical trauma or from metabolic depletion. The damage can occur both in normal healthy muscle and in structurally abnormal or metabolically altered states. The following discussion focuses on the effects of damage on previously healthy skeletal muscles, but reference will also be made to altered states.

Muscle contusion

The most common injury to muscle is contusion, caused by non-penetrating blunt trauma sustained during accidents or sports. In most cases of bruising and mechanical trauma, there is little damage to the muscle fibres themselves, but pain and swelling result from inflammation of the skin, subcutaneous tissue and supporting connective tissues. Major blunt muscle injury produces swelling, and bleeding leads to haematoma formation, which in turn causes an inflammatory response. Scar formation is normally associated with the subsequent repair process. Haematoma formation may further be complicated by the formation of bone tissue within the muscle. For example, 20% of quadriceps injuries are complicated by the development of myositis ossificans. Early surgical removal of this abnormal tissue is contra-indicated, as it frequently becomes resorbed with time.

Muscle damage in severe crush injury releases myoglobin into the circulation, and this can lead to serious complications, including renal failure. The particular enzymes that are liberated by the damage of the muscles are the muscle-specific isoenzymes of creatine kinase and lactate dehydrogenase. In addition to muscle injury, blunt trauma can also produce degeneration of the motor units. However, if the muscle basement membranes are intact, the motor endplates survive for considerable lengths of time and reinnervation can eventually take place.

Two important factors particularly influence the functional end results of muscle contusion: the age of the muscle and its functional activity (i.e. whether the muscle is mobilised or immobilised). In mobilised and younger-aged patients, the initial inflammatory reaction is intense but disappears rapidly, with more scar formation than occurs in immobilised muscle. The tensile strength also recovers faster after injury in mobilised muscle.

Laceration of muscle

Surgical procedures either themselves produce incisional lacerations or have to deal with lacerated muscle wounds. In experimental models, repaired lacerated muscle in an optimal neurovascular environment heals by the formation of a dense connective tissue scar. Some myotubules cross the bridge, but regeneration is by no means complete. The smaller the muscle involved the better the result. The repair and return of strength also varies according to the site of the muscle laceration. Mid-belly lacerations form more scars than those at the musculo-tendinous junction. Experimental studies where the lacerated gap is bridged by tendon graft have shown satisfactory recovery of 40% of the original grip strength and recovery to Medical Research Council (MRC) grades 4 and 5.

Recovery from the muscle damage also depends on the extent of revascularisation, reinnervation and reorganisation of its connective tissue basal lamina. Even in dead muscle fibres, the intact motor endplate and intact basal lamina can promote muscle regeneration, but the portion of the muscle isolated from the nerve will show evidence of denervation. Connective tissue proliferation in muscle damage can have detrimental effects on muscle repair.

Indirect muscle injury

Muscle tears may be complete or incomplete. Incomplete muscle tears are relatively common. Stretching of muscle can produce this non-disruptive damage, which most commonly results in a lesion near the muscle–tendon junction. There is an initial fibre disruption and haemorrhage. The repair process involves an inflammatory response that is followed by the formation of granulation tissue eventually replaced by the appearance of scar tissue. In the acute phase, the tensile strength of the muscle is decreased, but within weeks it returns to normal. In the lower limbs, a muscle crossing two joints (e.g. hamstring, gastrocnemius) is more prone to develop this type of injury. Magnetic resonance imaging (MRI) can detect damage of this kind through its detection of oedema and inflammatory changes.

Complete tears can occur at the muscle belly, musculotendinous junction or bone–tendon junction, but are most common close to the musculotendinous junction. The occurrence of a complete tear can vary when comparing activated or non-activated muscle. Slightly greater force is required to disrupt activated muscle: stimulated muscle can absorb more energy than a relaxed muscle, and through this mechanism can offer more protective support. During jumping and climbing down the quadriceps contracts eccentrically, and is required to absorb energy. On the other hand fatigued or weakened muscles can absorb less energy, and therefore are more prone to injury.

Muscle damage during exercise

Repeated high-force contractions can produce fatigue in skeletal muscles, and full recovery from this can take 1 or 2 days. This delay in recovery suggests that some cell damage may have occurred. However, there is no evidence to suggest that conventional everyday exercise produces any lasting damage.

Delayed muscle soreness manifests after a period of time following exercise (24–72 hours) and is clinically distinct from the discomfort experienced during exercise itself. The muscle is then swollen, and is tender or painful. It has a reduced isometric contraction strength (by up to 50% in the short term), but recovery usually takes place over around 10 days. Although naked-eye and light microscopic appearances do not demonstrate obvious changes, electron microscopic examination does reveal structural damage in delayed muscle soreness. The changes noticed are similar to those noticed in the metabolic depletion that may result in calcium entry into muscle cells: this changes the metabolic level and stimulates phospholipase, which causes cell membrane disruption. Furthermore, the oxidation of the free fatty acids liberates free radicals that cause further damage. The resulting structural disruption in delayed muscle soreness is most prominent in fast-twitch glycolytic (type IIb) fibres. There is a disorganisation of the A and Z bands, and of the myofibrils themselves. There are also associated changes in serum biochemistry, with increased plasma levels of the intramuscular enzymes and proteins such as creatine kinase, myoglobin and lactate dehydrogenase. There is also an increased excretion of urinary hydroxy-proline. MRI of the muscle demonstrates oedema.

EFFECTS OF MUSCLE DISUSE AND IMMOBILISATION OF MUSCLE

Immobilised muscles show changes in their size and structure, and in their physiological and metabolic properties (Pette, 1980). It is interesting to note that when the lower limb is immobilised in a long leg cast with the knee extended there is more wasting of the quadriceps than of the hamstrings. This is due to the fact that the quadriceps is immobilised in the resting shortened position, but the hamstrings are immobilised in a stretched condition. The latter allows tension and this appears to promote the maintenance of protein synthesis.

In muscles that are immobilised in the resting position, the first changes that take place are atrophy of the muscle fibres with loss of protein. There is a rapid initial weight loss and a reduction in muscle strength because of the diminished cross-sectional area. The other changes that take place include a reduced capacity of the muscle for prolonged work, increased fatiguability, low energy supply, a lowering of the cytosolic pH due to the accumulation of lactic acid and a diminished ability to use fatty acid in aerobic pathways. The rates of protein synthesis are also decreased, and insulin action at the cellular level in promoting the utilisation of carbohydrate is also diminished.

Immobilisation in a stretched position stimulates the synthesis of contractile proteins, so although the fibre cross-sectional areas are decreased, increases in length can compensate to some degree for the loss of muscle volume.

Muscle cramps

Cramps occur with the muscle involved in a shortened position and frequently follow fatigue, dehydration, long activity or even sleep. The spasmodic excitation of the muscle is unlikely to arise from a spontaneous contraction of the individual fibres but most likely results from the excitation of α-motor neurones. It is now well established that cramps usually occur in fatigued dehydrated muscle following the loss of water and sodium. They are also seen in renal failure. The distressing spasmodic contraction of cramped muscles can be relieved by stretching the antagonist muscle or by stimulating the sensory nerves of the skin. Thus calf muscle cramps are relieved by extension of the knee and dorsiflexion of the ankle. After cramps, the muscle shows evidence of fasciculation and altered excitability, but lasting damage occurs only with repeated cramps in metabolically depleted muscle.

MUSCLE PAIN

Muscles have a variety of sensory nerve endings with nociceptors. These are associated with type III small myelinated and type IV small unmyelinated nerve fibres. Their freely branching unencapsulated nerve endings are abundant in the myotendinous junctions and fascial sheaths. The nociceptors are polymodal and respond to mechanical, thermal and chemical stimuli. Tissue metabolites (e.g. lactic acid, bradykinin, serotonin, histamine and potassium ions) can stimulate such muscle receptors. Stimulation of type III nerve fibres gives rise to a short-lasting immediate sensation of localised pain. Type IV nerve stimulation results in a diffuse, longer duration, dull or burning pain.

Myalgic pain

Everyday clinical practice encounters patients presenting with pain or tenderness specially in muscles around the neck and shoulder; this can occasionally be of severe intensity and be associated with muscle stiffness. There are several hypotheses that attempt to explain the source of this phenomenon. Electromyographic (EMG) investigation has suggested an increased electrical activity at the site of the maximum tenderness. It has been suggested that this tenderness is localised mostly to the point of entry of the motor nerve in the skeletal muscle. Others have suggested that a nerve root lesion at the spinal level could produce such symptoms. There is also the possibility that local ischaemia produces reflex local muscle contraction, or of residual muscle damage after coxsackie 'B' virus infection. Local injections of anaesthetic agents or applications of heat massage are used to relieve symptoms, with uncertain results. Attempts should always be made to exclude spinal root lesions in these patients.

CLINICAL ASSESSMENT OF MUSCLE FUNCTION

Clinical examination of the size of a muscle may give indications concerning its use. Muscle hypertrophy is the result of a number of muscle diseases but an apparent increase in mass may also result from connective tissue proliferation. Atrophy may follow denervation or prolonged disuse. Abnormal spontaneous activity may produce visible fasciculations. It is also possible clinically to test muscle tone and the ability of a patient to control a muscle contraction. Tests of the associated spinal reflexes should also form part of the neurological examination as these provide indications of the function of the associated sensory receptors, afferent axons, spinal cord synapses, neuromuscular transmission and muscle contraction as a whole. Clinical assessment of muscle function involves the use of simple MRC muscle power grading, measurements of grip strength and functional evaluation of motor performance. These measures are supplemented by objective investigations that include EMG and radiological evaluation by ultrasonography and MRI.

Electromyography

The electrical signals that are produced in muscle may be detected by suitable electrodes, and amplification and analysis of these signals provides useful insight into muscle function. In orthopaedic practice, the most common uses of EMG are in the study of the kinetics of motion and in the assessment of muscle function following nerve injury. The electrical activity may be recorded either by surface electrodes placed on the skin or by needle electrodes inserted into the muscle. Surface electrodes are suitable for investigating large superficial muscles, but needle electrodes can be much more specific in defining precise sites of activity.

Two parameters are most commonly studied when analysing EMG signals. The first is the averaged integrated amplitude of the signal, and the second is the frequency of motor unit firing. *Figure 7.8* shows the averaged EMG amplitudes for the erector spinae, multifidus, rectus abdominis and external oblique muscles during flexion and extension of the lumbar spine. The magnitude of the EMG signal depends on the firing frequency, but a simple relationship between EMG amplitude and muscle force does not exist as this is also influenced by the number of motor units that are recruited. Measurements of EMG activity in conjunction with particular functional activities nevertheless help enormously in determining the particular muscles that are active during a given activity, and additionally give some indication of the extent of such muscle activity. Thus, the figure clearly demonstrates the times at which particular muscle groups become active during the flexion–extension cycle.

Analysis of the frequency of muscle stimulation is useful in the study of muscle fatigue and for the diagnosis of neuromuscular disorders. In general, when a muscle is activated to a constant force, the averaged EMG amplitude increases with time, but mean frequency decreases. The latter decrease in frequency is a good indicator of muscle fatigue.

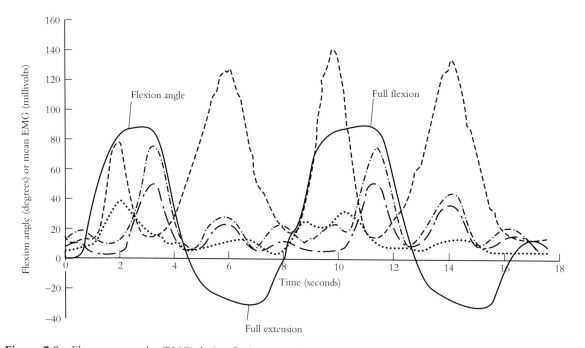

Figure 7.8 Electromyography (EMG) during flexion–extension. Integrated EMG for the erector spinae (– · – ·), multifidus (— · — -), rectus abdominis (– – –) and external oblique (· · ·) muscles during two repeats of moving from standing into full flexion and full extension. Kindly provided by Dr A McGregor and Mr H Ridha. Department of Orthopedic Surgery, Imperial College School of Medicine, London.

Ultrasonography

Ultrasonography is a valuable non-invasive dynamic investigative tool to delineate muscle morphology. As muscle strength is proportional to cross-sectional area, morphological measurements of muscle can detect muscle wasting and predict weakness.

Magnetic resonance imaging (MRI)

MRI is superior to computerised tomography and other forms of radiological investigation for visualising normal or injured muscles. The excellent cross-sectional anatomical evaluation of the skeletal muscles and surrounding tissues by MRI can detect minimal inflammatory changes more clearly than can isotope scans. Even the minimal changes induced by exercise can be identified by MRI. The changes resulting from intracellular water retention producing oedema are detected through changes in the T2 relaxation time in MRI.

DISEASES OF MUSCLE

A detailed discussion of muscle disease is beyond the scope of this chapter, and the reader is referred to more detailed sources elsewhere (for example, Walton, 1987). Muscle weakness is a frequent manifestation of muscle disease, and is generally the result of a primary defect in the muscle (myopathy) or in the nerves innervating the muscle (neuropathy). Excessive fatiguability may have several causes.

1 **Myopathies** can be either atrophic, where the fibres decrease in cross-sectional area, inflammatory, where muscle fibres are destroyed through autoimmune processes, or dystrophic, where the fibres are also destroyed often by a pathological process that can be attributed to a genetic defect. Atrophic myopathies are normally secondary to some other condition (e.g. hypothyroidism, osteomalacia, alcoholism) and are normally reversible if the underlying condition is treated. Duchenne muscular dystrophy is the most serious of the dystrophies. It is associated with defects in a gene for dystrophin, a protein found associated with the plasma membrane of muscle fibres (Emery, 1987).

2 Changes in muscle can be associated with **neurogenic** changes in three sites. Changes in the anterior horn cells occur in spinal muscular atrophies and motor neurone disease. Axonal lesions may occur as a result of peripheral nerve injury. Finally, myasthenia gravis illustrates an autoimmune process that involves the motor endplate.

3 In **metabolic** disorders increased fatiguability of muscle is normally the consequence of disorders of glycolytic metabolism (e.g. McArdle's disease, Tauri's disease) in muscle. At rest, muscle strength is frequently normal in such conditions, but function deteriorates rapidly with sustained demand.

REFERENCES

Adrian RH, Peachey LD (eds). *Handbook of Physiology. Section 10: Skeletal Muscle.* Bethesda, Maryland: American Physiological Society, 1983.

Emery AEH. *Duchenne Muscular Dystrophy.* Oxford: Clarendon Press, 1987.

Goldspink D. (ed.) *Development and Specialization of Skeletal Muscle.* Cambridge: Cambridge University Press, 1980.

Gordon AM, Huxley AF, Julian FJ. The variation in isometric tension with sarcomere length in vertebrate muscle fibres. *J Physiol* 1966; **184**: 170–192.

Huang CL-H. *Intramembrane Charge Movements in Striated Muscle.* Oxford: Clarendon Press, 1993.

Huxley AF. *Reflections on Muscle.* Princeton: Princeton University Press, 1978.

Hill AV. *First and Last Experiments on Muscle Mechanics.* Cambridge: Cambridge University Press, 1970.

Kedes LH, Stockdale FE (eds). *Cellular and Molecular Biology of Muscle Development.* New York: Alan R. Liss, 1989.

Lamb JF, Ingram CG, Johnston IA, Pitman RM. *Essential Physiology,* 2nd edn. Oxford: Blackwell Scientific, 1984.

Martonosi AN. Mechanisms of calcium release from sarcoplasmic reticulum of skeletal muscle. *Physiol Rev* 1984; **64**: 1240.

Peachey LD. The sarcoplasmic reticulum and transverse tubules of the frog's sartorius. *J Cell Biology* 1965; **25**: 209–231.

Pette D. (ed.) *Plasticity of Muscle.* New York: de Gruyter, 1980.

Reddy H, White MF. Metabolic processes. In: Glasby MA, Huang CL-H (eds) *Applied Physiology for Surgery and Critical Care.* Oxford: Butterworth–Heinemann, 1995: 93–98.

Squire JM (ed.). *Molecular Mechanisms in Muscle Contraction.* London: MacMillan, 1990.

Walton JN (ed.) *Disorders of Voluntary Muscle,* 4th edn. Edinburgh: Churchill-Livingstone, 1981.

Woledge RC, Curtin N, Homsher E. *Energetic Aspects of Muscle Contraction.* London: Academic Press, 1984.

Section II

Disorders of the Musculoskeletal System

8

Infection and Immune Responses in Prosthetic Joint Replacement

Anthony G Gristina, Thomas C Schuler and Girish Giridhar

INTRODUCTION

Infection

There are 25 million major surgical procedures performed in Europe each year, and an approximately equivalent number in the United States (Graves, 1991). All surgery involves the temporary or permanent use of biomaterials; these materials and traumatised tissues are ideal substrata for bacterial colonisation and are more readily infected by smaller microbial inoculi than are healthy tissues. Biomaterial-centred infections, regardless of the biomaterial or the tissue site, are extraordinarily resistant to antibiotic treatment. Major artificial organs (the total artificial heart), intravenous catheters, peritoneal dialysis catheters and urological devices rarely escape infection if left indwelling for any length of time (Dougherty and Simmons, 1982b; Bandyk et al, 1984; Dankert et al, 1986). Infection of a total joint or vascular prosthesis may result in reoperation, osteomyelitis, amputation, or death. Rates of death or amputation in infected abdominal and extremity vascular prostheses may exceed 30%.

The rate of infection in major surgery, even with prophylactic antibiotics, is between 0.5% and 6% (Dougherty and Simmons, 1982a,b; Muller et al, 1991). Musculoskeletal trauma with devitalisation of tissues, vascular injury, exposed bone and contamination raises infection rates from 2.5% to 15% and higher. In polytrauma, septic complications contribute to more than two-thirds of late mortality. Major spine surgery using instrumentation and bone grafts has a 7% rate of infection. And, finally, similar conditions and even higher rates of infection apply to artificial organs and allograft procedures (Dougherty and Simmons, 1982a,b; Molnar and Burke, 1983; Burwell et al, 1985; Christensen et al, 1987; Gristina et al, 1989a; Heller et al, 1992; Gristina, 1994; Karsch and Taffet, 1994).

Inflammation

Implant failure at even higher rates occurs due to a chronic continuum of inflammation, even in the absence of infection. The inflammation may be caused by cellular immune responses generated at the tissue implant interface by the presence of a biomaterial 'foreign body' surface and is amplified significantly by the wear-generated particulate biomaterial debris, as occurs in total hips and breast implants. Progress in the development and use of biomaterials and artificial organs has been delayed, therefore, by the failure of tissue integration caused by chronic inflammation secondary to biomaterial particulate debris, as well as by microbial adhesion and resistant infection.

Higher animals have not been programmed by evolution to tolerate foreign bodies or biomaterial implants.

MICROBES, TISSUES AND BIOMATERIAL SUBSTRATA

Microbial adhesion to biomaterials and damaged tissue surfaces is the first step in colonisation and infection. It is important to note that, in nature and disease, the major portion of bacterial biomass exists as microbial aggregates in a protective **biofilm slime layer**, adherent to surfaces. The biofilm resists environmental antagonists and optimises metabolism. Nutrients are concentrated at surfaces, and free energy for molecular interactions is also available.

Pathogenesis of biomaterial-centred resistant infection

At most sites of contamination, host defence systems normally eliminate transient bacterial colonisation unless: (1) the inoculum size exceeds specific threshold levels; (2) host defences are impaired; (3) tissue surfaces are traumatised; (4) a foreign body (e.g. biomaterial) is present; or (5) the tissue involved is relatively acellular or devitalised (e.g. bone, cartilage and traumatised tissues) (Gristina et al, 1985; Gristina, 1987; Voytek et al, 1988).

Artificial organs, biomaterials, devitalised tissues, bone and cartilage are essentially inanimate composites which, for pathogenic and some non-pathogenic microorganisms, resemble surfaces in nature. The interactions of these surfaces with certain bacteria may transform usually commensal organisms into virulent pathogens. The continuing presence of inanimate substrata and the biofilm mode of adherent infection results in the alteration of bacterial phenotypes for increased antibiotic resistance, the conversion of commensal organisms to slime and biofilm-protected pathogens, and thus persistent and resistant infection.

Biomaterial and devitalised or acellular tissue substrata must be removed to treat infection successfully, because they present loci for adherent biofilm-type resistant infection (*Figure 8.1*).

Features of bone, cartilage, biomaterial and traumatised tissue biofilm infection

The pathogenesis of biomaterial–foreign body-centred or damaged tissue–biofilm infection can best be understood as a unique process by cataloguing its common features:

- Adhesive biofilm-forming bacterial colonisation of substrata
- A biomaterial, damaged tissue, or relatively acellular tissue substratum (bone or cartilage)
- Smaller bacterial inoculi capable of initiating an infection
- Bacterial resistance to host defence mechanisms and antibiotic therapy
- The presence of characteristic bacteria such as *Staphylococcus aureus*, *S. epidermidis* and *Pseudomonas aeruginosa*

- The transformation of non-pathogens or opportunistic pathogens into virulent organisms by the presence of a biomaterial substratum
- Infections are frequently polymicrobial
- Related specificity of phenomena (biomaterial, organisms, host location)
- Persistence of infection until implant (substratum) removal
- The presence of inflammation, tissue cell damage and necrosis at the implant–tissue interface (the immuno-incompetent fibroinflammatory zone)
- Absence of tissue integration at the biomaterial interface
- Incompetence of host cellular and humoral immune responses secondary to biomaterial and microbial effects

Biomaterials

Biomaterials are not biologically inert, although they are inanimate and reasonably stable. At an atomic level, however, they are physically and chemically active at their surfaces, and may directly modulate molecular events such as cellular adhesion, integration, inflammatory and immune responses, receptor–ligand interactions, weak and strong chemical forces, and thermodynamic interactions. An ideal biomaterial of the future should be appropriately bioreactive and should have, in addition to desired architectural, mechanical and functional properties, surface properties designed to interact favourably with the host environment. That is, depending on the tissue systems involved, a biomaterial surface may be designed to encourage or discourage eukaryotic cell and matrix protein adhesion.

MOLECULAR MECHANISMS OF MICROBIAL ADHESION

Surface adhesion of bacteria, and to some extent of tissue cells, is dependent on the general and relatively long-range (15–100 nm) and short-range (< 15 nm) physical characteristics of the bacterium (cell), the fluid interface and the substratum. Ultimately, adhesion to biomaterial surfaces is based on time-dependent specific and non-specific adhesion–receptor interactions, in addition to charge and physical forces (Bayston and Penny, 1972; Fletcher, 1980; Gibbons and van Houte, 1980; Gibbons et al, 1985; Gristina, 1987).

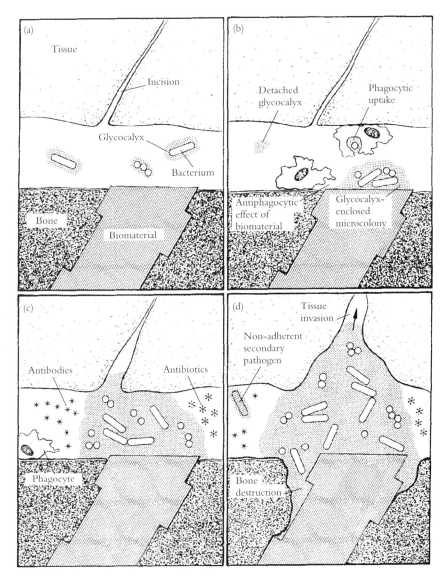

Figure 8.1   Diagrammatic evolution of an infection associated with a prosthetic biomaterial. (a) Initially, bacteria are introduced into the wound. (b) They express their natural tendency to adhere to an inert surface, on which they are protected by the antiphagocytic effect of the biomaterial and on which they form as microcolonies within a biofilm which protects them from phagocytic uptake and from non-immune antibacterial serum factors. (c) When the bacterial microcolony has burgeoned to a greater size, the ion-exchange function of its glycocalyx affords a measure of protection from antibiotics and appears to protect the bacteria from bactericidal and opsonising antibodies. (d) In the later stages of infection, the pathogens may cause destruction of bone and other tissue changes, and the colonies may shed secondary pathogens which, being for some reason less adhesive, are not necessarily representative in number, type or pathogenicity of the adhesive colonies, and may therefore confuse the diagnostic picture by dominating aspirates and other routine microbiological samples. From Gristina and Costerton (1984), with permission.

All surfaces exposed in a biological environment spontaneously acquire a conditioning film of glycoproteins such as albumin, collagen, fibronectin and fibrinogen. Molecular coatings of matrix proteins and tissue environmental debris are undoubtedly not confluent, or a consistent monolayer. Colloidal science suggests that particles of bacterial size initially attach reversibly to surfaces by van der Waals' forces and charge-related

interactions. Hydrophobic microbial and biomaterial surface components have also been demonstrated, and play a
role in more secure adhesion. The attractive magnitude of
hydrophobic interactions usually exceeds forces of repul-
sion at nanometre distances. In addition, many microorganisms possess specific outer cellular or extracapsular
polysaccharides and glycoprotein components (glycoca-

lyx, slime, adhesions, fimbriae) that may function in non-
specific and specific adhesion to the bare biomaterial
surface or to surface-linked matrix proteins (*Figure 8.2*).

   We have suggested that microorganisms essentially
attach and adhere to surfaces by means of one or more of
three types of cell-to-surface interactions. **Class 1** interactions are physical forces involving particle charge, van

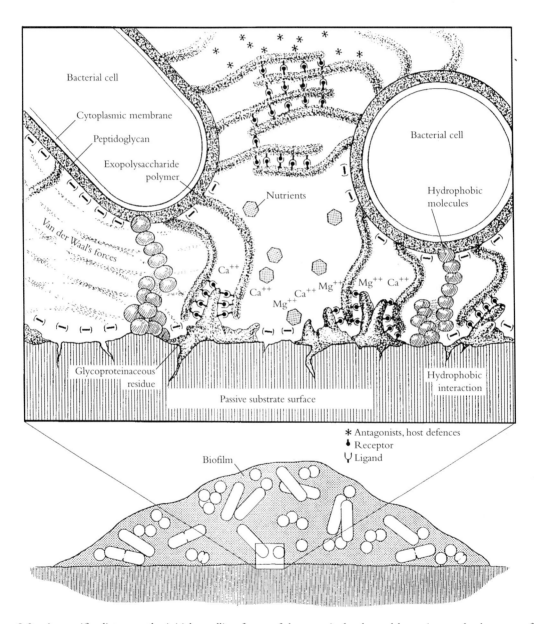

Figure 8.2   At specific distances, the initial repelling forces of the negatively charged bacterium and substrate surface are
overcome by attracting van der Waal's forces. There are also hydrophobic interactions between molecules (class I). Under
appropriate conditions, an extensive exopolysaccharide polymer develops (class II), facilitating ligand–receptor interactions
(class III) and bacterial attachment and adhesion to the substrate. From Gristina (1987), with permission.

der Waals' forces and hydrophobic interactions (the general, initial and sometimes reversible attachment of many organisms to biomaterial surfaces). **Class 2** involves non-specific chemical binding to exposed biomaterial or tissue substratum surfaces or to other bacteria by means of covalent, polar or hydrogen bonding interactions not involving receptor ligand configurations. Examples are the slime polysaccharide chemical binding to available sites on tissue, or matrix protein molecules at the biomaterial surface or to available atomic binding sites directly on the biomaterial surface (Gristina, 1987, 1994). **Class 3** involves specific bacterial receptor to surface protein ligand interactions as caused by bacterial receptor surface molecules and respective protein ligand or lectin molecules (an example would be fibronectin or fibrinogen molecules already adherent to the biomaterial surface). The latter mechanisms represent a portion of the evolved strategies of symbiotic and pathogenic organisms (e.g. *S. aureus* binding to collagen fibrils in osteomyelitis and to articular cartilage in intra-articular sepsis, or to conditioning films of matrix proteins on biomaterials) (Gristina, 1994).

Extracellular polymers: the glycocalyx 'slime' and biofilm

Biofilm

Shortly after attachment and adhesion (3–4 hours or less), as bacterial growth and propagation accelerate and if colony conditions are optimal, extracellular polysaccharide polymers are produced. Exopolymers enhance adhesion to surfaces and function in the co-aggregation of daughter cells or cells of other microbial species in consortial formation and pathogenically in polymicrobial infection. The production of polysaccharides and their function varies with the species, growth phase and nutrient conditions (*Figure 8.2*).

The biofilm slime matrix formed by the exopolysaccharide polymers not only serves as an adhesive mechanism but also appears to be related to virulence. Biofilm has been shown to confer resistance to host defence mechanisms by steric interference with phagocytosis, the muting of antigen presentation, and by impeding the effective penetration or function of antibiotics, antibodies and phagocytic cells. Accumulated biofilm and organisms may eventually fragment secondary to haemodynamic forces, trauma or friction, and detach in bacterial showers

forming distant abscesses. Pathogens present in biofilm represent a source of inoculum and can cause septic haematogenous emboli, distant seeding, secondary infection, exotoxin production and septic shock (Bayston and Penny, 1972; Govan, 1975; Baltimore and Mitchell, 1980; Beachy, 1981; Gristina and Costerton, 1984; Gristina et al, 1985, 1987).

Biofilm and antibiotic resistance

Studies have indicated that, as organisms adhere to biomaterials in a biofilm, their resistance to antibiotics increases and that this response is biomaterial specific (Gristina et al, 1989a,b, 1994a). Organisms adhering to polymers are extremely resistant to antibiotic treatment compared with their susceptibility in suspension. Resistance to antibiotic therapy is increased to a lesser extent on metal surfaces. Recent reports have discounted a biofilm diffusion barrier to antibiotics and have indicated that bacteria within isolated regions of biofilm have decreased metabolic rates and undergo phenotypic changes that may influence resistance and virulence. Studies have demonstrated, however, that 100-fold higher levels of antibiotics are required to kill surface-adherent bacteria, even if they are not slime biofilm producers (Gristina et al, 1989).

'The race for the surface': microbial adhesion versus tissue integration

The fate of an implant, biomaterial, damaged tissue or bone graft surface may be conceptualised as a 'race for the surface' between macromolecules, bacteria and tissue cells. Adhesive or integrative phenomena for bacteria or tissue cells, respectively, are interrelated and based on similar molecular mechanisms. Organic and ionic adsorbates and the atomic nature of surfaces result in a highly altered, reactive interface. When tissue cells (for example, in repair of damaged bone, or the integration of a total joint implant surface to bone) establish a secure bond at a surface, bacteria are confronted by living, integrated cells which are resistant to bacterial colonisation through intact cell membranes, extracapsular polysaccharides and functioning host defence mechanisms (Gristina et al, 1990).

However, bacteria are relatively ubiquitous in biological environments and may be the first to colonise a surface, resulting in infection and preventing tissue integration and repair. Bacterial cells, as evolved by

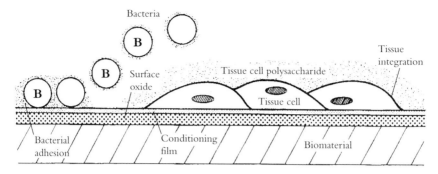

Figure 8.3 The race for the surface. Upon insertion, the outer atomic layers of a biomaterial surface interact instantly with the juxtaposed biological environment. Macromolecules, bacteria and tissue cells compete for surface domains at this reactive interface. Bacteria have the right of eminent domain. Tissue cell integration would tend to prevent bacterial adhesion and infection. From Gristina (1987), with permission.

natural selection, colonise generally inanimate substrata in nature. For most implant or damaged tissue surfaces, the colonisation potential by bacteria is higher than that of tissue cells, and tissue cells are generally unable to displace pioneer bacterial colonies. Therefore, biomaterial, compromised tissue surfaces, or exposed dead bone, represent the 'eminent domain', primarily of organic and inorganic molecules, and of bacteria rather than tissue cells (Gristina et al, 1988) (*Figure 8.3*).

In summary, bacteria have been programmed by evolution for integration to biomaterials. The race for the surface is a crucial competition between microbes, tissue cells and matrix proteins for available biomaterial, outer atomic layer, binding sites. The atomic composition of the biomaterial surface is critical, and the initial deposition of matrix proteins or ionic species may direct future events in which bacteria have a primitive and aggressive advantage (Gristina et al, 1994b).

BIOMATERIALS AND THE IMMUNE SYSTEM

Surgery and the implantation of biomaterials and tissue transplants both stimulate and disrupt host defence and immune mechanisms. Biomaterial surfaces and their wear-generated particulate debris increase susceptibility to infection, active host defences and stimulate release of inflammatory mediators, cytokines, oxygen radicals, enzymes and metalloproteinases. These actions lead to tissue protein damage and chronic local inflammation,

fibrosis, osteolysis and implant failure, as for breast implants, total joints and major vascular devices. Tissue damage may be further aggravated by bacterial activities and by their exotoxins. Bacterial exopolysaccharide slime and biomaterial particulates pre-empt macrophage oxidative responses (Zimmerli et al, 1982, 1984; Sugerman and Young, 1984; Gristina et al, 1989, 1991).

The immuno-incompetent fibro-inflammatory zone (cell-mediated immunity, macrophages and wear particles)

Billions of phagocytosable particulates in submicron to multiple micron sizes are derived from components of biomaterial implants such as silicone, high-density polyethylene, methylmethacrylate and metal alloys (see Chapter 16). The presence of biomaterial particles or surfaces tends to create an immuno-incompetent fibro-inflammatory zone at the implant tissue interface, within which chronic inflammation persists and where macrophage oxidative and killing potential is exhausted. Bacteria may find receptive ligands and nutrients for proliferation, and healthy tissue cells in adjacent areas are damaged and unable to integrate with the biomaterial surface (*Figure 8.4*). In part, this zone of chronic inflammation is the result of the natural tendency for local and recruited macrophages to attempt to phagocytose and digest the particulate debris, which is chemically resistant to enzymatic processes. In effect, this process produces cycling inflammation, protein denaturisation, tissue destruction and device failure, mediated by cellular, cytokine and

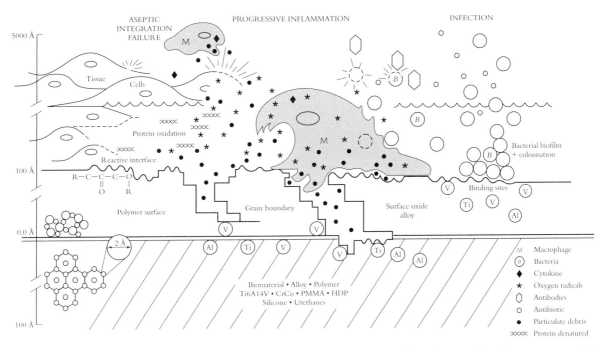

Figure 8.4   The immuno-incompetent fibro-inflammatory zone. To a greater or lesser degree, all implants are surrounded by an inflammatory zone. Macrophages encounter particulate debris at a biomaterial surface. Reactive oxygen intermediates and cytokines are released. The continuing activation of neutrophils and macrophages results in oxidative tissue damage and microbicidal incompetence, integration failure, immune exhaustion and, in the presence of bacteria, biofilm production. Antibiotics and host defences are less effective against biofilm-coated bacteria. Prosthetic tissue interface failure may then occur by aseptic chronic inflammation or by increased susceptibility to infection. From Gristina (1994), with permission.

enzymatic mechanisms. An enlarging immunoincompetent zone develops about implants, which features tissue damage and increased susceptibility to infection, and septic or aseptic failure of the implant, as exemplified by fibrosis about breast implants and osteolysis at the interface of total joint replacements, or by resistant infection about biomaterial devices (the artificial heart, vascular grafts, catheters and orthopaedic devices) (Bandyk et al, 1984) (*Figures 8.4* and *8.5*).

IMMUNITY AND THE IMMUNE SYSTEM

Higher animals have established very effective immune defence mechanisms against microbes. Invading bacteria are rapidly identified, via complement and immunoglobulin (natural antibodies), phagocytosed and destroyed by neutrophils and macrophages. Host immune responses are usually initiated after bacteria have attached to tissues or implants and begin to develop mechanisms to resist host defences (biofilm, antigen masking, replication, toxins). The first events (within a few hours) usually involve the migration of polymorphonuclear phagocytes to sites of bacterial colonisation. If immunoglobulins specific for the microorganisms also arrive at the wound site in adequate concentration, the bacteria will be opsonised and, in simple wounds, may be phagocytosed and killed. If bacteria continue to multiply and become shielded in biofilm, infection can develop. Within a few hours (peak activity at 3–4 days), macrophages are deployed to the site of infection and attempt to phagocytose the microorganisms. Specific antibodies (immunoglobulins) with opsonic (antibacterial) activity are also required by macrophages for phagocytosis and killing.

During the early period (1–4 days), macrophages encounter and process antigens derived from the infecting bacteria, and trigger multiplication of T and B lymphocytes (defence cells), which results in the synthesis of immunoglobulins specific for the surface antigens (telltale bacterial molecules) of the invading microorganisms.

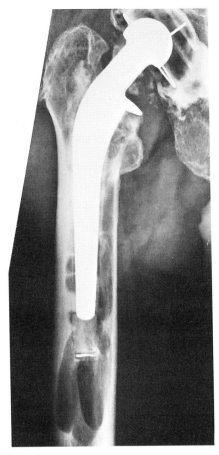

Figure 8.5 Radiograph of total hip prosthesis demonstrates widening peri-implant zone of osteolysis and loosening, the immuno-incompetent fibro-inflammatory zone. Reprinted with permission of Charles Engh, Anderson Orthopedic Clinic, Arlington, Virginia, USA. From Gristina (1994).

These events require at least 7–21 days. During the time required for peak immune activities, serious infection may become established, especially in traumatised tissues, biomaterial implants and immunocompromised patients. The presence of tissue damage (such as burns), foreign bodies (such as biomaterials) and bacterial biofilm significantly diminishes effective immune responses.

Human immune responses may be conceptualised as: (a) cell-mediated immune responses which are immediate, non-specific and non-memory based (e.g. macrophages and neutrophils rapidly respond to small particles such as invading bacteria and viruses by phagocytosis and oxidative or enzymatic destruction of the organism): and (b) humoral immune responses, which are memory-

based, antigen-specific, antibody responses and are delayed (7–21 days). The immunoglobulin (IgG, IgM, IgA, etc.) classes are composed of groups of antibodies perfectly designed by the immune system for high-affinity antimicrobial, antiviral and antitumour activity.

Immunotherapy

As host defence mechanisms have co-evolved with microbial virulence factors, it has seemed likely that amplified and directed natural immunotherapeutic strategies might provide effective counter-measures to the emerging problems of biomaterial-centred and resistant infections.

We have proposed two novel strategies for infection prophylaxis and treatment, based on the amplification, timing, focusing and targeting of natural host immune responses. They are (1) cell-mediated immune response amplification and (2) passive local immunotherapy.

Cell-mediated immune amplification

Although the chronic presence of large numbers of non-biodegradable particulate debris particles adjacent to the implant generates cycling destructive inflammation and implant failure, the short-term presence of phagocytosable (microbe sized) biodegradable particles is the first step in the upregulation of non-specific cell-mediated immunity for enhanced microbicidal activity (Corradin et al, 1991; Hsieh et al, 1993; Myrvik et al, 1993). Significantly, in studying these responses, we have discovered that the intratracheal or intravenous administration of both non-antigenic and antigenic particulates rapidly (1–3 days) upregulates or primes rabbit alveolar macrophages for a 100-fold increase in oxidative response when subsequently elicited by phagocytosed bacteria (Myrvik et al, 1993). This priming is non-specific and declines by 1 week after injection, indicating that specific antigen expanded T-cell clonal and memory-based immunity are not involved (Myrvik et al, 1993).

The effects have been observed in animal models to have a 7-day duration, and peak at 3 days for maximum bactericidal impact. In preclinical trials, immuno-amplified rabbits were observed to be highly resistant to closed abscess intradermal infection due to *S. aureus* and *P. aeruginosa*. Immune-amplified animals remained healthy without signs of adverse side-effects, whereas non-treated control animals developed major infections. Preliminary studies indicate that the mechanism of immune amplification is cell mediated, involving neutrophils, macrophages, T helper 1 cells and natural killer (NK) cells, and involves a cytokine cascade in which interleukin (IL) 12 is the likely initiator cytokine and interferon (IFN) γ is the effector cytokine:

Particles $\rightarrow$ macrophage $\rightarrow$ IL-12 $\rightarrow$ $T_H 1$ cells
$+$ NK cells $\rightarrow$ IFN-γ $\rightarrow$ macrophage priming and activation

This particle-dependent and, in part, non-receptor-mediated mechanism is believed to represent the response of primitive invertebrate immune cells (coloemocytes) to particles and microbes conserved by evolution.

This novel system upregulates macrophage and possibly neutrophil microbicidal activity, and amplifies cellular immunity non-specifically and broadly. It could be administered in anticipation of exposure to infectious agents or surgery, and may represent an effective prophylaxis or pretreatment (independent of antibiotic resistance) to prevent sepsis associated with wounds, biomaterials and disease (Giridhar et al, 1994, 1995a).

Passive local immunotherapy

Gristina and co-workers have developed novel prophylactic methods and compositions for the prevention of wound infection secondary to trauma, burns, surgery and biomaterials. Microbes are preopsonised locally with a full repertoire of immunoglobulins to prevent microbial adhesion and colonisation of tissue surfaces and biomaterials. By preventing adhesion to surfaces and by opsonising bacteria on arrival or shortly afterwards, bacteria are identified, made vulnerable and targeted for neutrophil and macrophage phagocytosis while numbers are low. Reproduction, release of toxins, destruction of tissue and formation of protective biofilms are all blocked. This process also assists antibiotic strategies as bacteria are more vulnerable before attachment to surfaces.

The use of applied coating concentrates of globulins to tissue, mucosal and biomaterial surfaces allows high dosages, including IgG, IgA and IgM, to be delivered directly to the wound. IgA and IgM components may therefore be included as needed without risk of side-effects. IgA specifically blocks bacterial adherence and neutralises viruses. Macrophages and complement arrive naturally at wound sites and are available to respond to the bacteria opsonised by the locally administered polyvalent globulins. The generation of immune complexes

and inflammatory mediators, as occurs with high intravenous doses of globulin preparations, is diminished or prevented by local delivery.

In summary, wound or biomaterial surface pretreatment, at time of surgery or shortly after trauma, would allow the effective use of a full repertoire of globulins including IgG, IgA and IgM, at high concentrations without side-effects before microbial colonisation and infection begin.

Gristina's team has used pooled human immunoglobulins (IgG) containing antibodies to contemporary pathogenic clinical isolates of *S. aureus* and other microbes as passive local immunotherapy to prevent bacterial infection in a closed abscess rabbit model. The closed abscess was standardised by intradermal injection with 10^6 colony-forming units of bacteria suspended in $100\,\mu l$ saline, which produced characteristic lesions 1 day after infection. Nutrient agar cultures of lesions excised from the infection sites showed numerous bacterial colonies. The lesions treated with locally injected human IgG (0.5 mg per site) demonstrated considerably reduced severity of infection in challenges by four pathogenic clinical isolates of *S. aureus*, and produced fewer bacterial colonies on nutrient media. Local injection of IgG also prevented polymicrobial (two clinical isolates of *S. aureus* injected at the same site) infection in the model. In additional studies, human IgG effectively prevented foreign body-associated infection (titanium wire implant). Similar studies utilising hyperimmune rabbit antiserum in the rabbit model sterilised the bacterial challenge (*S. aureus* and *P. aeruginosa*). These results suggest that the prophylactic, direct, local application of IgG to wound and biomaterial surfaces opsonises contaminating bacteria before microbial adhesion and biofilm formation, and may be utilised to prevent antibiotic-resistant, surgical and biomaterial implant infections (Giridhar et al, 1995b).

FUTURE THERAPEUTIC STRATEGIES

The key to the 'race for the surface' is the programming of surfaces at an atomic scale to eliminate particulate debris and to discourage cellular hyperinflammatory responses. If host cellular immune responses could be normalised, then the tendency to chronic inflammation, immunoincompetence and resistant bacterial infection would be eliminated. The key cell in the process of integration and inflammation is the macrophage. Biomaterials that encourage appropriate macrophage activity or a normalised healing and implant integration, rather than the chronic activation of cellular immune responses, should be most resistant to infection, rejection and failure (Gristina, 1994). Normalisation of macrophage response allows appropriate antibacterial activities, healing and integration. Microbial adhesion and infection can best be prevented by encouraging integration of tissue cells (the race for the surface) and the development of appropriate antibodies, vaccines and blocking analogues.

It is disappointing that the search for surface treatments to prevent microbial adhesion has not yet yielded effective coatings to prevent microbial adhesion or to encourage tissue integration. Insight and discovery emerge from the observation that, whilst evolution has granted microbes eminent domain over all known surfaces, there has been concomitant evolution of effective antimicrobial mechanisms in higher creatures from which therapeutic strategies may be developed.

EPILOGUE

All implants and all devitalised tissues are foreign bodies and their extrusion, driven by inflammatory responses, macrophage activation and cytokine cascades, is programmed by evolution. If extrusion is impossible and if the biomaterial surface area, or the quantity of implant debris, is sufficient, then a chronic and destructive hyperinflammatory response is the result. At the immuno-incompetent inflammatory interface, host tissues are also 1000-fold more vulnerable to infection. Biomaterial-generated inflammation or infection tends to be irreversible and will ultimately result in implant fibrosis, failure or systemic sepsis.

Surfaces of the future should be programmed at an atomic scale, specifically for a 'normalised' host matrix protein response and 'normalised' cell-mediated immune responses. 'Programmed biochip surfaces' should be designed to be essentially invisible to bacteria and to allow tissue integration, normalised host defence and antibiotic activity. The control of cell-mediated immunity is the critical factor in the race for the surface.

REFERENCES

Baltimore RS, Mitchell M. Immunologic investigations of mucoid strains of *Pseudomonas aeruginosa*: comparison of susceptibility to opsonic antibody in mucoid and nonmucoid strains. *J Infect Dis* 1980; **141**: 238–247.

Bandyk DR, Berni GA, Thiele BL et al. Aorta femoral graft infection due to *Staphylococcus epidermidis*. *Arch Surg* 1984; **119**: 102–108.

Bayston R, Penny PR. Excessive production of mucoid substances in *Staphylococcus* SIIA: a possible factor in colonization of Holter shunts. *Dev Med Child Neurol* 1972; **14**: 25–28.

Beachy EH. Bacterial adherence: adhesion–receptor interactions mediating the attachment of bacteria to mucosal surfaces. *Infect Dis* 1981; **143**: 325–345.

Burwell RG, Friedlaender GE, Mankin HJ. Current perspectives and further directions: The 1983 Invitational Conference on Osteochondral Allografts. *Clin Orthop* 1985; **197**: 141–157.

Christensen GD, Baddour LM, Simpson A. Phenotypic variation of *Staphylococcus epidermidis* slime production *in vitro* and *in vivo*. *Infect Immun* 1987; **55**: 2870–2877.

Corradin SB, Buchmuller-Rouiller Y, Mauel J. Phagocytosis enhances murine macrophage activation by interferon-γ and tumor necrosis factor-α. *Eur J Immunol* 1991; **21**: 2553–2558.

Dankert J, Hogt AH, Feigen J. Biomedical polymers: bacterial adhesion, colonization and infection. *CRC Crit Rev Biocompat* 1986; **1**: 219–301.

Dougherty SH, Simmons RL. Infections in bionic man: the pathobiology of infections in prosthetic devices, Part II. *Curr Probl Surg* 1982b; **19**: 265–319.

Dougherty SH, Simmons RL. Infections in bionic man: the pathobiology of infections in prosthetic devices, Part I. *Curr Probl Surg* 1982a; **19**: 221–264.

Fletcher M. Adherence of marine microorganisms to smooth surfaces. In: Beachey EF (ed.) *Bacterial Adherence: Receptors and Recognition*, series B, Vol. 6. London: Chapman and Hall, 1980: 345–374.

Gibbons RJ, van Houte J. Bacterial adherence and the formation of dental plaques. In: Beachey EH (ed.) *Molecular Mechanisms of Microbial Adhesion*, series B, Vol. 6. London: Chapman and Hall, 1980: 63–104.

Gibbons RJ, Etherden I, Moreno EC. Contribution of stereochemical interactions in the adhesion of *Streptococcus sanguin* C5 to experimental pellicles. *J Dent Res* 1985; **64**: 96–101.

Giridhar G, Shibata Y, Kreger AS, Myrvik QN, Gristina AG. A novel system of particle-induced immune augmentation to prevent bacterial infection. 30th National Meeting of the Society for Leukocyte Biology. *J Leukoc Biol Suppl* 1994: 33 (abstract).

Giridhar G, Shibata Y, Kreger AS, Myrvik QN, Gristina AG. Cell mediated immune response amplification for the prevention of biomaterials-associated bacterial infection. *Transactions of the 21st Annual Meeting of the Society for Biomaterials* 1995a; **18**: 195.

Giridhar G, Shibata Y, Kreger AS, Gristina AG. Passive local immunotherapy: *in situ* human immunoglobulins to prevent bacterial infections in a closed abscess rabbit model. 31st

National Meeting of the Society for Leukocyte Biology: Host Defence Against Infections and Cancer. 1995b: 26 (abstract).

Govan JRWW. Mucoid strains of *Pseudomonas aeruginosa*: the influence of culture medium on the stability of mucus production. *J Med Microbiol* 1975; **8**: 513–522.

Graves EJ. Detailed diagnosis and procedures, National Hospital Discharge Survey 1989. National Center for Health Sciences. *Vital Health Stat* 1991; **13**: 108.

Gristina AG, Naylor PT, Myrvik QN. Mechanisms of musculoskeletal sepsis. *Orthop Clin North Am* 1991; **22**: 363–371.

Gristina AG, Webb LX, Barth E. Microbial adhesion, biomaterials and man. In: Coombs R, Fitzgerald R (eds) *Infection in the Orthopaedic Patient*. London: Butterworths, 1989a: 30–42.

Gristina AG. Implant failure and the immuno-incompetent fibro-inflammatory zone. *Clin Orthop* 1994; **298**: 106–118.

Gristina AG, Oga M, Webb LX, Hobgood C. Bacterial colonization in the pathogenesis of osteomyelitis. *Science* 1985; **228**: 990–993.

Gristina AG. Biomaterial-centered infection: microbial adhesion versus tissue integration. *Science* 1987; **237**: 1588–1595.

Gristina AG, Costerton JW. Bacterial adherence and the glycocalyx and their role in musculoskeletal infection. *Orthop Clin North Am* 1984; **15**: 517–535.

Gristina AG, Hobgood CD, Barth E. Biomaterial specificity, molecular mechanisms and clinical relevance of *S. epidermidis* and *S. aureus* infections in surgery. In: Pulverer G, Quie PPG, Peters G (eds) *Pathogenicity and Clinical Significance of Coagulase-Negative Staphylococci*. Stuttgart: Gustav Fischer, 1987: 143–157.

Gristina AG, Giridhar G, Gabriel BL, Naylor PT, Myrvik QN. Cell biology and molecular mechanisms in artificial device infections. *Int J Artif Organs* 1994a; **16**: 755–764.

Gristina AG, Jennings RA, Naylor PT, Myrvik QN, Barth E, Webb LX. Comparative *in vitro* antibiotic resistance of surface colonizing coagulase-negative staphylococci. *Antimicrob Agents Chemother* 1989b; **33**: 813–816.

Gristina AG, Naylor PT, Myrvik QN. Musculoskeletal infection, microbial adhesion, and antibiotic resistance. *Infect Dis Clin North Am* 1990; **4**: 391–406.

Gristina AG, Dobbins JJ, Giammara B, Lewis JC, DeVries WC.

Biomaterial-centered sepsis and the total artificial heart. *JAMA* 1988; **259**: 870–874.

Gristina AG, Giridhar G, Myrvik QN. Bacteria and biomaterials. In: Greco RS (ed.) *Implantation Biology: The Host Response and Biomedical Devices*. Boca Raton: CRC Press, 1994b: 131–148.

Heller JG, Whitecloud TS III, Butler JC et al. Complications of spinal surgery. In: Rothman RH, Simeone FA (eds) *The Spine*, Vol. II. Philadelphia: WB Saunders, 1992: 1817–1837.

Hsieh CS, Macatonia SE, Tripp CS, Wolf SF, O'Garra A, Myrphy KM. Development of T_H1 CD4$^+$ through IL-12 produced by *Listeria*-induced macrophages. *Science* 1993; **260**: 547–549.

Karsch R, Taffet R. Infection in open tibial fractures. *Orthop Trans* 1994; **18**: 903 (abstract).

Masur H, Johnson WD Jr. Prosthetic valve endocarditis. *J Thorac Cardiovasc Surg* 1980; **80**: 31.

Mears DC. *Materials and Orthopedic Surgery*. Baltimore: Williams and Wilkins, 1979.

Molnar JA, Burke JF. Prevention and management of infection in trauma. *World J Surg* 1983; **7**: 158–163.

Muller E, Takeda S, Goldmann D, Pier G. Blood proteins do not promote adherence of coagulase-negative staphylococci to biomaterials. *Infect Immun* 1991; **59**: 3323.

Myrvik QN, Gristina AG, Giridhar G, Hayakawa H. Particle-induced *in vivo* priming of alveolar macrophages for enhanced oxidative responses: a novel system of cellular immune augmentation. *J Leukoc Biol* 1993; **54**: 439–443.

Sugarman B, Musher D. Adherence of bacteria to suture materials. *Proc Soc Exp Biol Med* 1981; **167**: 156–160.

Sugarman B. *In vitro* adherence of bacteria to prosthetic vascular grafts. *Infection* 1982; **10**: 9–14.

Sugerman B, Young EJ (eds). *Infections Associated with Prosthetic Devices*. Boca Raton, Florida: CRC Press, 1984.

Voytek A, Gristina AG, Barth E et al. Staphylococcal adhesion to collagen in intra-articular sepsis. *Biomaterials* 1988; **9**: 107–110.

Zimmerli W, Lew PD, Waldvogel FA. Pathogenesis of foreign body infections: evidence for a local granulocyte defect. *J Clin Invest* 1984; **73**: 1191–1200.

Zimmerli W, Lew PD, Waldvogel FA. Pathogenesis of foreign body infections: description and characteristics of an animal model. *J Infect Dis* 1982; **146**: 106–118.

9

The Biology of Fracture Repair

Allen E Goodship, Timothy J Lawes and Luise Harrison

INTRODUCTION

Bone, both as a tissue and an organ, fulfils a number of roles, and these are often divided into mechanical and biological. The major mechanical role of the skeleton is to provide structural support for the body, whereas the predominant biological role is frequently given as being the reservoir for calcium and associated control of calcium homoeostasis. In fact, it is difficult to separate the two traditional roles, because the biological and mechanical aspects of the living skeleton are inseparable under normal circumstances.

The bones of the skeleton also provide a system of strong levers upon which muscles act to produce movement of skeletal segments. In addition to the axial compression of the bones from gravitational loading, muscles induce bending and torsional moments in the diaphyses of the long bones with predominantly compressive forces at the metaphyses and epiphyses. The mechanical requirements are reflected in the morphology of the individual bones. For example, the long bones comprise a tubular shaft with cortex forming the walls of the tube and the medullary cavity, containing marrow and fat, forming the core of the tube.

The overall diameter and cortical thickness are related to the strength of the bone in bending and torsion. Each individual bone is loaded in a particular manner that will result in specific axes of deformation. In bending one cortex will be in tension and the opposite cortex in compression. In many bones, such as the tibia and femur (*Figure 9.1*) there is a considerable torsional component of loading and in this situation the tension axis is at approximately 45° to the longitudinal axis of the bone (Goodship, 1992). The relevance of the pattern of loading of the long bone diaphysis is related to the optimal method of fracture fixation. For example, the use of internal fixation with plates is best applied to bones loaded predominantly in bending, with a tension axis aligned to the longitudinal axis of the bone, the plate being applied on the tension surface aligned with the tension axis.

At the extremities of the long bones or in short bones the bone is loaded in compression and the structure comprises a thin cortical shell supported by an internal mesh of cancellous bone. The plates and struts of the

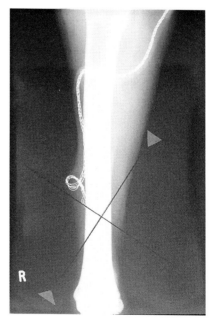

Figure 9.1 Radiograph of ovine tibia with rosette strain gauge attached to diaphysis showing principal tensile strain at approximately 40° to long axis of the bone. Strain data from the tibia show a high degree of torsional deformation during locomotion.

cancellous bone are arranged in a strategic manner; the solid elements are aligned with the principal trajectories of tensile and compressive stresses (*Figure 9.2*).

Unlike inert supporting structures such as bridges, where the mechanical demands together with an appropriate safety margin form the design specification, the skeleton must have the capacity to adapt its architecture to accommodate changes in loading demands associated with different levels of activity throughout life, a process termed functional adaptation. In addition, the skeleton has to maintain its integrity over long periods of cyclical loading, which will induce fatigue damage that, without repair, would accumulate and lead to a catastrophic failure of the structure (i.e. a fatigue fracture of the complete bone).

The mechanical integrity of the skeleton is achieved and maintained by biological processes in which the removal and deposition of bone are the prime means of both repair of micro-damage and adjustment of tissue and organ architecture. These biological processes are termed modelling and remodelling. In both cases the sequence of events is similar, namely the activation of the bone-resorbing cells, osteoclasts, followed by bone removal then bone formation by the osteoblasts. If the removal and formation of tissue occur at different sites at the same time, the gross morphology of the bone is changed and the process is termed 'modelling'. If, however, the removal of bone is followed by formation at a later time but at the same site, the process is known as remodelling, as is seen in the formation of a secondary osteon (*Figure 9.3*).

The initial stimulus for these two processes may be mechanical or hormonal (Lanyon, 1994). In response to mechanical changes it is now thought that the osteocyte is an important cell in the coordinated change in skeletal architecture; the osteoblast is thought to be the cell that allows the resorbing cells access to the bone surface. Evidence of repair of micro-damage by internal remodelling can be seen by the presence of secondary osteons within the bone cortex.

Changes in mechanical loading in terms of magnitude or direction on a repeated basis will act as a stimulus for an adaptive response (Rubin and Lanyon, 1987); sudden single overload events may be accommodated without gross fracture by virtue of the inbuilt safety factors. However, load levels that exceed the safety factor will result in fracture of the bone. The main consequence of fracture is a reduced functional loading of the limb. The application of a device to stabilise the fracture will further reduce the load carried by the bone and decrease the resulting deformation of the bone tissue. Thus the mechanical stimulus for bone formation is diminished, leading to a drive to reduce bone mass at a time when an osteogenic stimulus is required.

The mechanical conditions at the fracture site will influence the pattern and rate of repair. There are

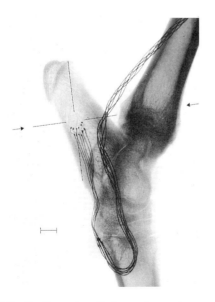

Figure 9.2   Radiograph of the ovine calcaneus with rosette strain gauge attached to lateral cortex. Principal tensile strain outlined with underlying plantar trabecular arcade. From Lanyon (1973).

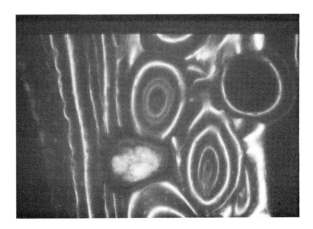

Figure 9.3   Transverse section of ovine radius demonstrating secondary osteonal remodelling of the primary bone structure. This is similar to the osteonal remodelling in 'direct' fracture repair. Normally, this remodelling may be associated with repair of micro-damage within the cortex.

predominant patterns of bone repair termed direct (primary) and indirect (secondary) bone healing. Following fracture, bone shows a remarkable ability to mount a repair process that not only restores mechanical integrity but also restores the anatomical configuration with little or no evidence of scar tissue, as would be seen following injury in other musculoskeletal tissues. It is said that high-velocity fractures cleave the microstructural elements of bone such as secondary osteons, whereas in low-velocity fractures the fracture line passes around such structures. Initially, fracture compromises the functional use of a limb or part of the skeleton; as healing progresses, function is gradually regained. The relationship between the progression of healing and increased use of the limb is poorly understood and will be considered later.

PATTERNS OF BONE HEALING

Conventionally there have been two major patterns of bone healing, as stated above: direct and indirect repair. However, it is probably reasonable to consider a third pattern of repair, that seen in distraction osteogenesis. In techniques such as limb lengthening and bone transport, the osteotomy or corticotomy is subjected to controlled distraction regimens that induce axial tension in the repair tissue. In this process it has been reported that intramembranous ossification occurs to form a type of callus termed the 'regenerate'.

Direct fracture repair

The different biological patterns of repair are associated with the mechanical environment at the fracture site. When the fracture fragments are stabilised with rigid fixation there is little or no interfragmentary motion. The fragments are compressed such that in places the bone matrix of one is in direct contact with that of the apposing fragment. The high level of rigidity allows secondary osteons to remodel the bone across the fracture line. The mechanisms that induce this process are poorly understood. As in any intracortical remodelling sequence the bone-resorbing cells are first activated, a 'cutting cone' of osteoclasts is formed that resorbs a tunnel of bone along the longitudinal axis of the bone across the fracture line. Immediately behind the cone of osteoclasts

are active osteoblasts and a vascular bud. The osteoblasts deposit circumferential bone lamellae behind the cutting cone to form the typical osteon (*Figure 9.4*). The secondary osteon can be distinguished from a primary osteon by the punched-out appearance and a 'cement line' that separates the outermost lamella from the surrounding lamellae. On microradiographs the secondary osteons remain less radiodense than the surrounding tissue for some weeks after formation. Gradually the fracture line is obliterated by the formation of many secondary osteons.

In direct fracture repair there is little or no periosteal response in the form of a bridging callus.

The process is slow and takes months or years to complete. Much of the work to illustrate the histological features was conducted in experimental situations using a simple transverse osteotomy. In clinical fractures the accurate reduction and thus apposition of fragments under compression is more difficult to achieve. In these situations it is likely that point contact will be made between the fragments, leaving some gaps. The gaps are filled with woven bone which will then be remodelled.

The most common method of achieving the levels of interfragmentary stability that induces direct bone healing is by the use of rigid internal fixation. In this technique a metal plate is attached to the bone, on the tension surface, usually with the application of compression across the fracture site (Perren, 1979).

However, the fracture plate not only stabilises the fracture site but also provides a load-sharing path to

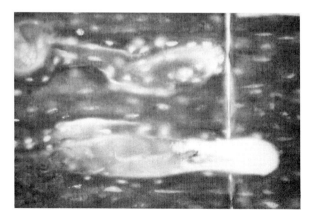

Figure 9.4 Longitudinal section of a 'cutting' core of osteoclasts crossing a fracture line and progressive osteonal remodelling across the fracture line. Courtesy of Stephen Perren.

reduce further the load taken by the bone, and consequently decreases the deformation or functional surface stain beneath the plate. Thus both the injury effects and the application of a plate decrease the mechanical signal that is thought to be responsible for inducing the cellular activity involved in maintaining bone mass (*Figure 9.5*). This apparent paradox may be relevant to the control of the healing process. Perren (1979) reported an observation of intracortical porosity beneath the fracture plate, initially thought to be due to strain protection. Later studies by the AO group suggested that this effect might also be attributed to vascular occlusion of periosteal vessels compressed by the overlying plate. Our studies show that customary bone strain is reduced by up to 30% beneath a commercial fracture plate. This reduction in strain was accompanied by an increase in intracortical porosity.

To differentiate between vascular and mechanical effects, a plate was modified to include a low-rate spring in the mid-section (*Figure 9.5*). The experimental (spring) and control (standard dynamic compression plate (DCP)) plates were applied to the dorsal aspect (tension surface) of the ovine radius for a period of 12 weeks. The spring plate was applied with the spring extended (under tension). Histology revealed the expected intracortical porosity and also evidence of endosteal resorption. The spring plate, in which near-normal loads were carried through the cortex with physiological strain magnitudes, showed little intracortical or endosteal bone loss beneath the spring (*Figure 9.6*). It could be argued, however, that the contact profile of the plates differed and the vascular factor may still

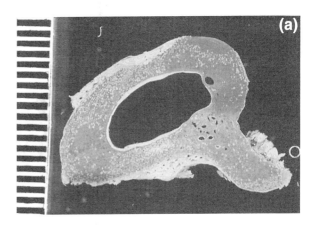

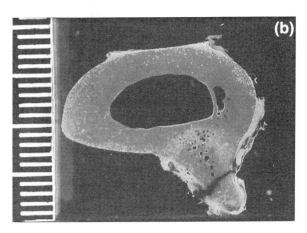

Figure 9.6 (a) Porosity beneath a load sharing rigid fixation plate. Bright areas represent areas of resorption resulting from the presence of the plate. The predominant regions of loss are the endosteal surface and intracortical porosity. (b) Similar section from an experimental plate in which a spring section under tension transferred the load to the bone only. Note little or no osteopenia occurs where there is no significant strain protection.

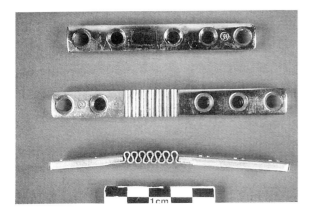

Figure 9.5 Plates used to investigate the effects of strain protection osteopenia.

account for remodelling differences. It is known that changes in vascular dynamics may influence bone formation. Stimulation of new bone formation distal to a venous tourniquet has been reported by Kruse and Kelly (1974).

Rubin showed that strain protection in the avian ulna preparation resulted in bone loss by both endosteal resorption and intracortical porosity (Rubin and Lanyon, 1987). In this model the surgical isolation inevitably produces a vascular disturbance; thus there are two potential influences on bone cell activity: first, a change in haemodynamics and, second, a reduction in customary strain. The influence of strain protection in bone modelling can be evaluated without concurrent vascular impingement by the use of external fixation.

O'Doherty and colleagues (1995) studied the influence of strain protection by applying bilateral external fixators with identical anatomical location and frame configuration. The experimental tibia was protected by an intact frame, and in the control the fixator bar was discontinuous to allow functional loads to be carried by the tibia. Strain gauge measurements showed the functional tibia strains were reduced to 50% by the presence of the intact fixator, but in the discontinuous fixator normal strain patterns were retained. Over a period of 16 weeks bone mass was decreased in the protected tibia. The loss of bone was a result of endosteal resorption and consequential thinning of the cortices (*Figure 9.7*). There was no

evidence of intracortical porosity or increased intracortical remodelling. Thus, these data would support a modelling change to optimise mass and structure of the bone for a decrease in functional demand. In addition it could be postulated that intracortical resorption may be induced by changes in haemodynamics.

Interfragmentary motion in areas of small fracture gaps would create high strain fields that would inhibit bone formation; thus direct repair can occur only under conditions of rigid fixation. Because strain is a change in length as a function of original length, small deformations of a very small gap may provide strains too high to sustain bone as a material. As bone will fail at strains greater than 2%, bone union is not possible if this level of deformation is exceeded.

Although there are advantages of direct repair in terms of restoration of anatomical integrity, and this may be required in intra-articular fractures, the process is a lengthy one taking months to years to complete with possible complications of implant failure if loosening occurs. Removal of the plate after union will also induce the potential for refracture at the junction of the strain-protected area of the bone, with a thinned and possibly porotic cortex, and the adjacent normal cortex.

Rigid internal fixation is also dependent on a knowledge of biomechanics of the bone. In some cases an appropriate axial tension axis may not exist; for example, in the tibia the physiological principal tension axis is at 40° to the longitudinal axis of the bone. Thus it is not possible to align the plate with the principal tension axis.

Indirect (secondary) bone healing

The second type of bone healing, indirect repair, involves the formation of 'callus' to provide a biological splint that stabilises the fracture. This type of repair is relatively rapid, with bony union being achieved in weeks to months. During this type of healing, bone forms in a number of places. The periosteum and endosteum produce 'hard' callus by activation of the osteogenic layer of the periosteum, which forms by intramembranous ossification. In this process bone matrix is deposited on a fibrous tissue scaffold. The level of activity is greatest adjacent to the fractured end of the fragment. The morphology of the periosteal hard callus is related to the mechanical environment of the fracture.

The second type of callus is found between the fragments beneath the bridging periosteal hard callus and

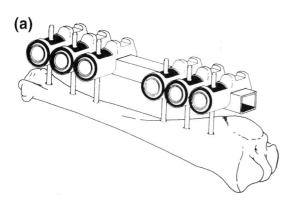

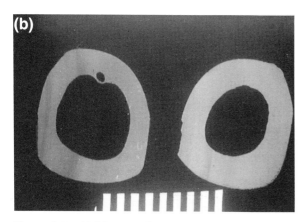

Figure 9.7 (a) Diagram of external fixator on intact tibia. (b) Microradiographs to show reduction of cortical cross-sectional area by endosteal resorption resulting from a 50% strain reduction.

is sometimes termed the 'soft' callus. This comprises a mixture of tissues which change as a function of time but may also be related to the mechanical environment of the fracture site. The soft callus is initiated by the haematoma that occurs at the fracture site. The fracture haematoma then undergoes a cascade of tissue differentiation. The haematoma is replaced with granulation tissue; this differentiates to fibrous tissue and then to fibrocartilage and hyaline cartilage. The hyaline cartilage is then invaded by vascular buds and the process of endochondral ossification occurs, resulting in the formation of woven bone, which remodels to the definitive tissue of lamellar bone. The woven bone is characterised by coarse collagen fibres arranged in a haphazard fashion and large osteocyte lacunae. This process, which is very similar to the endochondral ossification that occurred in the development of the appendicular skeleton, gives rise to the term endochondral repair, which can also be used to describe this type of healing.

Thus indirect repair is a complex array of biological processes; the periosteal callus initiated on each fragment progresses and forms a bridge between the fragments as the soft callus differentiates (*Figure 9.8*). The cellular and molecular mechanisms that control the process are poorly understood, although there is a time-dependent sequential expression of messenger RNA for proteins characteristic of the tissues seen in indirect bone repair.

Frequently there is intracortical porosity and remodelling of the cortices of the fracture fragments adjacent to

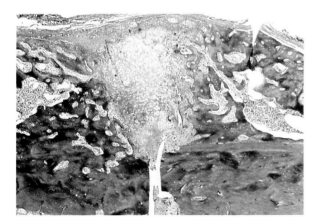

Figure 9.8 Longitudinal section through an osteotomy healing by indirect repair to show periosteal bone formation of bridging or 'hard' callus and differentiating tissue within the gap at the stage of chondral repair (the 'soft callus').

the fracture; sometimes this is termed cancellisation of the cortex. This process integrates the bony callus with the original cortical tissue.

Following the initial bony union there is a prolonged phase of callus remodelling to restore the anatomical morphology of the bone.

Although the initial repair and restoration of mechanical integrity is rapid, in indirect repair the contour of the bone shows the bulge of callus for the protracted period of remodelling (McKibbin, 1978).

Indirect fracture repair is sensitive to both biological and mechanical factors. The mechanical environment imposed by the fixation device, be it cast brace, external fixation or intramedullary nail, influences both the mass and distribution of callus. The mechanical properties of the healing bone are determined by the mass and distribution of the callus. Sarmiento has shown that bone healing by bracing techniques results in greater torsional strength than plating, largely as a function of the support provided by the callus (Sarmiento et al, 1977).

The cascade of differentiation of callus is also related to the mechanical environment, although it is not clear whether the specific genes for the different macromolecules characteristic of each connective tissue are activated by a particular mechanical regimen, or whether the progression of repair is impeded by the ability of a particular tissue to exist in the prevailing mechanical environment. Rahn (1982) showed that each of the different tissues seen in the process of endochondral fracture repair can be deformed to a level where it will return to its original dimensions when the load is removed. This is termed elastic deformation. However, if the deformation continues beyond this point, the tissue will be damaged and will not return to its original dimension when the load is removed; this point is termed the yield strain. If the tissue continues to be deformed it will eventually break at a level of deformation termed the ultimate strain.

As the soft callus differentiates, each sequential tissue has both a lower ultimate strain and a higher modulus of elasticity (stiffness). Consequently, the interfragmentary movement is reduced as healing progresses. However, if the loads across a healing fracture are too great then progression to the next tissue is impeded or the tissue is damaged. A lack of adequate stability can, therefore, lead to a hypertrophic non-union with excessive periosteal hard callus but a cartilaginous endpoint at the fracture line. This situation can be rectified by increasing the stability of the fracture. Alternatively the progression of healing may be impaired by too high a level of stability, in which case the amount of callus is reduced; in this situation the formation of callus can be stimulated by reducing the level of stability.

The biological process is acutely sensitive to very subtle changes in fixation stability that result in small changes in deformation at the fracture site leading to significant changes in the biological progression of healing. This was demonstrated in an experiment in which a standard osteotomy was stabilised using a single-sided fixator with constant anatomical location and frame geometry except for one variable, namely the offset distance between the fixator bar and the bone. A difference of only 10 mm in this one construct variable induced a significant difference in the rate of mineralisation in the osteotomy gap and also in the rate of increase in fracture stiffness index.

In addition, the different stiffness values of the frame influenced the ground reaction force of that limb. The stiffer frame induced a greater ground reaction force in the early stages, which remained relatively constant thereafter, whereas a lower frame stiffness resulted in a low initial ground reaction force but a progressive increase during the healing period. This suggests the presence of a mechanosensory biofeedback system to control weight-bearing on the fractured limb and, as a consequence, deformation of the fracture site (Goodship et al, 1993b).

Distraction osteogenesis

With the current interest in limb lengthening and bone transport, pioneered by Ilizarov (1989), it is appropriate to consider a third type of repair that occurs under conditions of distraction. Perhaps the conventional patterns of bone healing should now be revised to include this process, which involves repair by intramembranous bone formation. There is direct bone formation on a fibrous scaffold of type I collagen.

In both bone lengthening and the transport of a segment of bone within a limb, there is usually an elective osteotomy or corticotomy. In the case of corticotomy, the objective is to divide the bone matrix of the cortex with minimal damage to the periosteum and endosteum, leaving the intramedullary blood vessels intact. After a period of approximately 2 weeks the fragments are separated by distraction using one of a number of external fixation systems. The distraction can also be performed over an intramedullary nail. There are various regimens of distraction, ranging from two periods per day to experimental systems of continuous distraction. It is usual for approximately 1 mm total distraction to be achieved in a 24-hour period. The newly formed bone is often termed the 'regenerate' and comprises an area similar in diameter to the original diaphysis, unlike the bulging callus seen in indirect bone repair.

It has been shown by Einhorn that there is a coincident increase in gene expression for vascular endothelial growth factor (VEGF), with distraction (T. Einhorn, personal communication, 1996). Perhaps this indicates a link between the application of tensile forces and a stimulus for vascularisation.

At the end of the lengthening of a bone or the transport of a segment of bone to manage a large defect, there is a period of 'consolidation' in which the regenerate becomes more mineralised and the new cortices and medullary cavity can be recognised. In addition to this process being seen in traumatic fracture, it also forms the basis of bone regeneration during leg lengthening and bone transport procedures.

BIOLOGICAL MECHANISMS IN BONE REPAIR

Growth factors and cytokines

Bone repair is a complex biological process, which under normal circumstances will lead to the restoration of both morphological and mechanical integrity of the bone. In all the different patterns of repair there is complex control of cell activity. Interactions between cells and also between cells and their extracellular matrix can be influenced by mechanical and mechanically related signals. Cell–cell and cell–matrix interactions may be mediated by small peptides called growth factors; indeed, bone is an extremely rich source of these molecules. Another group of molecules that may act in the regulation of cellular processes occurring in fracture healing are the cytokines.

In a review of growth factors, Lind (1996) proposes three groups of cytokines that affect bone cells: the colony-stimulating factors, the tumour necrosis factors and the interleukins. He suggests that these are involved primarily in the osteoblast–osteoclast interactions associated with modelling and remodelling. The cytokines are mainly regulators of immune responses secreted by haematological cells. However, they may also regulate bone cell function. It is suggested that interleukins are produced during the fracture repair process and also that these molecules have been shown to influence chondrocytes, both in joint degeneration and also in chondrocyte transplantation when the cells are covered by perichondrium or periosteum. Thus there is a possible paracrine influence of the periosteal osteogenic cells on the underlying chondral tissue of the soft callus.

Growth factors

The major growth factors associated with bone are the transforming growth factor (TGF) β superfamily, which includes the bone morphogenetic proteins, of which a number have been sequenced, the acidic and basic fibroblast growth factors, platelet-derived growth factors and the insulin-like growth factors, of which there are two main types, IGF–1 and IGF–2. In fracture repair and remodelling these growth factors and some others play an important role in stimulating the proliferation and differentiation of the tissues that lead to bony union of the fragments.

They are found in the non-collagenous protein fraction of the extracellular matrix of bone, where, although they represent less than 1% of this fraction of the matrix, they are potent regulators of bone metabolism, both in remodelling and in control of the repair process. Other non-collagenous proteins play a role in the cell–matrix interactions, regulating mineralisation, organisation of the collagenous component and cell–matrix binding. One of the first growth factors to be found in bone was discovered by Urist, who observed that demineralised bone placed subcutaneously would induce a bony ossicle. The protein involved in this bone induction was termed bone morphogenetic protein (BMP).

Since this discovery a number of different BMPs have been sequenced. These growth factors belong to a superfamily of transforming growth factors, the TGF-β family. Growth factors in this group can stimulate cell proliferation, differentiation and synthesis of proteins. The BMP group of growth factors is responsible for the stimulation of differentiation of stem cells to chondroblasts and osteoblasts. These factors are also involved in the process of endochondral ossification. TGF-β itself is present as a number of types and is found not only in bone, but is also abundant in platelets. Thus, after fracture, the ensuing

haematoma with the degranulation of platelets and also the associated resorption of the fragment ends both provide a rich source of TGF-β. Bolander (1992) suggests these factors are involved in the initiation of the early stages of fracture repair.

The platelets are also a source of platelet-derived growth factor which, together with TGF-β, is thought to initiate the repair process by stimulating both the proliferation of mesenchymal cells in the periosteum and also the subsequent differentiation of these cells. In the periosteal callus the stimulation is greatest near the fracture site and decreases with distance away from the fracture. The reason for this is not clear. The cells within the bone close to the fracture site are often necrotic and there is subsequent resorption of the matrix in this area. The resorption may also be related to the inevitable reduction in the mechanical loading of the bone at the fracture site. It is possible that the resorption of bone releases growth factors that may then act locally on the adjacent periosteum, with greatest activity adjacent to the fracture site.

As healing progresses the haematoma differentiates to granulation tissue which is richly vascularised; fibroblast-derived growth factors play a role both as potent mitogens but also in the process of angiogenesis. The osteoblasts can also synthesise fibroblast growth factor (FGF). The basic form of this growth factor is present in the bone matrix in much higher proportions than the acidic form; thus matrix resorption will also release FGFs.

There are also other growth factors that are associated with the vascularisation of the early callus. VEGF has been demonstrated in the early callus; Einhorn and co-workers (T. Einhorn, personal communication, 1996) have demonstrated the presence of VEGF in the callus associated with endochondral repair and have also shown that there is an upregulation of VEGF some 8 hours after each increment of lengthening in distraction osteogenesis. The granulation tissue differentiates further into fibrous tissue, fibrocartilage and then to the avascular hyaline cartilage of the soft callus. The hyaline cartilage resembles that seen in the early cartilage anlage of the skeleton.

Indirect fracture repair has many similarities to the process of endochondral ossification during skeletal development. Stafford et al (1994) has reported that the phenotypic hypertrophying chondrocytes, seen as the process of endochondral ossification commences, are capable of synthesising osteoblast marker proteins such as type I collagen and bone sialoprotein. This may be suggestive of a change in cell type. However, Einhorn et al. (T. Einhorn, personal communication, 1996) suggest that the DNA fragments and Bcl2 indicative of apotosis (programmed cell death) can be demonstrated in indirect fracture repair; this would suggest that the chondrocytes are replaced by cells of an osteoblast lineage. Thus the mechanisms that control the transition of one tissue type to the next are not clear.

The process continues with the calcification of the hyaline cartilage matrix followed by release of matrix vesicles and subsequent vascularisation, ossification and replacement with woven bone, which is then replaced by lamellar bone and is remodelled and modelled towards the original architecture of the bone before fracture. This process consolidates the 'soft' callus and may take place beneath a bridge of bone formed by the periosteal 'hard' callus from each of the fragments. In some cases of delayed union or hypertrophic non-union, the cartilaginous component of the callus extends completely across the fracture site. The magnitude and distribution of the periosteal callus may be influenced by various factors, including soft tissue damage, local blood supply, magnitude and pattern of the interfragmentary micromovements or fragmentary bone strain, and periosteal integrity.

IGFs, also synthesised by osteoblasts, may play a role in both the process of ossification and the subsequent remodelling phases. The most abundant form in bone is IGF-2. This growth factor has been associated with mechanically stimulated bone formation by Lanyon (1994); there is also a link with prostacyclin synthesis in the transduction of mechanical signals to cellular activity in strain-induced bone formation. IGF-1 is synthesised in response to the action of growth hormone and acts on the cartilage of the growth plate to control longitudinal growth; again the similarity with the process of endochondral ossification in bone growth is interesting.

The histological sequence of tissue differentiation as a function of time has been described in the rat femoral fracture model of Bonnarens and Einhorn by Jingushi (1992). These workers also characterised the gene expression for the different extracellular matrix molecules associated with the tissues of fracture callus as a function of location and time following fracture. They found that gene expression patterns for the structural proteins of cartilage (type II collagen and proteoglycan core protein) and bone (type I collagen) and for markers of chondrogenesis and osteogenesis (osteonectin, osteocalcin and

alkaline phosphatase) differed between the regions of hard and soft callus, and changed as healing progressed to correlate with the histological picture.

Eicosanoids as mediators of endochondral repair

Eicosanoids have also been shown to be linked to both mechanically induced bone formation and endochondral fracture repair (Goodship et al, 1993a). Nordin suggested that exogenous prostaglandin E_2 increased both cell proliferation and the rate of differentiation in endochondral fracture repair (Norrdin and Shih, 1988). Indirect evidence of the role of prostanoids is provided by studies that show a downregulation of mechanically induced bone formation and the rate of indirect bone repair under the influence of indomethacin, a prostaglandin synthetase inhibitor.

Role of hormones in bone repair

Hormones may also influence the rate of endochondral bone repair. Bolander demonstrated oestrogen receptors in fracture callus and showed that the gene for this receptor was expressed at all time points but peaked at 14 days in the rat femoral fracture model (M.E. Bolander, personal communication, 1994). He also found that ovariectomy reduced the rate of healing in this model. Exogenous oestrogen supplementation enhanced the rate of healing but not to the level seen in intact controls. The mechanisms for these effects have not been elucidated but may have some relevance in relation to fracture repair in postmenopausal osteoporosis. Bolander (personal communication, 1994) has also suggested that diabetes mellitus delays indirect fracture repair, characterised by a small callus with a low volume of cartilage.

Once the control and combined actions of these signalling peptides and hormones is understood more fully, it may be possible to enhance fracture repair by pharmacological means (Einhorn, 1995). In this way some of the management problems associated with the use of fixation devices may be overcome without the need for specialist biomechanical understanding. However, until such time it is possible to influence the fracture healing process by changing the biochemical environment at the fracture site.

MODULATION OF BONE REPAIR BY THE MECHANICAL ENVIRONMENT

What are stress and strain, and why are they relevant to fracture healing? When a load is applied to a structure stresses are generated within the material and as a consequence the structure deforms. The deformation represents a change in dimension compared to the original dimension and is termed 'strain'.

The mechanical environment at the fracture site in terms of interfragmentary strain is dependent on a number of factors. Perhaps the most important are the loads applied by the patient and the characteristics of the fixation device. The tissues differentiating at the fracture site will also contribute to the level of micro-motion at the fracture gap. There is a complex interaction between the level of strain induced at the fracture site and the progression of healing, in that only certain types of tissue can exist in areas of specific strain magnitude (Blenham et al, 1989).

Most fractures stabilised by various forms of external fixation and intramedullary nailing undergo indirect healing, in which the fragments are stabilised by the formation of external periosteal callus. The fracture gap is initially occupied by the postfracture haematoma, which then differentiates through granulation tissue, fibrous tissue and fibrocartilage to woven and lamellar bone. The mechanical properties of each of these tissues are different. The stiffness increases with the progression from granulation tissue to bone; the ultimate tensile strain decreases (*Table 9.1*).

This means that each tissue can be deformed to a critical level before it fails. Granulation tissue can be extended to 100% of its original length before damage occurs; however, bone can be deformed only up to 2%

without risk of failure. If the loads applied to the fracture gap produce strains in excess of the safe level for the tissue present, then damage occurs and the healing process may be adversely affected. At safe levels of loading the change in tissue type with associated increase in stiffness results in a decrease in the amount of deformation at the fracture site. Thus it would appear that the level of strain occurring at the fracture site is critical to the progression of healing and restoration of mechanical integrity of the fractured bone.

If fracture management is to advance, then it is important not only to understand the biology of bone healing but also to be able to monitor and control the process in a relevant manner. Because restoration of mechanical integrity is the obvious goal for both patient and surgeon, perhaps the relevant aspect to control and monitor is strain at the fracture site, in order to be able to determine progressive changes in fracture stiffness.

There is some debate in relation to the correlation of fracture stiffness with ultimate strength, as in mechanical terms these two variables are quite different. However, it is not possible to determine the ultimate strength of a fracture in patients, whereas there are a number of techniques for assessing the change in fracture stiffness. On an empirical basis it has been shown that attainment of a defined axial and bending stiffness indicates that the fracture will tolerate functional loading. These stiffness values may not represent those of the intact normal bone but after removal of the supporting fixator the osteogenic mechanical stimulus will result in further adaptive hypertrophy and bone remodelling in which a near-normal gross and microscopic bone architecture will be restored.

As indicated above the displacement at the fracture site is determined by both the loads applied by the patient and the type of device used for fixation. The biomechanical characteristics of fracture fixation devices in general and external skeletal fixators in particular have been determined in the laboratory. Although such data are available, it is difficult for the surgeon to utilise this information because the exact requirement for optimal healing has not been established. However, with the recent increase in popularity of the external fixators, it is possible to use these devices both to control and to monitor the mechanical environment at the fracture site.

For a given patient the strain levels at the fracture can be controlled in two ways, firstly by adjustment of the inherent stiffness of the frame. This can involve variables fixed at surgery such as pin spacing, pin numbers, pin

Table 9.1 Tissue differentiation in endochondral repair with material properties of the defined tissue types.

Tissue	Ultimate strain (%)	Elastic modulus (N/mm^2)
Haematoma	Negligible properties	Negligible properties
Granulation	100	0.05
Fibrous	5–17	16.7–100
Fibrocartilage	10–13	20–800
Compact bone	2	10 000

diameter and fixator geometry (unilateral, bilateral, triangular, etc.) or factors that can be adjusted during healing such as the offset distance between bars and bone, or destabilisation during healing by a reduction in the number of bars. Secondly, the stress and consequent strain at the fracture site can be controlled independently of the type of frame or the loads applied by patients, by attachment of an actuator to the fixator to provide a controlled actively applied micro-motion to the fracture fragments.

Both these approaches can influence significantly the progression of healing. Experimental studies have shown that alteration in frame stiffness, effected solely by small differences in the distance between the bar and the bone, results in a significant difference in the rate of mineralisation of the fracture gap and in the rate of increase in fracture stiffness (Goodship et al, 1993b). The radiological assessment confirmed that a less rigid configuration promotes interfragmentary strain and promotes callus formation, whereas the more rigid configuration with the bar closer to the bone inhibits periosteal callus formation (*Figure 9.9*).

In the clinical situation the level of applied load is more variable and the stiffness of the frame has to be determined in relation to the level of activity and confidence of the individual patient. To date, such adjustment of the frame geometry is attempted in only relatively few centres. In the fracture clinic the correct matching of frame stiffness and rigidity to patient activity in absolute terms using engineering formulae is impossible. However, by an application of the mechanics and biology of fracture healing, together with a monitoring system, it is possible for the surgeon to utilise the natural biofeedback and make appropriate changes to the frame to maximise healing potential.

It has been shown that the process of fracture healing can also be modified by very short periods of applied intermittent deformation (*Figure 9.10*). Some stimulation regimens can enhance healing (Goodship, 1989; Goodship and Kenwright, 1985; Kenwright and Goodship, 1989), and this allows the possibility to utilise a very rigid frame and then superimpose an actively applied mechanical stimulus to induce cyclical strains at the fracture site and within the developing callus. This allows the osteogenic benefits of a flexible frame together with the improved pin–bone and pin–skin interfaces seen with frames of high rigidity. Furthermore, the ability to impose a mechanical stimulus to the healing fracture indepen-

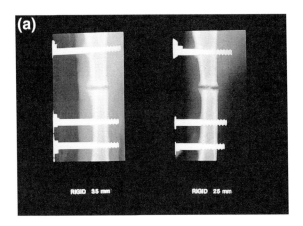

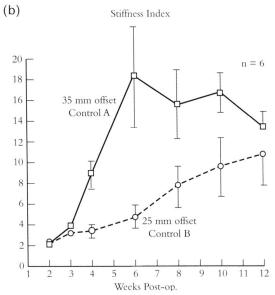

Figure 9.9 (a) Radiographs and (b) stiffness plots of the effect of fixator bar offset distance on the progression of healing in a standard osteotomy.

dently of patient weight-bearing provides the means to enhance repair of fractures in non-ambulatory patients or those with psychological inhibition of normal weight-bearing. In such cases the absence of self-imposed mechanical stimulation may in itself result in a net bone loss remodelling and reduction in callus formation, resulting in local osteopenia and delayed union.

Although there is increasing evidence that dynamisation of external fixators can be used to enhance the rate of fracture repair, the decision on the time to apply dynamic stimulation has been based largely on empirical judgement rather than a scientific understanding of the process of fracture healing and its relationship to mechanical

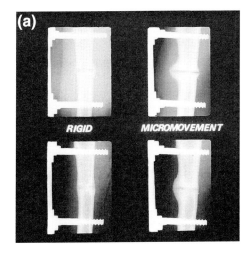

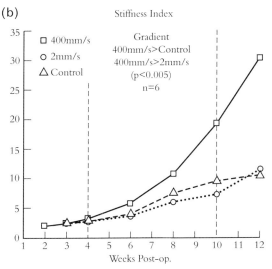

Figure 9.10   (a) Radiographs and (b) stiffness plots of the effect of applied intermittent deformation on the progression of healing in a standard osteotomy.

environment. The time of application, duration and character of stimulus may all affect the repair process. Our work on controlled fractures has shown that not only is the healing process extremely sensitive to very short periods of mechanical stimulation, but it is also influenced by the nature of the stimulus. The magnitude of applied force, deformation and the rate of deformation may all affect the rate of repair.

Dynamisation

As has been indicated above, the mechanical conditions applied to a fracture will modulate the pattern of repair.

The mechanical environment at the fracture site will be dependent both on the method of fixation and on the activity of the patient. For any fixation device the application of load that is shared by the fracture and the device will result in either interfragmentary movements or deformation of the bone of the fragments when in contact under load. Thus there will always be a dynamic change of strain at the fracture site when the patient loads the limb, either during locomotion or with muscle contractions. This can be termed inherent dynamisation.

The fracture may also be subjected to changes in mechanical stimulation by applying a load via the fixation system to induce movement and/or strain at the fracture site; this is also a dynamic stimulus and can be thought of as active or applied dynamisation.

Inherent (passive) dynamisation

The combination of a fracture fixation device and functional activity results in a dynamic interfragmentary micromovement and/or deformation of the bone tissue of the fragments adjacent to the fracture. The characteristics of such motion, or strain if the fragments are apposed, will depend on the device and magnitude of loading imposed by the individual. In the early stages of healing such motion may be minimal; indeed, unless the patient is ambulatory, the mechanical stimulation may be insufficient to induce bone formation.

The magnitude and pattern of this self-induced mechanical stimulus will influence both the rate of repair and the amount and distribution of callus. Preliminary data indicate that the orientation of an external fixator with respect to the anatomical axis of the bone may induce a local mechanical environment that can influence the distribution of callus.

In an experimental model a single-sided fixator was applied in two groups with an angular difference of approximately 90° with respect to the long axis of the tibia. The axes of the ellipse of callus in the two groups also differed by approximately 90°. This suggests that a knowledge of the biology and biomechanics could be used to plan the most effective position for a device to induce callus at a particular site, within the anatomical and clinical constraints of a particular fracture.

In some systems the fixator is fixed in a 'rigid' mode for the first few weeks of the healing period, then the body of the fixator is released to allow enhanced dynamic mechanical stimulation of the fracture. The validity of such a concept depends on the ability of the device to allow unrestricted cyclical motion between the fragments and the control of deformation of the healing tissues, such that the ultimate strain values are not exceeded. In some studies these devices merely allow collapse of the fragments rather than a true cyclical dynamisation. The sudden change in mechanical conditions may not only damage the developing callus but would also require a change in structure and distribution to accommodate the new loading magnitudes and directions.

Active (applied) dynamisation

In many cases of fracture the patient will be non-ambulatory in the early postoperative period. Particularly in conjunction with external fixation, it is possible to apply mechanical stimulation to the fracture by means of an attached actuator. The rationale behind this type of mechanical stimulation is that the repair process in bone is also acutely sensitive to short periods of cyclical deformation. Furthermore the characteristics of such stimulation are critical to the rate of progression of the repair process.

Early experimental work showed that a short period of cyclical interfragmentary micro-motion applied to a midshaft ovine tibial osteotomy for 500 cycles at 0.5 Hz resulted in an increase in the rate of healing in terms of mineralisation and fracture stiffness index. These early data provided the basis for a clinical trial on human fractures where, again, the early application of mechanical stimulation resulted in a significant increase in the rate of healing. It is perhaps more appropriate to consider that the osteogenic mechanical stimuli override the inhibition to repair resulting from the strain protection of the fixation device.

Subsequently it has been shown that the tissues are also sensitive to the specific characteristics of the mechanical signal within the short period of applied stimulation.

Biological responses to specific mechanical stimuli

Different mechanical characteristics result in specific responses, even though the stimulus is applied only for a very short period of approximately 17 minutes each day. Some stimuli may decrease the rate of healing, others have little effect, and others enhance the repair process. Small differences in the magnitude of displacement, rate

of displacement and applied force will all influence the pattern of tissues present in the repair process.

Results from experimental studies indicate that small displacements applied with a low force using a high rate of deformation provide the most osteogenic signal. The effect of a high rate of displacement is interesting in relation to a similar effect of high strain rates in intact bone, resulting in consistent high-amplitude electrical signals attributed to streaming potentials caused by ionic fluids flowing through the small porosities of bone.

Thus there is a relationship between the patient's activity, the mechanical stiffness of the device and the progression of the repair process. Inadequate stabilisation may result in excessive deformation of the repair tissues and thus prevent the differentiation to bone and consequent restoration of mechanical integrity. Alternatively too great a level of stabilisation will reduce the osteogenic stimulus and suppress periosteal callus formation. Using external fixation the fixator stiffness can be adjusted to an individual patient's level of activity and body-weight in a number of ways, for example by changing the offset distance of the fixator bar.

Although the progression of healing is often monitored by sequential radiography, this may not provide adequate objective information regarding the restoration of mechanical stiffness. As indicated above, the stiffness of the fracture will depend on the material properties of the tissues within the callus, the mass and distribution of callus in relation to the loading magnitude and direction.

There are now systems available for the measurement of an index of stiffness of the healing fracture for use with external fixations systems. On an empirical basis it has been shown that values of bending stiffness above 15 Nm per degree indicate a minimal risk of refracture following removal of the fixator in tibial fractures.

Timing of mechanical stimulation of fracture repair

It has also been shown that the early application of the applied osteogenic stimulus is important. When the same stimulus is applied later in the period of repair, the effect may be to inhibit the process, perhaps due to cellular activity to accommodate to a new mechanical environment requiring a reorganisation of mass and distribution of callus. The tissues involved in endochondral repair appear to follow the concepts proposed by Wolff in relation to bone, in terms of adjustment of mass and distribution in relation to prevailing mechanical demands. Thus when the pattern of deformation is changed, the tissues have to remodel to reform in a distribution appropriate to optimise resistance to the new loading pattern.

The use of mechanical stimulation could also be applicable in situations where the time for bone union and consolidation of callus is preplanned. Such an application could be in limb lengthening, where an osteotomy is made to allow the soft tissues to be extended. During this process the fracture callus is also distracted but the rate of distraction that is optimal for viscoelastic soft tissues is not the same as that for fracture callus. Thus it may be possible to use applied inhibitory regimens of large cyclical deformation at high loads, and low rates to retard healing until the required additional limb length has been attained, then to change the regimen to induce rapid bone union and consolidation.

It is interesting to note that many reports on limb lengthening and bone transport suggest that the distracted callus or regenerate bone undergoes intramembranous ossification; some studies have, however, suggested the presence of cartilaginous areas of ossification in some models (e.g. sheep). This may be caused by the response of the tissues to other distraction stimuli with a superimposed inherent dynamisation.

During the repair process a cascade of connective tissue differentiation occurs. Each tissue has different material properties, thus there is an increase in stiffness and a consequent decrease in displacement at the fracture site. The factors controlling these events have not been established. Delayed or non-union may result from an inappropriate mechanical environment for the tissue present, thus damaging the extracellular matrix.

Using applied mechanical stimulation it has been shown that some stimuli are inhibitory; this effect may be as a result of tissue damage. In cases where the stimulus enhances the rate of repair, the mechanical signal may be 'driving' the process of callus differentiation. Displacement is also controlled by the feedback process that influences loads applied to the limb. There may be a possibility of utilising the sensitivity of the process to mechanical signals to provide a further enhancement of the rate of repair.

Again using our model we applied a programmed stimulus in which the magnitude of displacement was reduced as a function of time and compared this to a group in which a similar initial stimulus was used throughout the period of healing. Results indicated that

the rate of differentiation of callus was enhanced further, leading to a significant increase in the bending and axial stiffness of the fracture. Histologically the callus appeared more consolidated and with greater proportions of ossified bone than in the group in which a self-adjustment of the stimulus had occurred.

This provides additional evidence that the biological patterns of repair can be influenced by using appropriate mechanical signals. The tissues present in a fracture or osteotomy gap can be 'engineered' by controlling the local mechanical conditions. An understanding of the general relationship between mechanical conditions and specific biological tissues is essential for the future development of orthopaedic implants and treatment methods for fractures.

TRANSDUCTION MECHANISMS FOR MECHANICAL MODULATION OF BONE REPAIR

The mechanisms of transduction of the mechanical signal to cellular activity are not clear. As with mechanically induced bone formation there are a number of possible transduction pathways, including direct mechanical deformation of cells and indirect stimulation from electrical streaming potentials. In intact bone, prostanoids have been implicated in the transduction pathway.

It has been shown that the adaptive response to mechanical loading is downregulated under the influence of indomethacin (a prostaglandin synthetase inhibitor). Prostacyclin and nitric oxide have been shown to be present within a very short time after mechanical loading and after a few hours IGF-2 can be demonstrated (this is a potent mitogen). The link between these events is, however, still unclear. In fracture repair indomethacin also inhibits the rate of repair. In addition it has been reported that exogenous prostaglandin E_2 increases the proliferation and differentiation of callus.

We have shown that, in our ovine model, the levels of endogenous prostaglandin E_2 are significantly different in groups stimulated with specific short periods of applied interfragmentary micro-motion (Goodship et al, 1993a; *Figure 9.11*). The different levels of prostaglandin E_2 associated with the specific stimulatory and inhibitory regimens of applied micromovement are evident within 2 weeks of the commencement of mechanical stimula-

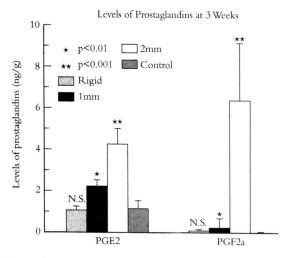

Figure 9.11 Histograms to show the tissue levels of prostaglandins from the callus of osteotomies healing under different types of specific mechanical stimulation.

tion. This provides further evidence that conditions in the early stages of the repair process may be critical in determining the progression of the healing process. These data may also suggest a common role for prostanoids in the strain transduction pathway in bone repair.

Recent work on recording streaming potentials *in vivo* from fracture callus has shown differences in signal with time. Again, the significance is not clear but streaming potentials may also play a role in the transduction mechanism. The field of electrical and electromagnetic stimulation is complex and will not be discussed here.

BIOLOGICAL AND PHARMACOLOGICAL MODULATION OF FRACTURE REPAIR

Various biological agents have been used in an attempt to enhance fracture repair, in particular the bone morphogenetic proteins (Urist, 1965; Reddi et al, 1987). The effect of medication for concurrent conditions may also influence the repair process, but often in an inhibitory manner.

As growth factors are involved in the fracture repair process, their use as exogenous agents to enhance repair has been used in various ways in both experimental and clinical situations.

Integration of callus with the fracture fragments and the remodelling of the callus itself to form a scar-free repair involves a remodelling process that requires coupling between osteoblasts and osteoclasts. Agents that influence the activity of this process will also modulate the final stages of fracture repair. In some cases this can produce different effects in terms of the biomechanical and biological outcome; this demonstrates the importance of evaluating the true scenario resulting from the use of agents being developed for modification of bone remodelling and repair.

In our model we studied the effect of pamidronate (a bisphosphonate) on the repair process. Pamidronate influences the activity of osteoclasts when these cells attack bone matrix in which the drug has been incorporated. In comparing treated and control groups it was seen that the effect of the drug was to increase the mass of callus. The enhanced callus resulted in a greater torsional strength of the fracture. On histological examination, however, it was evident that there had been no remodelling of the fragment ends nor was there any incorporation of the callus with the original cortical bone. This would suggest that only a short-term benefit in terms of mechanical strength would be obtained, with a risk of accumulation of fatigue damage and long-term failure.

CONCLUSIONS

Bone is a tissue that has a great capacity for repair; the healing process results in a restoration of both morphology and mechanical integrity. This repair process is acutely sensitive to biological and mechanical influences. However, it is likely that management of fractures is often the cause of delayed or inhibited healing, rather than inherent biological deficiencies. It is therefore important to appreciate the complexities and interactions of the biology and mechanics of fracture healing to be able to monitor and control factors that will modulate the repair process.

REFERENCES

Blenham PR, Carter DR, Beaupre GS. Role of mechanical loading in the progressive ossification of a fracture callus. *J Orthop Res* 1989; **7**: 398–407.

Bolander M. Regulation of fracture repair by growth factors. *Proc Soc Exp Biol Med* 1992; **200**: 165–170.

Einhorn T. Enhancement of fracture-healing. Current concepts reviews. *J Bone Joint Surg* 1995; **77A(6)**: 940–956.

Goodship AE. The measurement of bone strain *in vivo*. In: *Strain Measurement Biomechanics*. Miles AW, Tanner KE (eds) London: Chapman and Hall, 1992: 70–87.

Goodship AE. Experimental studies of micromotion. In: *External Fixation and Functional Bracing*. Coombs R, Green S, Sarmiento A (eds) London: Orthotext, 1989: 105–111.

Goodship AE, Kenwright, J. The influence of induced micromovement upon the healing of experimental tibial fractures. *J Bone Joint Surg* 1985; **67B(4)**: 650–655.

Goodship AE, Norrdin R, Francis M. The stimulation of prostaglandin synthesis by micromovement in fracture healing. In: *Micromovement in Orthopaedics*. Turner-Smith AR (ed.) Oxford: Clarendon Press, 1993a: 291–295.

Goodship AE, Watkins PE, Rigby HS, Kenwright J. The role of fixator frame stiffness in the control of fracture healing. An experimental study. *J Biomech* 1993b; **26(9)**: 1027–1035.

Ilizarov G. Experimental studies of bone elongation. In: *External Fixation and Functional Bracing*. Coombs R, Green S, Sarmiento A (eds) London: Orthotext, 1989: 375–379.

Jingushi S. Genetic expression of extra-cellular matrix proteins correlated with histologic changes during fracture repair. *J Bone Mineral Res* 1992; **7**: 1045–1055.

Kenwright J, Goodship AE. Mechanical stimulation of tibial fractures. *Clin Orthop* 1989; **241**: 36–47.

Kruse RK, Kelly PJ. Acceleration of fracture healing distal to a venous tourniquet. *J Bone Joint Surg* 1974; **56A(4)**: 730–739.

Lanyon LE. Mechanically sensitive cells in bone. In: *Biomechanics and Cells*. Lyall F, El Haj AJ (eds) Cambridge: Cambridge University Press, 1994: 178–186.

Lanyon LE. Analysis of surface bone strain in the calcaneus of sheep during normal locomotion. *J Biomech* 1973; **6**: 41–49.

Lind M. Growth factors: possible new clinical tools – a review. *Acta Orthop* 1996; **67(4)**: 407–417.

McKibbin B. The biology of fracture healing in long bones. *J Bone Joint Surg* 1978; **60B(2)**: 150–162.

Norrdin RW, Shih MS. Systemic effects of prostaglandin E$_2$ on vertebral trabecular remodelling in beagles used in a healing study. *Calcif Tissue Int* 1988; **42**: 363–368.

O'Doherty DM, Butler SP, Goodship AE. Stress protection due to external fixation. *J Biomech* 1995; **28(5)**: 575–586.

Perren SM. Physical and biological aspects of fracture healing with special reference to internal fixation. *Clin Orthop* 1979; **138**: 175–196.

Rahn BA. Bone healing: histologic and physiologic concepts. In: *Bone in Clinical Orthopaedics*. Sumner-Smith G (ed.) Philadelphia: W.B. Saunders, 1982.

Reddi AH, Wientroub S, Muthukumaran N. Biologic principles of bone induction. *Orthop Clin North Am* 1987; **18**: 207–212.

Rubin CT, Lanyon LE. Osteoregulatory nature of mechanical stimuli: function as a determinant for adaptive remodelling in bone. *J Orthop Res* 1987; **5**: 300–310.

Sarmiento A, Schaeffer JF, Beckerman L, Latta LL, Enis JE. Fracture healing in rat femora as affected by functional weight bearing. *J Bone Joint Surg* 1977; **59A**: 369–375.

Stafford HJ, Roberts MY, Oni OOA et al. Localisation of bone-forming cells during fracture healing by osteocalcin immunocytochemistry: an experimental study of the rabbit tibia. *J Orthop Res* 1994; **12**: 29–39.

Urist MR. Bone: formation by autoinduction. *Science* 1965; **150**: 893–899.

10

Host Defences and Trauma

Latif Khan and Oleg Eremin

INTRODUCTION

Since the original suggestion early this century, a substantial body of evidence has accumulated showing that trauma (external, surgery) induces a variable degree of suppression of host defences (Biebuyck, 1990). More recently, there has been an increasing awareness of the possible detrimental clinical effects of this inhibition of host defences by trauma and, in particular, of the likely consequences of perioperative immune suppression for surgical practice. It has been suggested that suppression of the immune system by surgery, external trauma, sepsis or inflammatory-induced tissue necrosis is an adaptive physiological response which downregulates the host's immune reactivity against the body's autologous proteins, which have been released as a result of the organ damage and tissue necrosis. However, inhibition of host defences in patients undergoing surgery has been shown to be associated with an increased incidence of postoperative morbidity and mortality (Guillou, 1993).

Despite the recent advances in surgical practice and anaesthetic techniques, more ready availability of intensive care facilities, improvements in patient care and the development of a wide range of new antibiotics, sepsis continues to be a major cause of morbidity in patients following trauma. It has been estimated that up to 80% of the late deaths in such patients are due to multisystem organ failure, in which sepsis is considered to play a significant part. Furthermore, it has also been demonstrated that, in patients with malignant disease, surgical resection of the tumour is associated with an increased 'shedding' of tumour cells into the circulation. This occurs at a time of inhibition of anticancer host defences and, therefore, may facilitate metastatic tumour cell dissemination and subsequent establishment of systemic disease.

IMMUNE SYSTEM

The immune system can be divided functionally into two major but overlapping components (*Table 10.1*). The

Table 10.1 Classification of the immune system.

Component	Innate system	Acquired system
Non-specific	Mechanical: epidermis, endothelium Physiological: ciliary motion and propulsive flow, mucus, HCl and HCO_3	
Humoral	Acute-phase proteins, lysozyme, complement components, kallikrein and related kinins, prostanoids and cytokines	Immunoglobulins (IgG, IgM, IgD, IgA and IgE)
Cellular	Mononuclear cells, NK and LAK cells, monocytes and macrophages	T- and B-cell subsets (helper, cytotoxic) and macrophages (antigen presentation, cytotoxic)

cellular component is mediated by the integrated action of different types of cells responsible for innate (natural killer (NK) and lymphokine-activated killer (LAK) cells, macrophages, etc.) and adaptive immunity (T-lymphocyte subsets), whereas the humoral component is mediated by soluble factors (e.g. antibodies, acute-phase proteins and complement components). However, it should be emphasised that there are overlapping and often integrated interactions between the two components, and both are modulated and regulated by a complex cascade of interactive humoral factors (e.g. cytokines, prostanoids) (Eremin and Sewell, 1992).

CELL-MEDIATED IMMUNITY

T lymphocytes

Lymphocytes recognise and interact with foreign antigens on exposure at surface–environment interphases or through internal contact following entry into the tissue environment of the host. The antigens may present as simple or complex molecules or as part of a defined structure (e.g. cell membrane). T lymphocytes, responsible for the generation of cell-mediated immune responses, can be divided into functionally distinct but morphologically less well defined subsets with either regulatory or effector functions: T helper, cytotoxic and suppressor cells. These functional subdivisions should not be interpreted too rigidly. T helper cells (broadly defined phenotypically by the cluster of differentiation (CD) antigens) are key regulators of the immune response. The $CD4^+$ cells interact with antigens, closely linked to the major histocompatibility complex (MHC) class II receptor, which is located on the surface of antigen-presenting cells (macrophages and dendritic cells).

Two populations of T helper cells (T_H1 and T_H2) have been identified and characterised. T_H1 cells secrete interferon (IFN) γ, tumour necrosis factor (TNF) β and interleukin (IL) 2, whereas T_H2 cells produce IL-4, IL-5 and IL-10. The former provide the necessary help (through cytokine release) with initiation and activation of cell-mediated immunity. T_H2 cells (through cytokine release) augment the differentiation of B cells and production of immunoglobulin (Ig) G. IL-10 plays a key role in inhibiting the activity of T_H1 function. T cytotoxic ($CD8^+$) effector cells are activated by interaction with an antigen–MHC class I receptor and release cytolysins,

which are able to induce target cell membrane damage and subsequent lysis. T suppressor cells ($CD8^+$, $CD11b^+$), on the other hand, play an important role in the inhibition of immune responses, by as yet poorly defined mechanisms (Eremin and Sewell).

Following surgery, there is a significant reduction in the total number of circulating lymphocytes and their various subsets, in particular, $CD4^+$ T helper and $CD8^+$ suppressor lymphocytes. The reduction in the number of $CD8^+$ cells, however, is less pronounced than the fall in $CD4^+$ cells, and hence the ratio of $CD4^+$ to $CD8^+$ cells is reduced. This may be responsible, in part, for aspects of the well-documented perioperative immune suppression. The reduction in the circulating levels of these T-lymphocyte subsets is related to the degree of surgical trauma (e.g. extent of tissue damage and duration of surgery), and may last up to 2 weeks or more after operation. Furthermore, there is a variable disturbance of lymphocyte function following surgery and trauma. For example, there is in general a reduction of lymphocyte reactivity (assessed *in vitro* by lymphocyte transformation and proliferation by polyclonal mitogens, such as phytohaemagglutinin (PHA)). Also, the ability to interact with and respond to allogeneic cells (mixed lymphocyte culture *in vitro*) is depressed. Thus, general lymphocyte reactivity, as well as the ability to respond to specific antigens, is inhibited. These pathophysiological changes are believed to predispose to defective responses to environmental pathogens (e.g. viruses) and to lead to an enhanced risk of postoperative or post-traumatic sepsis.

Natural killer cells

NK cells are predominantly large granular lymphocytes (some are small agranular cells) which lack cell surface immunoglobulins characteristic of B lymphocytes but express a complex array of CD cell surface markers (predominantly CD16 and CD56, but lacking CD3). NK cells are non-adherent non-phagocytic cells and are characterised *in vitro* by spontaneous non-MHC-restricted cytolytic activity against a variety of tumour cells, cells infected with viruses and certain normal cells. NK cells are believed to play an important role in the destruction of malignant cells.

Experimental studies in animals have demonstrated that NK cells prevent the metastatic dissemination of tumour cells. Their role in the prevention of metastatic spread in humans has been less well characterised. However, in NK deficiency states (e.g. pharmacological immune suppression in transplant recipients), there is an increased incidence of malignant disease, many of the tumours (e.g. lymphomas) probably being virally induced.

Studies have also shown that the NK cell activity of peripheral blood lymphocytes is reduced in patients with a range of malignancies (e.g. prostate, melanoma, ovary, pancreas, head and neck). It is not clear whether the low level of NK cell activity predates the malignant process or is a consequence of progressive tumour growth. In addition, NK cells are involved in the control of microbial infections (viruses, parasites, fungi and bacteria) and take part in the regulation of haematopoiesis (Brittenden et al, 1996).

The effects of surgery on NK cell activity have been well documented. Although a small number of studies have shown an increase in NK cell activity following surgery, the majority of investigations have demonstrated a marked impairment of NK cell cytotoxicity (*Figure 10.1*) in the perioperative period (Khan et al, 1995). The duration of reduced NK cell activity varies with the extent of surgical trauma; it can be quite pronounced and last for up to 2 weeks after major surgery.

Not only is NK cell function depressed, but there is also a reduction in the circulating number of NK cells in the immediate postoperative period; NK cell levels in blood subsequently return to preoperative levels. This reduction in the number of NK cells is not related to the amount of intraoperative blood loss or other operative factors. However, haemorrhage and hypovolaemia, and infusion of allogeneic blood (see later sections), can all inhibit natural cytotoxicity. Changes in the levels of catecholamines, corticosteroids and prostaglandins in the perioperative period have all been suggested as possible mediators for these changes.

Irrespective of the inducing mechanisms, the inhibition of NK cell activity may partly explain the frequent incidence of infection and likelihood of severe sepsis following major surgery or trauma, and highlights the risk of possible tumour cell dissemination and establishment of metastatic disease with major resectional cancer surgery.

Lymphokine-activated killer cells

LAK cells are believed to be derived from NK cells or their precursors following stimulation by IL-2, and have a wider cytotoxic repertoire and increased activity against a range of tumour cells, including autochthonous cancer

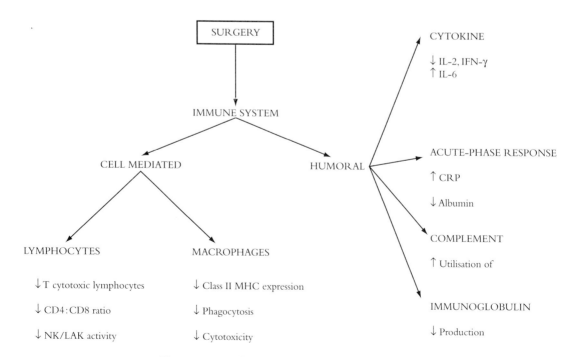

Figure 10.1   Effects of surgery on the immune system.

cells. LAK cells express CD16, CD56 and various other cell surface markers. Animal studies have demonstrated the effectiveness of LAK cells in destroying a wide range of metastatic and advanced malignancies (carcinomas, sarcomas), with both immunogenic and non-immunogenic tumours. However, in humans, the precise role of LAK cells in the destruction of tumour cells has not been fully elucidated. Some patients with malignant disease have been demonstrated to have reduced levels of LAK activity in peripheral blood, whereas in other patients LAK activity does not appear to be reduced.

LAK cells, produced *in vitro* after harvesting of peripheral blood lymphocytes and incubation with recombinant IL-2, have been used in the treatment of human malignant disease (with and without other cytokines). Such forms of therapy have produced a variable degree of efficacy in destroying metastatic tumour deposits, most notably in the treatment of melanoma and renal cell cancers (Heys et al, 1993).

The effects of surgery on LAK cells are not well studied and variable findings (inhibition, no change) have been documented. The interpretation of these results is open to debate and is further complicated by the fact that certain tumours can produce substances that inhibit LAK cell generation.

Monocytes and macrophages

Macrophages play a key role in host defences by functioning as antigen-presenting cells. They ingest and partially degrade the antigen, re-expressing it on the cell surface in its modified form (closely linked to the class II MHC antigens) to $CD4^+$ T helper cells (T_H1), inducing the release of IL-2 and other cytokines. In addition, they regulate the immune response by acting as either activators or suppressors of immune processes. During infection, trauma and surgery, macrophages are activated through the release of macrophage-activating factors from T lymphocytes specifically sensitised to antigens. These factors include the important regulatory cytokines IFN-γ and IL-2, as well as the granulocyte–macrophage colony-stimulating factors (Ennen et al, 1986). The activation of macrophages results in the release of various secretory products, such as stromal degradation enzymes and cytokines (e.g. IL-1, IL-6 and TNF-α), which induce an acute-phase response, as well as prostanoids (e.g. prostaglandin (PG) E_2), which suppress host defences (Boraschi et al, 1984).

Although surgery increases the absolute number of circulating monocytes (*Table 10.2*), it inhibits significantly various macrophage functions (phagocytosis, chemotactic motility, release of lytic enzymes and free radicals, etc.). This is due to an increase in the secretion of inhibitory prostanoids (e.g. PGE_2) and concomitant reduction in the secretion of enhancing cytokines (e.g. IL-1, IL-2), as well as diminished expression of human leucocyte antigen (HLA)-DR expression (Hershman et al, 1990).

Inappropriate and uncontrolled release of humoral mediators by macrophages in trauma and sepsis is believed to be an important mechanism of this immune suppression, and is supported by extensive work done both in animal models and in the clinical setting. The production of excessive TNF-α and arachidonic acid metabolites (such as PGE_2) by macrophages following trauma, inhibits the release of IL-2 by T_H1 lymphocytes. The inhibition of IL-2 release downregulates T-cell expansion and proliferation, and also inhibits the expression of T-cell IL-2 receptors.

The secretion of IFN-γ by T_H1 lymphocytes is also reduced. This produces two variable effects on macrophages. Firstly, it acts as a negative feedback on macrophage activation and secondly, the lack of IFN-γ further promotes the release of PGE_2, while the secretion of IL-1 by macrophages is reduced.

The factors that induce the macrophages to become inhibitory are not fully characterised. The presence of

Table 10.2 Effects of surgery on the number and functions of macrophages and neutrophils.

Monocytes and macrophages	Neutrophils
1. **Monocytosis**	1. **Neutrophilia**
2. **Function**	2. **Function**
Decreased	*Decreased*
Chemotaxis	Chemotaxis
Phagocytosis	Phagocytosis
Release of free radicals	Release of free radicals
Lysosomal production	Lysosomal production
Downregulation of MHC class II antigens (HLA-DR expression)	Respiratory burst
	Myeloperoxidase activity
	B_{12}-binding protein activities
	Superoxide production
	Release of LTC_4
	Increased
	Production of LTB_4

excessive amounts of immune complexes or complement components (*in situ* or in the circulation) may play an important role in the overproduction of prostaglandins and dysregulation of cytokine release by macrophages. These various disturbances of macrophage function induced by trauma and tissue damage are believed to predispose to sepsis, cachexia and delayed rehabilitation, particularly if this dysfunction is pronounced and prolonged (weeks).

Neutrophils

Although neutrophils are not part of the cell-mediated immune response, they are key cells involved in the non-specific but very important host defence against bacterial infections. They rapidly ingest and dispose of bacteria by generating intracellular free radicals (superoxide, hydrogen peroxide, hydroxyl moieties). They also produce and release other chemical mediators that are important in the inflammatory response. For example, they generate leukotriene (LT) B_4, which is a potent chemo-attractant for neutrophils, and LTC_4 and LTD_4, which increase microvascular permeability to other inflammatory cells.

Following surgery, there is a leucocytosis in peripheral blood, with an increased proportion of neutrophils and monocytes and a reduction in the number of circulating eosinophils and lymphocytes. Despite this increase in the numbers of neutrophils, there is impairment of various neutrophil functions following major surgery and severe trauma. For example, the following defects have been documented: impaired chemotaxis, defective phagocytosis, reduced lysosomal enzyme content, decreased myeloperoxidase activity and defective superoxide production (Utoh et al, 1988). All of these functions play an important role in the antimicrobial activity of neutrophils. Leukotriene production is also altered in the postoperative period, with an enhanced production of LTB_4 and a decreased release of LTC_4.

This significant impairment of neutrophil function in the perioperative period and following severe trauma is partly due to a change in the circulating neutrophil subpopulations: an increased number and proportion of immature neutrophils. Enhanced catecholamine and glucocorticoid output following trauma may play an important part in the impairment of various aspects of neutrophil function, leading to defective handling of endogenous organisms and environmental pathogens. Drugs and anaesthetic agents, used in treating such injured patients and those undergoing major surgery, may also contribute to this disturbance of circulating neutrophil numbers and functions.

HUMORAL IMMUNITY

Humoral immunity is mediated by a variety of soluble factors (e.g. acute-phase reactants, complement components and immunoglobulins). B lymphocytes, which respond to foreign antigens (with or without the help of T lymphocytes) by developing into antibody-producing plasma cells, play a central role. Humoral immunity is the principal defence mechanism against extracellular pathogens and their toxins because antibodies can bind to these and assist in their inactivation and subsequent removal. Until recently, the effect of surgery on humoral immunity was poorly investigated.

B lymphocytes

B lymphocytes contain cell surface receptors (immunoglobulins) for antigens and MHC class II molecules, which they use to recognise and interact with foreign antigens present on the surface membrane of mononuclear cells. B lymphocytes are stimulated to proliferate by IL-4 (produced by activated T_H2 lymphocytes), and are transformed into either antibody-producing plasma cells or memory cells by IL-5 (secreted by T_H2 cells) and IL-6 (produced by macrophages). The antibodies bind to microorganisms, allogeneic and tumour cells, and facilitate their inactivation, ingestion and destruction through complement-mediated lysis, phagocytosis by macrophages or antibody-dependent cellular cytotoxicity by killer (K) lymphocytes or monocytes. However, antibody production can be inhibited by T suppressor cells.

Studies evaluating the effect of surgery on circulating B-lymphocyte numbers have yielded variable results, with either no change, an increase or a decrease in the number of circulating B lymphocytes being reported to occur in the postoperative period (Mollitt et al, 1984).

The effects of surgery on B-lymphocyte function also have not been fully elucidated. Some studies have found an enhanced antibody response or no alteration, whereas others have documented a depressed antibody response following surgery. However, it has been demonstrated that surgery results in a reduction in the antibody concentration in the circulation. Factors that have been suggested to be responsible for this include haemodilution, extravascular loss of proteins and immunoglobulin consumption.

The antibody response by B lymphocytes to various polyclonal mitogens (e.g. pokeweed mitogen [PWM]) and antigens (*Staphylococcus aureus* Cowan I) has also been studied *in vitro* in patients who have undergone surgery. These studies have shown that surgical trauma depresses both the proliferative response and the antibody-producing response (IgG, IgM, IgA) to T cell-dependent mitogens but does not alter the production of antibodies to T cell-independent mitogens. This suggests that a T-cell defect may be responsible for this aspect of suppression of the immune response following major trauma.

Cytokines

Cytokines are endogenous peptides secreted by a variety of cells (lymphocytes, macrophages, Langerhans cells, fibroblasts, tumour cells) in response to stimuli such as surgery, trauma, infection and malignancy. They are involved in the control and regulation of the immune response, inflammation and tissue repair (Eremin and Sewell, 1992). The functions of a selected group of cytokines, IL-1β, IL-2, IL-6, IL-8, IL-10, IFN-γ and TNF-α, and changes in their serum concentrations following surgery, are discussed below.

Interleukin 1β

IL-1β is secreted primarily by cells of the monocyte–macrophage lineage in response to various injurious stimuli. It is required for activation and proliferation of T helper and cytotoxic cells, expression of IL-2 receptors, activation and chemo-attraction of neutrophils, and synthesis of acute-phase proteins by hepatocytes (Dinarello, 1984). The effects of IL-1β can be inhibited by IL-4, IFN-γ, IL-1 itself, PGE$_2$ and histamine. IL-1β levels increase within 2–4 hours after surgery and, in uncomplicated cases, return to normal within 12 hours. The serum concentration of IL-1β, however, is variable and is influenced by the presence of different plasma antagonists. Also, less than 20% of the total synthesised IL-1β is released into the circulation in the active form.

Interleukin 2

This is produced by T$_H$1 cells and increases the activity of cytotoxic T lymphocytes, NK and LAK cells, against both tumour cells and infective agents. Following surgery, serum levels of IL-2 have been reported to be decreased (Akiyoshi et al, 1985) and this impaired production of IL-2 has been correlated with an increased risk of sepsis and mortality (Wood et al, 1984). A reduced concentration of this key regulatory cytokine is a major disadvantage in the traumatised host, particularly with extensive tissue damage. Not only is the ability to mount an effective immune response compromised, but so is the control of inappropriate macrophage release of pro-inflammatory cytokines (e.g. TNF-α).

Interleukin 6

IL-6 is secreted by activated monocytes and macrophages in response to tissue injury and other inflammation-associated cytokines (IL-1, IL-3, TNF-α, platelet–derived growth factors, GM-CSF, etc.). IL-6 controls the transcription of hepatic cell production of acute-phase proteins, is involved in the differentiation of B lymphocytes into antibody-secreting plasma cells, and also stimulates various T lymphocyte subsets with subsequent production of IL-2 and cell proliferation. Moreover, in association with IL-2, it plays an important part in the generation and activation of NK and LAK cells. Plasma IL-6 concentration rises within 8 hours of trauma and may remain raised for up to 48–72 hours.

Interleukin 8

IL-8 is a major proinflammatory cytokine produced by lymphocytes, monocytes and epithelial cells. It belongs to a group of peptides termed chemokines, which are able to induce circulatory leucocytes to home into damaged and inflamed tissues. IL-8 is a selective chemo-attractant for neutrophils. Although its role in normal biological processes is poorly defined, several studies have documented the effects of IL-8 in various pathological conditions (Marty et al, 1994). High levels of IL-8 have been reported in chronic inflammatory conditions of skin (psoriasis) and joints. In patients with septic shock, the circulating levels of IL-8 correlate with the degree of insult and serum IL-6 concentrations. Thus, IL-8 probably does have an important role in tissue response to injury.

Interleukin 10

This is an important cytokine produced by T_H2 cells. It inhibits a range of immune responses, through suppression of T_H1 activity and modulation of the output of the key cytokine IL-2. There is some evidence to suggest that part of the immune suppression induced by trauma is due to activation of T_H2 cells and increased production of IL-10.

Tumour necrosis factor α

TNF-α is produced by macrophages and has selective anabolic effects on the liver. It stimulates production of acute-phase proteins, including C-reactive protein (CRP), hepatic uptake of amino acids and hepatic lipogenesis. It also has an effect on blood flow in the microcirculation of tissues. Uncontrolled and prolonged secretion of TNF-α is important in the induction of skeletal muscle protein breakdown, weight loss, inanition and delayed rehabilitation that not infrequently occurs after major trauma.

Interferon γ

IFN-γ is produced by T_H1 cells in response to various stimuli (e.g. IL-2, polyribonucleotides, viruses). IFN-γ activates the microbicidal activities of macrophages and increases the expression of their MHC class II antigens. It also activates NK cells and regulates antibody production by B cells, and increases the production of IL-1, TNF, IL-4 and IL-10. Following major surgery, there are decreased levels in the serum of IFN-γ. The reasons for this are not well established, but highlight the disordered capacity of host defences to mount an effective response as a result of major trauma.

A marked increase in the serum concentration of the above cytokines, however, may be detrimental to the host. For instance, very high levels of IL-1 may induce adult respiratory distress syndrome, TNF may cause cardiovascular collapse and death, and a serum IL-6 concentration over $400 \, \text{pg ml}^{-1}$ is associated with a high incidence of major postoperative complications. The serum levels of these cytokines, therefore, are regulated by a number of cytokine antagonists; these include antagonists for TNF and IL-1 receptor (IL-1ra). High levels of IL-1ra have been detected in serum after elective surgery, although its functions remain to be fully clarified.

Complement

The complement system comprises a series of plasma and cell membrane proteins, which are involved in host defence against microbial infections and in the pathogenesis of immunologically mediated diseases. Complement components are secreted by hepatocytes and macrophages into the serum and mediate the non-specific component of humoral immunity.

The complement system can be activated either by antibodies ('classical' pathway) or by various antibody-independent mechanisms ('alternative' pathway). Complement has a wide range of biological functions; these include opsonisation and lysis of invading microorganisms and abnormal cells, mediation of the inflammatory process, chemotactic activities and solubilisation of immune complexes.

The complement system is activated by trauma either via the classical or the alternative pathway. This leads to a reduction in the circulating levels of various complement components, as a result of their increased consumption and the appearance of the products of complement activation in the systemic circulation. These reductions in the levels of complement components have been shown to be associated with an increased risk of sepsis (Heideman et al, 1982). In patients following trauma or with major burns, the degree of depletion of the proteins of the complement system has been correlated with the severity of the injuries. Various factors have been proposed to be responsible for this reduced complement activity. These include activation by released products of tissue damage, denaturation and loss of plasma proteins, and the use of polyanions such as heparin during and after surgery.

The acute-phase response

The acute-phase response is a non-specific humoral response occurring as a result of trauma, surgery, sepsis and malignancy. This is characterised by alterations in the serum concentrations of specific plasma proteins termed the acute-phase proteins (APPs), which have a wide range of biological functions. The APPs are believed to be important in restricting tissue damage, by scavenging and neutralising oxygen free radicals and released proteolytic enzymes, and in aiding with phagocytosis and removal of antigens and microorganisms (Pepys and Baltz, 1983). They take part in promoting resolution of tissue damage and enhancing tissue repair, and are believed to modulate both non-specific and specific components of host defences. More recently, it has been suggested that one of the APPs, CRP, may enhance lymphocyte proliferation and modulate NK cell activity. The synthesis of some of the APPs is upregulated (e.g. CRP and α_1-antitrypsin), whereas that of others is reduced (e.g. albumin, prealbumin, transferrin) following severe trauma and major surgery. The hepatic production and release of these APPs is controlled by various cytokines (IL-1, TNF-α and IL-6), although it is now believed that both IL-1 and TNF-α mediate this action predominantly through IL-6.

Changes in the circulating levels of APPs following surgery have been well documented and CRP concentration shown to be a sensitive marker of both the timing and magnitude of trauma. In addition, serial measurements of CRP may be helpful in the early detection and monitoring of postoperative complications. Serum levels of CRP begin to rise approximately 6 hours after surgery; they peak at 48 hours and then fall towards preoperative levels by the third day after operation. A delay of up to 24 hours occurs before the initiation of a rise in the serum level of other proteins; for example, α_1-antitrypsin reaches a peak at 72–96 hours and falls by the fourth day after operation. Serum concentrations of these mediators accurately and sensitively reflect the temporal course of tissue inflammation and/or necrosis, and persistently high values beyond the third day after surgery suggest a continued source of inflammation.

ASSOCIATED FACTORS IN TRAUMA-INDUCED IMMUNE SUPPRESSION

In addition to the immunosuppressive effects of physical trauma, a number of other factors may also induce immunosuppression in the perioperative period or following trauma. Some of these factors are discussed below.

Anaesthesia

As early as 1903, it was documented that experimental animals subjected to anaesthesia had a reduced resistance to infection. Over the past two decades, extensive research has been carried out to elucidate the effects of anaesthesia (general, regional), analgesia and other drugs on host defences. Although it is difficult to isolate the effects of anaesthesia from those of surgery, there is convincing evidence that anaesthesia *per se* induces immune suppression, albeit with a transient effect. In the clinical setting, this immune dysfunction may be more important in patients receiving prolonged anaesthesia, as in intensive care units.

The adverse effects of anaesthesia on the host immune response may be due either to the mechanical ventilation or to the anaesthetic drugs used. The former include the depressed mucociliary function due to tracheal intubation and the systemic effects associated with ventilation (such as impaired mobilisation of lymphocytes and reduced thoracic duct lymph flow), which impairs bacterial clearance. The effects of anaesthetic agents on the immune system have been investigated by means of *in vitro* experiments assessing drugs on cellular function. Anaesthesia has been shown to suppress a variety of cell-mediated immune responses (Salo, 1982). Natural cytotoxicity is downregulated by anaesthetic agents such as halothane and isoflurane.

Even when anaesthetic agents spared baseline NK cell activity, they reduced interferon-inducible cytotoxicity. However, when interferon was administered to an animal before anaesthesia, NK cell cytotoxicity was unaffected. This highlights the importance of interferon in the regulation of NK cell cytotoxicity and the potential of augmenting NK cell activity in immunocompromised patients undergoing surgery. B-cell function also may be impaired by anaesthetic agents. IgG production is first reduced and, with increasing concentrations of the anaesthetic drugs, there is reduction in IgM and subsequently IgA.

General anaesthesia would be expected to induce a greater depressive effect upon host defences than regional anaesthesia. Clinically, regional anaesthesia is associated with reduced blood loss, shortened postoperative stay and smaller incidences of pulmonary infection and thromboembolic episodes. Epidural analgesia reduces the endocrine-mediated metabolic response to stress and, thus, is less likely to induce significant immune suppression, compared with general anaesthesia.

These clinical differences have not always been reflected in concurrent alterations of immune reactivity assessed *in vitro*. In patients undergoing total hip arthroplasty, there was no difference in the postoperative leucocytosis and lymphopenia in those who received regional, compared with general, anaesthesia. Similarly, no differences were found in the type IV hypersensitivity responses or in circulating T-cell subsets in patients undergoing major abdominal surgery. The severity of anaesthetic-induced immunosuppression is related directly to the duration of the anaesthesia. The mechanism of cell-mediated immunity depression is not clear but it has been suggested by several *in vitro* studies that a number of anaesthetic agents (e.g. halothane, nitrous oxide, diethyl ether) are antimitotic and inhibit both RNA and protein synthesis.

Blood loss

Haemorrhage and hypovolaemia are frequently associated with trauma and surgery. It is not easy, therefore, to dissociate the effects of haemorrhage from those of the accompanying tissue damage. Consequently, various animal species have been studied to evaluate the adverse effects of blood loss on the host immune response.

Studies in experimental animals have shown that haemorrhage depresses both the cell-mediated and humoral immune responses (Chaudry et al, 1989). The proliferative responses of peripheral blood lymphocytes *in vitro* to various antigens and mitogens, and the secretion of cytokines such as IL-1, IL-3, IL-6 and IFN-γ, which modulate both cell-mediated and humoral immunity, are impaired by haemorrhage. Various studies have also provided direct evidence of suppression of B-lymphocyte function, macrophage activation, and alteration in cytotoxic T-cell and NK cell function. The antigen-presenting function, the expression of Fc or C3b receptors, and the cytotoxicity of macrophages are also depressed by haemorrhage. Interestingly, however, the cytotoxicity and cytokine secretion by hepatic Kupffer cells (*in situ* macrophages) are not impaired, but are in fact enhanced. This may be due to bacterial translocation across the gut and delivery to the liver via the portal circulation.

The factors responsible for immune suppression induced by haemorrhage remain elusive. However, a number of possibilities have been suggested. These include bacterial translocation across the gut and associated endotoxaemia, enhanced production of PGE_2, alteration in calcium homoeostasis, decreased cellular levels of ATP due to regional hypoxia, and enhanced secretion of hormones (e.g. catecholamines and corticosteroids).

Blood transfusion

The transmission of infection (viral, bacterial, protozoal) and fluid overload with subsequent cardiac failure are well-recognised complications of blood transfusion. The detrimental effects of blood transfusion on the host immune system have also been increasingly documented. Following the original report in 1973 of enhanced renal allograft survival in patients receiving blood transfusion, a number of studies have implied that the intravenous administration of blood transfusion leads to immune suppression in the host (Agarwal et al, 1993). Evidence is available that multiply transfused patients have low NK cell activity, abnormal immunoglobulin levels and impaired *in vitro* T-lymphocyte responses to foreign antigens. In addition, these patients also have defective phagocytosis and complement-mediated killing capacity. The generalised immunosuppression following transfusion appears to be related to an increased synthesis of PGE_2 and non-specific stimulation of suppressor T lymphocytes. This impaired immune system has been associated with an increased incidence of tumour recurrence and poor prognosis in patients with cancer. However, the vast majority of these studies were retrospective. More recently, findings from prospective studies have failed to confirm the retrospective observations. On the other hand, there are convincing data from prospective studies of an increased incidence of sepsis (wound, chest) in patients undergoing major resectional surgery for malignant disease.

MECHANISMS INDUCING IMMUNE SUPPRESSION

The precise nature of the mechanisms responsible for the immune suppression induced by trauma and surgery remains unclear, although several factors have been studied extensively to provide an explanation. Studies in humans and animals have produced conflicting results

Table 10.3 Mechanisms involved in trauma-associated immune suppression.

Cellular components	*T helper cells*: reduced numbers and activity (T_H1); abnormal activity (T_H2) *T suppressor cells*: increased numbers and activity ($CD8^+$) *Monocyte–macrophage suppressor cells*: increased numbers and activity ($CD14^+$); defective antigen presentation
Humoral components	*Abnormal cytokine production*: reduced levels (IL-1, IL-2, IFN-γ); increased levels (IL-6, IL-10, TNF-α) *Abnormal prostanoid production*: increased levels (PGE_2, PGF_2, thromboxanes, leukotrienes) *Exaggerated hormone release*: increased levels (catecholamines, glucocorticoids, prolactin, growth hormone) *Abnormal proteolytic enzymes and free radical release*
Gut barrier	*Bacterial translocation and endotoxaemia*: abnormal cytokine cascade activation; complement and acute-phase protein consumption

about the role of stress-induced hormones (e.g. cortisol, catecholamines, prolactin and growth hormone). Animal studies, however, suggest a possible role for the hypothalamopituitary axis and hypothalamic releasing factors. Immune suppression induced by trauma is a complex biological process, involving the differential activity of various helper and suppressor cells (lymphocytes, macrophages) and the release (often inappropriate and uncontrolled) of a range of humoral mediators (*Table 10.3*).

Suppressor cells

T suppressor cells are thought to be a distinct class of regulatory T cells whose interactions are probably mediated by soluble suppressor factors. They express the CD8 cell surface markers, although not all $CD8^+$ T lymphocytes are suppressor cells. The role postulated for T suppressor cells in trauma is to regulate and facilitate the rapid removal of autologous cellular constituents, thus minimising the risk of potentially antigenic proteins inducing autoimmune damage to the injured host. The uncoordinated and prolonged overactivity of these suppressor cells is believed to be a key factor inducing the severe and protracted inhibition of host defences documented following trauma, major surgery, burns, sepsis, etc. However, there appears to be a close association and integration with $CD4^+$ T helper cell activity. The ratio of T helper to T suppressor cells ($CD4^+ : CD8^+$) is regarded by some as an indicator of immune competence in a variety of diseases. Although not confirmed in all studies, a significant body of evidence suggests that major tissue damage results in the reduction of both T helper and suppressor cells, but with a differential inhibition in the number of circulating $CD4^+$ lymphocytes, with a result-

ing shift of the immunoregulatory system towards suppression.

T helper cells

Inappropriate production of IL-2 by T_H1 cells may be an important factor in the immune suppression associated with trauma, surgery and burns. Diminished IL-2 production has been documented in patients with moderate to severe injury and following extensive burns (Wood et al, 1984; Akiyoshi et al, 1985). The reduction in IL-2 production appears to be directly proportional to the severity of the trauma. In burned patients, low IL-2 production has been correlated with decreased *in vitro* lymphocyte blastogenesis to both PHA and concanavalin A.

The factors responsible for reduced T_H1 activity and IL-2 production are not well defined and are probably multifactorial. These factors include stress-related corticosteroid and catecholamine release, complement activation following trauma, and generation and activation of suppressor mechanisms (T cells, macrophages). As previously discussed, reduced IL-2 production may be due to inhibition of secretion of IL-1 by macrophages, possible sequestration of circulating $CD4^+$ cell subsets or excessive downregulation of T_H1 activity by IL-10 (see *Table 10.3*).

Macrophages and humoral mediators

Activated macrophages secrete a number of eicosanoid products including PGE_2, 6-keto-PGF_1, thromboxane B_1, PGF_2 and the leukotrienes. PGE_2 has well-recognised inhibitory effects on a range of immune functions (e.g.

NK cell cytotoxicity). High levels of PGE_2 (and its derivatives) have been found in patients with major burns. These raised values ($1000-3000\,pg\,ml^{-1}$) correlated with depressed *in vitro* lymphocyte responsiveness and were reversed with anti-PGE antibody.

Following trauma, a reduction in IL-2 production by blood lymphocytes, for 5–10 days after the severe injury, has been documented. This was shown to coincide with significantly raised levels of PGE_2 over the same temporal sequence. PGE_2 downregulates T_H1 activity (with intermittent inhibition of IL-2 production) and the expression of MHC class II antigens on monocytes (with resultant defective antigen presentation) (Faist et al, 1987).

In addition, PGE_2 inhibits the production of IL-1 by macrophages and reduces TNF-α synthesis and release by interfering with gene transcription. This appears to be a feedback mechanism as both IL-1 and TNF-α directly induce the release of PGE_2. The nature of the injury, to some degree, determines the eventual cytokine output. For example, trauma induces an increased production of PGE_2 with a concomitant fall in the level of IL-1, whereas thermal injury may produce a reversed pattern of cytokine production. However, in many instances of trauma, particularly with persistence of severe injury, uncoordinated and abnormal secretion of cytokines (IL-1, IL-2, IL-6, TNF-α, etc.) can occur and may have little correlation with PGE_2 levels in serum.

A potent regulator of monocyte function is IFN-γ, produced by activated T cells. Trauma, both thermal and direct injury, has been shown to reduce circulating levels of IFN-γ. Failure of production of IFN-γ can lead to defective expression of HLA-DR antigens (and thus antigen presentation), defective phagocytosis and release of proinflammatory cytokines by monocytes and macrophages.

Gut barrier

In addition to the functions of digestion, absorption and secretion, the intestine acts as a major protective barrier against the intestinal bacterial flora and their various toxins. The importance of the immune function of the gut-associated lymphoid tissue in the intestinal wall is evidenced by the presence of a rich network of lymphocytes, macrophages, Peyer patches and mesenteric lymph nodes, supported by the large volume of Kupffer cells in the liver and the major lymphoreticular organ, the spleen. The intestinal mucosa may be transgressed by bacteria and

toxins in conditions associated with defective splanchnic blood flow, loss of enterocyte integrity and impaired gut-associated host defences, such as occurs in major surgery, severe trauma, extensive burns and serious sepsis (Wilmore et al, 1988). Hypovolaemia with selective redistribution of organ blood flow and defective splanchnic microcirculation is believed to be an important initiating factor. Bacterial translocation may also occur when the gut mucosa is physically disrupted and in conditions of intestinal bacterial overgrowth, such as occurs in intestinal stasis, with long-term antibiotic therapy, etc.

The loss of the intestinal mucosal barrier results in bacterial or endotoxin invasion, which may have substantial systemic immunosuppressive effects. Intestinal endotoxin has been shown to induce the proliferation of suppressor T cells, which may inhibit both specific and non-specific immune responses (Deitch et al, 1991). The resultant suppression of host defences and uncontrolled and inappropriate release of various humoral mediators (PGE_2, TNF-α, kinins, etc.) can result in multiorgan failure.

REFERENCES

Agarwal N, Murphy JG, Cayten G et al. Blood transfusion increases the risk of infection after trauma. *Arch Surg* 1993; **128**: 171–177.

Akiyoshi T, Koba F, Arianga S et al. Impaired production of interleukin-2 after surgery. *Clin Exp Immunol* 1985; **59**: 45–49.

Biebuyck JF. The metabolic response to stress: an overview and update. *Anaesthesiology* 1990; **73**: 308–327.

Boraschi D, Censini S, Tagliabue A. Interferon reduces macrophage suppressive activity by inhibiting prostaglandin E₂ release and inducing interleukin 1 production. *J Immunol* 1984; **133**: 764–768

Brittenden J, Heys SD, Ross, J, Eremin O. Natural killer (NK) cells and cancer. *Cancer* 1996; **77**: 1226–1243.

Chaudry IH, Stephen RN, Harkema JM et al. Immunological alterations following simple haemorrhage. In: Faist E, Ninnemann J, Green D (eds). *Immune Consequences of Trauma, Shock and Sepsis*. Berlin: Springer, 1989: 363–373.

Deitch EA, Dazhong Xu, Lu Qi et al. Bacterial translocation from the gut impairs systemic immunity. *Surgery* 1991; **109**: 269–276.

Dinarello CA. Interleukin-1 and the pathogenesis of acute phase response. *N Engl J Med* 1984; **31**: 1413–1418.

Ennen JM, Ernst M, Flad HD. Lymphokine-activated monocytes: role of interferon-γ and interleukin 2. *Immunobiology* 1986; **173**: 117.

Eremin O, Sewell H. *The Immunological Basis of Surgical Science and Practice*. Oxford: Oxford University Press, 1992.

Faist E, Mewes A, Baker CC et al. Prostaglandin E₂ (PGE_2)-

dependent suppression of interleukin-2 production in patients with major trauma. *J Trauma* 1987; **27**: 837–848.

Guillou PJ. Biological variation in the development of sepsis after surgery or trauma. *Lancet* 1993; **342**: 217–220.

Heideman M, Saravis C, Clowes GHA. Effect of nonviable tissues and abscesses on complement depletion and the development of bacteremia. *J Trauma* 1982; **22**: 527–532.

Hershman MJ, Cheadle WG, Wallhausen SR et al. Monocyte HLA-DR antigen expression characterizes clinical outcome in the trauma patients. *Br J Surg* 1990; **77**: 204–207.

Heys SD, Franks C, Eremin O. Interleukin-2 therapy: current role in surgical oncological practice. *Br J Surg* 1993; **80**: 155–162.

Khan AL, Heys SD, Eremin O et al. Polyadenylic–polyuridylic acid enhances natural cell-mediated cytotoxicity in patients with breast cancer undergoing mastectomy. *Surgery* 1995; **118**: 531–538.

Marty C, Misset B, Tamion F et al. Circulating interleukin-8 concentration in multiple organ failure of septic and nonseptic origin. *Crit Care Med* 1994; **22**: 673–679.

Mollitt DL, Steele RW, Marmer DJ et al. Surgically induced immunological alterations in the child. *J Pediatr Surg* 1984; **19**: 818–821.

Pepys MB, Baltz ML. Acute phase proteins with special reference to C-reactive protein and related proteins (pentaxins) and serum amyloid A protein. *Adv Immunol* 1983; **34**: 141–211.

Salo M. Effects of anaesthesia and surgery on the immune response. In: Watkins J, Salo M (eds) *Trauma, Stress and Immunity in Anaesthesia and Surgery*. London: Butterworths, 1982; 211–253.

Utoh J, Yamamoto T, Utsunomiya T et al. Effect of surgery on neutrophil function, superoxide and leukotriene production. *Br J Surg* 1988; **75**: 682–685.

Wilmore DW, Smith RJ, O'Dwyer ST et al. The gut: a central organ after surgical stress. *Surgery* 1988; **104**: 917–923.

Wood JJ, Rodrick ML, O'Mahony JB et al. Inadequate interleukin 2 production: a fundamental immunological deficiency in patients with major burns. *Ann Surg* 1984; **200**: 311–320.

11

Cartilage Changes in Osteoarthritis and Rheumatoid Arthritis

Mark F Brown

INTRODUCTION

The effects of osteoarthritis (OA) and rheumatoid arthritis (RA) account for the majority of the adult elective orthopaedic workload. One-third of all impairment in the population is as a result of OA or RA, 25% of general practice consultations are for joint and back pain, and about 40 000 hip joint replacements alone are performed per year in the UK for advanced disease. In elderly people the numbers are even greater: 50% of those aged over 65 years have symptomatic joint disease. The clinical features are familiar to all doctors, and to orthopaedic surgeons in particular: pain and loss of function of joints, frequently accompanied by swelling, and with warmth and redness completing Celsus' cardinal signs of inflammation, at some stage at least, in all cases of RA and in many cases of OA.

Macroscopically OA and RA are typically rather different, with OA being hypertrophic (osteophytes and subchondral sclerosis are typical) and RA being atrophic (cysts, erosions, osteopenia and muscle wasting). This difference was noted by Goldthwaite in 1897 (Dieppe, 1991). Idiopathic OA, as opposed to that following trauma or osteonecrosis, is a disease of middle age and onwards, which has led to the view of it as a matter simply of 'wear and tear'. It especially affects hands, hips, knees and lumbar zygapophysial joints, giving rise to pain and stiffness. RA, by contrast, has a peak incidence in the fourth decade of life, and affects all joints of the upper limb, especially hands and wrists, the cervical spine and knees.

The end result of both OA and RA is joint destruction, with loss of articular cartilage and ultimately bone changes. The pathogenesis of such cartilage loss is the subject of this chapter.

JOINT DISEASES: HISTORICAL ASPECTS AND NOMENCLATURE

Joint diseases have been recognised for a very long time, and have existed for as long as evidence is available, being demonstrable in palaeolithic and even Neanderthal human skeletons, and from even earlier in other mammals. Indeed, the preponderance of osteoarthritic changes in cave bears led Virchow to refer to it as *Hohlengicht* (cave gout). Osteoarthritic changes are widespread in Ancient Egyptian mummies. The earliest known reference to joint disease is found in the state letters of ancient Assyria, where gout is mentioned. The distinction between gout, OA and RA was not made clearly until Garrod's 1907 edition of *A System of Medicine*, although Hippocrates, Galen and Sydenham apparently recognised the difference between rheumatism and gout. The first description of RA as such was by Haygarth in 1805, under the title of *Nodosity of the Joints*. Heberden described OA of finger joints, and the nodes which now bear his name, in 1803.

It is often suggested that the correct term for OA is osteoarthrosis (see, for example, Chapter 5), because of the view that *-itis* implies inflammation, which, it is suggested, is not present in OA. This, it can be argued, is misguided. The word 'arthritis' was used for an affection of the joints long before concepts of inflammation were formulated; and 'osteoarthrosis' sounds as though it should have a similar etymology to such anatomical terms as diarthrosis, amphiarthrosis, etc., and refer to a type of articulation.

Theories of the aetiology have abounded: cold and damp in the eighteenth century, lactic acid in the nineteenth century, and the triad of infection, autoimmune disorder and genetic causes in the twentieth century. Infective agents suggested have been bacteria, mycoplasma, blue-green algae and viruses. Slow viruses (lentiviruses, one of three types of retrovirus) currently receive the most support (Kalden et al, 1991).

EPIDEMIOLOGY AND AETIOLOGY

Osteoarthritis

A degree of damage to cartilage is a normal ageing phenomenon. Only a proportion of these cases progress to symptomatic OA, and many factors seem to be involved. For example, hand and knee OA have a higher female preponderance than hip OA; obesity is closely correlated with hand and knee OA but not with hip disease, and so on. It would appear that genetic factors, age, sex, occupation, local joint factors such as injury, sporting activity, and so on, all combine to create clinical OA. It is clearly, however, more than just the 'wear and tear' it was once thought to be, with specific changes in numerous measurable markers. OA of relatively early onset can be associated with a mild chondrodysplasia, and in such cases there is a specific amino acid substitution in type II collagen (519 Arg → Cys) (Lohmander, 1994). The possibility remains that idiopathic OA may be genetically determined.

Rheumatoid arthritis

RA has even more specific accompanying changes. The theory of an infective aetiology has remained a possibility (Kalden et al, 1991), and the pathogenetic mechanisms are becoming clearer as large amounts of research are devoted to the subject. The aetiology certainly has a genetic element, and the association with the class II human leucocyte antigen (HLA) DR4 is well known. HLA-DR4 is more common in patients with severe disease, but there is no correlation with presence of rheumatoid factors. Similarly the autoimmune element to the aetiology is clear, with several characteristic auto-antibodies. It predominates in females, with a ratio of around 3 : 1, as is the case for many autoimmune diseases, and symptoms are frequently alleviated during the last trimester of pregnancy.

ARTICULAR CARTILAGE AND ITS STRUCTURE

To appreciate the changes that occur in disease, and in this context especially RA and OA, one must look at the biochemical and physical changes in terms of their effects on the function of cartilage. The only function of articular cartilage is as a bearing surface, to allow as nearly as possible friction-free movement between the bones involved in diarthrodial joints.

The structure of normal articular cartilage has been covered in detail in Chapter 5; the following summarises aspects of relevance to the changes observed with ageing and disease. Articular cartilage is unusual in several respects: its avascularity, absence of nerves, and absence of a basement membrane. Its cellularity is very low, a property shared only with the other two avascular tissues in the body, the intervertebral disc and the vitreous of the eye. The mechanical properties depend on the interrelationship between collagen fibres and ground substance (proteoglycan). Like most tissues, the greatest constituent of cartilage is water (65–80%), and if the matrix loses water as a result of losing proteoglycan, the mechanical properties are lost. The stresses within cartilage can be huge; during normal activity, pressures can rise to 10–20 MPa over short periods of time in small areas. This is probably the ultimate cause of breakdown in OA, although it would appear that high pressure is required for maintenance of a normal matrix (Urban, 1994).

The collagen fibres, predominantly type II (see below), of the matrix, are arranged in hoops, arising from the tide-mark (calcified zone) at the bone–cartilage junction, and peaking just below the surface. At or near the surface of the cartilage, the fibres run transversely (or more accurately, tangentially). Thus shear forces at the surface are experienced by the collagen fibres as tension (in which they are strong) rather than bending (in which they are weak). This zone of tangential collagen fibres, closely packed and with very little proteoglycan, is seen under phase contrast microscopy as a bright line – the lamina splendens. It is coated with a film of adsorbed

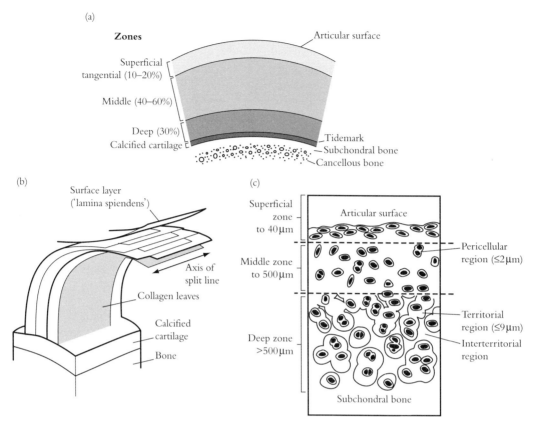

Figure 11.1   Topography of the collagen fibres in articular cartilage. From Sledge (1993), courtesy of Rockefeller University Press.

hyaluronan complexed to a glycoprotein, and probably important in lubrication. Deeper in the cartilage, the collagen fibres run more and more perpendicular, until they are 'gripped' by the calcified layer of cartilage at the tide-mark, thus completing the loop, and preventing the fibres from separating under the swelling pressure exerted by the proteoglycan (*Figure 11.1*).

The cellularity is greater in the middle of the cartilage, where proteoglycan turnover is higher (Stockwell, 1979); one can imagine that maintenance of the swelling pressure in the middle of the cartilage is the main function of the cells of normal adult cartilage. The surface of articular cartilage is not quite the 'smooth, polished, and covered with a membrane' surface that Hunter described in 1742–3. Apart from the well-known fact that it is not covered with a synovial membrane, neither is it smooth. It has been demonstrated that there are undulations, both of the order of 0.4–0.5 mm and also of 20–30 μm. These may be important in joint lubrication (see below).

MACROMOLECULES OF ARTICULAR CARTILAGE

Collagens

Articular hyaline cartilage (the cartilage of all diarthrodial joints except on bones ossifying in mesenchyme) contains two fibrillar and three non-fibrillar types of collagen. Type II is found in the greatest quantity (about 90%) and is the main structural collagen, providing tensile strength and acting as a check to swelling of the proteoglycan ground substance. It has a structural effect only when in tension, explaining why cartilage loses structural integrity when proteoglycan is removed, either as a temporary phenomenon (see reference to Thomas's experiments on rabbit ears in Chapter 5) or permanently in the arthritides. Loss of proteoglycan from the cartilage of a load-bearing joint quickly leads to loss of collagen by attrition. Type XI collagen is the other fibril-forming type; it is present in

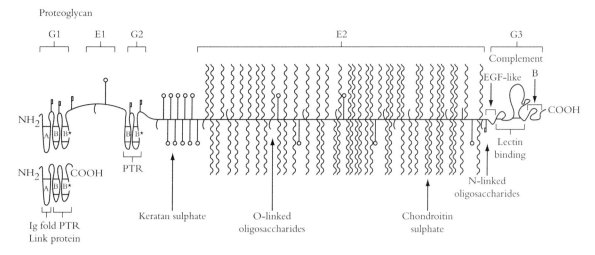

Figure 11.2   Structure of aggrecan, the large aggregating proteoglycan of articular cartilage. PTR, proteoglycan tandem repeat. From Hardingham et al (1992), with permission.

only small amounts and may be involved in control of collagen fibril diameter.

Type IX collagen is a short molecule that does not form fibrils, but has the unique property of being effectively both a form of collagen and a form of proteoglycan, and it can bind covalently to both type II collagen and to chondroitin sulphate. This suggests that its role may be to hold proteoglycan ground substance in the collagen matrix; it may also cross-link type II collagen and add to its strength. If forms about 1% of adult articular cartilage collagen (10% in the foetus). Type X collagen is present in small amounts in the deep calcified layer of mature cartilage, as well as in the growth plates of developing bones; it is synthesised only by hypertrophic chondrocytes. Its function is unclear. Type VI collagen is found in small amounts in articular cartilage, especially in the lacunae around chondrocytes, and aspects of its structure suggests that it may have cell adhesion properties.

Proteoglycans

This subject also has been described in detail in Chapter 5. The basic structure of the large aggregating proteoglycan or aggrecan, the main cartilage proteoglycan, is a central core protein (molecular weight 210 kDa) with side branches of the glycosaminoglycans chondroitin sulphate and keratan sulphate attached by link protein, of covalently linked oligosaccharides, and with a binding region at one end. The ratio of the two glycosaminoglycans varies with age and location, and also with disease, but in general up to about 100 molecules of chondroitin sulphate and 50 of keratan sulphate may be attached to each protein core (*Figure 11.2*).

The proteoglycans aggregate extracellularly by binding to a hyaluronic acid (hyaluronan) chain; there are several hundred proteoglycan molecules to each hyaluronan chain of molecular weight 1–3 MDa. The whole aggregate has a molecular weight of 5×10^7 to 5×10^8. Hyaluronan itself is a glycosaminoglycan, to which chondrocytes can bind by way of cell surface receptors. The minor proteoglycans decorin, biglycan and fibromodulin are described in Chapter 5. Decorin and fibromodulin are known to interact with type II collagen, and are found in greater amounts in the superficial layer of articular cartilage. The function of biglycan is unknown, but it has been shown that transforming growth factor-β (TGF-β) binds to both biglycan and decorin (Lohmander, 1994). The turnover of proteoglycans is, by contrast with that of collagens, quite rapid (half-life in the region of 1 year), and this is probably the reason for proteoglycan loss being at least initially reversible. They are degraded by various enzymes, notably the matrix metalloproteinases. The major glycosaminoglycans are highly sulphated, which gives the molecules an overall fixed negative charge. This leads to a higher concentration of cations (notably Na^+) within the matrix than in the fluid with which it is at equilibrium, according to the Gibbs–

Donnan equilibrium (see Chapter 5), and so a higher osmotic pressure. This pressure is balanced by the tension in the collagen fibrils, so maintaining cartilage structure. The swelling pressure of the aggrecan is such that, in water, it swells to about 50 times its dry volume; in healthy cartilage, however, the swelling is restricted to only 20% of this, by the collagen meshwork.

Other components of articular cartilage matrix

The other important components of the matrix are the non-collagen proteins fibronectin, chondrocalcin, cartilage oligomeric matrix protein (COMP), anchorin and tenascin. Fibronectin is a cell surface glycoprotein adhesion molecule, present in small amounts in normal articular cartilage and related to plasma fibronectin, previously known as cold insoluble globulin. It is found in greater amounts in the superficial layer of cartilage in RA (Shiozawa et al, 1992), where it is thought to be responsible for allowing extension of the pannus over the joint surface. Fibronectin concentration is also increased in osteoarthritic cartilage (Lohmander, 1994), where it may enhance release of metalloproteinases from chondrocytes; certainly, fibronectin fragments can cause chondrolysis in tissue culture. Anchorin and tenascin are also adhesion molecules, whose exact function is unclear. Tenascin, like COMP, is of interest mainly as a marker of joint destruction in the arthritic diseases, but it also has functions in wound repair. It has been shown to be present in greater amounts in arthritic cartilage and synovial membrane; this may represent a repair phenomenon (Salter, 1993).

CHONDROCYTES

The cells of cartilage are unusual in several respects. They are of a single type, they have an extremely low mitotic rate (in fact, in normal cartilage they probably do not divide at all) and because of the avascular nature of all articular cartilage they exist in a very hypoxic environment with a high lactate concentration. Their metabolism is largely anaerobic, and the cells are at a very low density. This is presumably because of the poor supply of nutrients and oxygen, although glucose concentration is diminished to a lesser extent than in that of oxygen. It can be

shown (Stockwell, 1979) that there is a constant relationship between articular cartilage thickness and cellularity, such that the number of cells under a unit surface area of cartilage is roughly constant, even over a very wide range of thicknesses. Incidentally, this may be a relationship that applies to all avascular tissues, as it also obtains for the intervertebral disc, with a thickness about another factor of 10 greater. As far as is known, the only function of chondrocytes is synthesis and control of the matrix, and to this end they synthesise the matrix macromolecules and also the growth factors and enzymes that are involved.

The hydrostatic pressure experienced by chondrocytes is also remarkable – up to 10–20 MPa (see above) – and such pressures are both necessary for normal chondrocyte metabolism (Urban, 1994) and may serve for mechanotransduction to allow modelling of cartilage to accommodate loads (Swann and Seedhom, 1993).

SYNOVIAL FLUID

Normal synovial fluid is a clear, slightly yellowish, viscous fluid, rather like egg white (hence its name). It is rich in hyaluronan, as well as having small amounts of glycoproteins and glycosaminoglycans, and has a sparse cellularity. These features all change in disease, with the characteristic rheumatoid fluid being less viscous (at least partly because of enzymatic degradation of hyaluronan) and more cellular. It is also rich in enzymes secreted by the rheumatoid pannus (cathepsins and metalloproteinases; see below) and in cytokines such as catabolin/interleukin-1 (IL) (see below). Osteoarthritic synovial fluid is typically present in greater amounts than normal, owing to a secondary synovitis, but is of normal viscosity. It is often mildly increased in cellularity, and often has debris from cartilage or bone attrition. It may contain crystals if, as often the case, there is an element of gout or pseudogout. Its function is nutritive to the cartilage and for lubrication of the joint.

Lubrication of the synovial joint

The friction in the normal synovial joint is remarkably low – similar to wet ice on wet ice – and this is maintained until senescence. This is a remarkable achievement, and is dependent on mechanisms of lubrication that are still not fully understood (Unsworth and Seedhom, 1993). Several types of lubrication are recognised, the main types of relevance being fluid film and boundary lubrication. Fluid film is the ideal form of lubrication, whereby the opposing surfaces do not touch, because of a continuous film of fluid between them. This film may be created by external pressure, as in the internal combustion engine (hydrodynamic), or by moving parts entraining the lubricant, as in wheel bearings (hydrostatic). Boundary lubrication relies on adsorbed lubricant to reduce the coefficient of friction of surfaces that do touch. Articular cartilage lubrication is much more complex, in which a biphasic model of lubrication can explain the frictional properties of joints (see Chapter 16).

The surface of articular cartilage is not quite smooth when viewed at high magnification, and this leads to trapping of the viscous synovial fluid, rich in hyaluronan, in the crevices formed as the two slightly irregular surfaces are forced together. The hydrostatic pressure exceeds the swelling pressure of the cartilage matrix, and water flows from fluid to cartilage. This leads to an increase in viscosity of the film of synovial fluid, until the pressures are equal. A gel is formed, preventing the cartilage surfaces from touching and providing very good lubrication. This process breaks down in RA, owing to the lower viscosity and lower hyaluronan content of the fluid, and secondary cartilage breakdown occurs.

CARTILAGE CHANGES WITH AGEING

To appreciate the changes in the arthritic diseases, they must be seen in the context of the normal changes with age. There are changes in cellular and matrix composition, and with these changes in the mechanical properties. The superficial chondrocytes are mostly lost, with a slight increase in those of deeper zones; the significance of this is unknown. Water content decreases, and the amount of keratan sulphate increases with age. Thus the keratan sulphate to chondroitin sulphate ratio increases. This leads to a greater compressive stiffness of the matrix and an increased transmission of stress to the subchondral bone. An exaggeration of this may be responsible for the sclerosis seen in the subchondral bone in OA; it is reasonable to suppose that such sclerosis might be effect

rather than cause of cartilage changes (Nuki, 1980; Swann and Seedhom, 1993). Chondroitin sulphate chain length is decreased, which may give rise to a reduced swelling pressure and so lead to the decreased water content. However, this is difficult to reconcile with the swelling observed in very early OA or chondromalacia (see next section).

There are changes in the content of minor proteoglycans and non-collagen proteins. Tenascin is not present in youth, but develops with age, and is present in greater amounts in both RA and OA (Salter, 1993).

Chondromalacia patellae

The condition of adolescents known as chondromalacia patellae, and the similar lesions found on femoral condyles and elsewhere, may represent an early form of degenerative change that may lead ultimately to frank OA. There are several stages, and the more advanced merge into early stages of OA; it has been suggested (Dandy, 1987) that when both joint surfaces are involved it can be called OA. In the early stages, there is characteristic softening of the cartilage, without disruption of the surface. Arthroscopically, such lesions can be recognised by the 'pitting oedema' of the surface: a probe makes a dent, which fills slowly, rather than springing back immediately. It is known that in such cases the proteoglycan chain length is reduced, and it is tempting to speculate that the proteoglycan–water mixture changes from a gel to a sol. Thus water is expressed on pressure, and flows back slowly. This is the so-called 'blister lesion'. It may progress by bursting, with exposure of fibrillated cartilage, loss of mechanical properties and relatively rapid progression to OA. Alternatively it may enlarge laterally, with fibrosis in the centre, leading to the so-called 'umbilicated blister'. This is probably relatively benign. When the surface breaks down, either as a consequence of the blister lesion or *de novo*, fibrillation is seen; this may be coarse or fine, and is an antecedent of OA.

Idiopathic chondromalacia occurs in cartilage that is thicker than normal, and it is possible that it is a nutritive phenomenon: if growth of the cartilage renders the nutrition of the deeper chondrocytes inadequate to maintain the matrix, then matrix macromolecules will be degraded. As proteoglycan turnover is much faster than that of collagen, the first manifestation of the loss of nutrition will be proteoglycan breakdown, as is seen. It typically occurs during adolescent growth spurts, when cartilage thickness increases and the demands put on the joint increase.

OSTEOARTHRITIS

Early OA is associated with increases in both degradative and reparative processes. It is only when the capacity for repair is exceeded by the rate of degradation that decompensation occurs and OA becomes progressive. Symptoms and signs of overt disease ensue. Increases in synthesis and deposition, as well as destruction, of type II collagen in early OA have been shown in animal models. An increase in messenger RNA for type II collagen has been shown, indicating that the increase in synthesis is a result of gene activation rather than, or at least in addition to, a post-transcriptional phenomenon (Lohmander, 1994). Type IX collagen is depleted, although synthesis may be increased as well as breakdown. In advanced OA, collagen types I and III are expressed – types not usually present in cartilage. Expression of type X collagen has been shown by *in situ* hybridisation in the deep layers of osteoarthritic cartilage, but not in normal cartilage. It has been identified in the fibrillated superficial layer of osteoarthritic cartilage (Aigner et al, 1993). Results from extraction of collagen from human OA specimens seem to follow these results from animal models.

Because of the radiographic appearance of osteoarthritic joints, showing sclerosis of subchondral bone, and because of the negative clinical correlations between osteoporosis and OA, and between OA of the hip and fracture of the femoral neck, it has been postulated that the fundamental change in OA is in the bone. Sclerosis, the theory suggests, leads to stiffening of the bone and consequently to a greater absorption of energy by the cartilage, with any stress on the joint. However, when examined microdensitometrically, this sclerosis is not seen in the Pond–Nuki model, and it has been shown that indeed osteopaenia can lead to OA (Brandt, 1991). This apparent paradox has not been resolved.

The result of all this – the structural changes of OA – can be classified in several ways. Histologically, early stages are characterised by loss of glycosaminoglycan staining of the matrix and clustering of chondrocytes around fissures, presumably reparative. Later, if fissures traverse the cartilage, there may be granulation tissue ingrowth and formation of fibrocartilage. Radiologically, several classification systems have been advanced, but these necessarily address only the bony changes of advanced OA, or imply cartilage changes from loss of joint space.

Macroscopic classifications that encompass early and late disease (i.e. operative findings) have risen to prominence with arthroscopy, and with the ability both to examine quickly many more joints than would be possible or appropriate by arthrotomy and to see easily the joint surface with a degree of magnification. The arthroscopic appearance of OA has been classified into four grades by Dandy (1987).

RHEUMATOID ARTHRITIS

Despite the continuing uncertainty about the aetiology of RA, the pathogenesis of the joint destruction is reasonably well understood. The primary process is synovial proliferation and inflammation, with an increase in cellularity, and even development of lymphoid follicles. The cellular infiltration is composed of T lymphocytes, dendritic cells and macrophages, fibroblasts and often plasma cells. The cells are activated, as shown by the presence of HLA class II antigens and cell adhesion molecules. It has been suggested that the antibody production by rheumatoid synovial membrane is equivalent to that of a stimulated lymph node. The cause of the immunological stimulation remains unclear (Roitt, 1988).

Several mechanisms lead to cartilage destruction. Enzymes are elaborated by the synovium and cause cartilage breakdown from the surface. Normal synovial fluid contains inhibitors of enzymes, in particular tissue inhibitor of metalloproteinase (TIMP) (Cawston, 1991), and the balance between enzyme and inhibitor is lost in RA. There is also direct destruction of the cartilage by the rheumatoid pannus (the proliferating synovium that invades the cartilage), and several mechanisms have been proposed to account for this invasion. It has been pointed out by Rich et al (1981) that, because of the fibronectin content of cartilage, it is more surprising that synovial cells normally do not migrate to the cartilage surface. Rich and co-workers showed that the proteoglycans of cartilage can inhibit this fibronectin-mediated adhesion, and so protect the cartilage. It may be that the early loss of proteoglycan in RA leads not only to loss of cartilage matrix integrity by its effect on swelling pressure, and consequent loss of tension in collagen fibres, but also to facilitation of synovial cell adherence to and invasion of the cartilage. A vicious circle indeed.

Cytokines are also involved. The experimental evidence for this started with the work of Fell and Jubb (1977), who showed that the tissue culture medium in which synovial membrane had been cultured was capable of stimulating the release of proteoglycan from the matrix of living, but not dead, articular cartilage. It was clear, then, that the chondrocytes themselves were causing the release, stimulated by a factor produced by the synovium. The factor was named catabolin, but has subsequently been shown to be identical to IL-1. It was shown that production was increased in RA (Brown et al, 1987), and this may explain one mechanism of cartilage breakdown in RA.

IL-8, a potent chemotactic factor for neutrophils and T lymphocytes, has been shown to be present in the majority of synovial lining cells in patients with RA or OA, but in only a small minority in healthy controls. The proportion of cells immunostaining for IL-8 deeper in the tissue was much lower. This provides evidence that IL-8 may be involved in the inflammatory process in arthritic diseases. Indeed, virtually all cytokines and growth factors have been identified in the rheumatoid synovial membrane, either by immunostaining or by *in situ* hybridisation (Brennan et al, 1991). It has recently been shown that a combination of IL-4 and IL-10 can prevent or even reverse cartilage destruction produced *in vitro* by mononuclear cells from rheumatoid synovial fluid or peripheral blood from patients with RA.

GROWTH FACTORS AND THEIR ACTIONS ON ARTICULAR CARTILAGE

Several growth factors are thought to be involved in the control of articular cartilage matrix turnover (Trippel, 1995). Those that have been most studied are insulin-like growth factor 1 (IGF-1), basic fibroblast growth factor (bFGF) and transforming growth factor β (TGF-β). IGF-1 stimulates cultured chondrocytes in both cell division and proteoglycan synthesis (more to synthesis that division at low concentration). Any growth factor acting on

articular cartilage must travel via the synovial fluid, and it has been shown that at least a part of the stimulatory effect of synovial fluid on sulphate incorporation by chondrocytes is attributable to IGF-1. Some research has suggested that serum IGF-1 levels are lower in OA than in normal controls, suggesting a possible link between IGF-1 deficiency and OA, but other studies have contradicted this. Both IFG-1 levels and chondrocyte responsiveness decrease with age, which may be linked with development of OA with ageing. Chondrocytes in patients with OA have been shown to possess not only a receptor for IGF-1 but also a binding site with no activity, thus effectively downregulating IGF-1 receptor affinity. Intra-articular administration of IGF-1 has been shown to augment the cartilage-preserving effect of intramuscular pentosan polyphosphate in the Pond–Nuki model of OA; it may have a therapeutic role.

bFGF seems to have varying effects depending on dose: it is a more potent mitogen than IGF-1 but has less effect on synthetic activity. Low concentrations of bFGF have been shown to have the effect of increasing synthesis and decreasing breakdown, whereas high concentrations have the opposite effect (Trippel, 1995).

TGF-β also has varying effects depending on the circumstances. It has been shown to have stimulatory and inhibitory effects on chondrocyte division and matrix synthesis. It is found in high concentrations in rheumatoid synovial membrane (Brennan et al, 1991), and is likely to have a major role in the cartilage changes of joint diseases.

Tumour necrosis factor α (TNF-α) induces prostaglandin E_2 and collagenase, leading to cartilage breakdown, activates osteoclasts, induces synthesis of IL-1 and has several other effects (Brennan et al, 1991). The rheumatoid pannus is rich in IL-1 and TNF-α, as well as in enzymes (see below), and it has been suggested that its central role in RA may provide a therapeutic target.

THE ENZYMES OF CARTILAGE TURNOVER AND DISEASE

Turnover of connective tissue matrices is a normal process, and it is only when breakdown exceeds repair that cartilage destruction ensues. The enzymes involved are those produced by chondrocytes; it is unlikely that enzymes from synovial fluid are involved in normal turnover, as in normal synovial fluid enzyme inhibitors outweigh enzymes. With disease, the levels of all the enzymes increase, and cartilage is lost. The main enzymes involved are the matrix metalloproteinases (MMPs), active at neutral pH in the pericellular space (Murphy et al, 1991). There are four classes of MMP: collagenases, gelatinases, stromelysins and an enzyme called punctuated metalloproteinase 1 (Pump-1). Other enzymes are also involved in disease: acid cysteine proteinases, serine proteinases and the lysosomal enzymes.

The most abundant enzymes in the rheumatoid pannus are collagenase, stromelysin and neutrophil elastase. Cartilage also undergoes degradation far from the junction with pannus; this must presumably somehow be mediated by synovial fluid (Larbre et al, 1994). Cartilage explants *in vitro* undergo degradation when exposed to rheumatoid synovial fluid, an effect antagonised by anti-IL-1 antibodies. Synovial fluid proteases are present in very variable amounts, and their effect is lost on storage of synovial fluid, which may explain the relative lack of reports in the literature. The proteases, elastase in particular, are derived partly from neutrophils present in rheumatoid synovial fluid (the role of neutrophils in joint destruction has been somewhat neglected and is probably more important than hitherto appreciated; see below). The proteases in question include elastase, collagenase, gelatinase, stromelysin, serine proteases and metalloproteases (Larbre et al, 1994).

Experimental chondrogenesis in mouse limb buds in tissue culture is inhibited by co-cultivation with rheumatoid synovial cells; if the rheumatoid synovial cells are added later on in the culture, formed cartilage matrix is broken down. This effect is thought to be the result of enzymatic activity and/or production of cytokines (catabolin/IL-1) or prostaglandins. This effect of the synovial cells is inhibited (i.e. chondrogenesis proceeds despite their presence) if certain enzyme inhibitors are added to the culture (Mohamed-Ali et al, 1993). Both released enzymes, in particular metalloproteinases, and membrane-bound enzymes on chondrocytes are secreted in a latent form and need to be activated by endoproteases such as plasmin. Plasmin arises from plasminogen, which is abundant in inflamed tissues, under the action of plasminogen activator. Plasmin has several roles in cartilage matrix breakdown: activation of procollagenases, stimulation of chondrocytes to produce collagenase and direct degradation of proteoglycans are probably the most important. It has been shown that addition of avarol (a

naturally occurring benzoquinone inhibitor of both cyclo-oxygenase and lipoxygenase), especially but not exclusively in combination with plasminogen activator inhibitor (PAI) 2, to co-cultures of rheumatoid synovium and articular cartilage antagonises the effect of the synovial tissue and prevents loss of cartilage matrix. This lends further weight to the importance of both prostaglandins and metalloproteinases in cartilage breakdown.

The normal balance between enzymes and their inhibitors has already been mentioned. The main inhibitors *in vivo* are probably α_2-macroglobulin, α_1-proteinase inhibitor, PAIs and the TIMPs (see above) (Cawston, 1991).

CELLULAR MECHANISMS IN MATRIX BREAKDOWN

In RA especially, proliferation of macrophages and fibroblasts, and their synovial counterparts the type A and type B synoviocytes respectively, leads to irreversible cartilage destruction. The contribution of the chondrocytes has been debated (see above); as well as the evidence from Fell, Dingle and others (Fell and Jubb, 1977; Dingle et al, 1979) that stimulated chondrocytes resorb the matrix, it has also been shown that IL-1-stimulated chondrocytes in culture produce proteases that degrade collagens II, IX and XI. The role of polymorphonuclear leucocytes has been discussed above (Larbre et al, 1994), and it is clear that many cell types contribute both to the normal turnover of articular cartilage and, especially, to cartilage breakdown in both OA and RA.

MARKERS OF ARTHRITIS AND JOINT INJURY

It is reasonable to assume that, if one is to avoid joint destruction of OA, the disease must be detected at the preclinical stage (the stage of compensation; see above). A large amount of research into arthritis, therefore, involves identification of and studies on serum and synovial fluid markers that can be used to follow the course of early disease (Lohmander, 1994). These fall into two categories: products of degradation of the actual structural components of cartilage, and others including cartilage constituents whose functions are unknown, and markers not originating in cartilage. Looking at the structural components has obvious attractions; loss of these is clearly related directly to impairment of cartilage function, but it can be difficult to ensure cartilage specificity (many are involved in bone turnover as well) and several more sensitive probes have been described.

Monitoring release of collagen cross-links is attractive; the peptide-bound ones are type-specific, and should provide a measurement of turnover. Measuring release of the peptide liberated by the conversion of procollagen to collagen (Shinmei et al, 1993) may provide a measurement of synthesis. Measurement of the pyridinoline cross-link is well described, but is not cartilage specific, being liberated from bone collagens as well.

Aggrecan can be found released into synovial fluid; it is cleaved in the E1 domain between the G1 and G2 domains (see *Figure 11.2*) by stromelysin and aggrecanase, and this fragment (G2 to the end) is found in early OA.

The intact aggrecan molecule, including the hyaluronan-binding domain, is released only in advanced disease. These markers may provide a measure of disease progression. Another domain of aggrecan has recently been reported as a potentially useful marker of breakdown in RA. It has immunoreactivity with epidermal growth factor (EGF), and can be analysed by an assay for EGF. Levels of keratan sulphate within cartilage are useful if cartilage specimens are available; this tends to limit its use to study of advanced disease or occasionally at autopsy. Levels are increased in OA with the change in aggrecan composition already described, and in RA keratan sulphate levels correlate with C-reactive protein level (as a marker of an acute-phase inflammatory response). There is poor correlation in OA.

Probably the largest amount of research on markers of cartilage breakdown concerns COMP and chondrocalcin (see section on cartilage constituents above). COMP is specific to cartilage, especially articular, and is a normal trace constituent of serum. Levels are increased in OA (Malemud, 1993), and serum levels may be useful as a non-invasive monitor of disease progress. Chondrocalcin, which is the C-terminal propeptide of type II collagen, is found in synovial fluid in OA – greatest in moderate disease and reduced again in advanced OA as cartilage is lost. Link protein has a possible use as a marker, and is particularly interesting in the aetiology of OA and use of animal models, because human link protein is much more

readily degraded by proteolysis than the equivalent protein from other species studied; this may explain to some extent why humankind is so susceptible to OA (Malemud, 1993).

The neuropeptides nerve growth factor and substance P, found in low concentration in the synovial membrane in OA, are found in greater amounts in RA, and their presence may be related to pain production in RA. Finally, one must consider assay of the cytokines possibly related to the pathogenesis of the disease. Levels of IL-1 vary with disease, as has been discussed (Brown et al, 1987), and it has been shown that IL-8 levels also vary. Osteoarthritic synovial fluid was found to contain IL-8 rarely (7% of cases), by contrast with RA (32%). In conclusion, many molecules that have been studied can be seen as markers of joint breakdown; the ideal specific markers of RA and OA that can be assayed easily from peripheral blood are yet to be found.

ANIMAL MODELS OF OSTEOARTHRITIS

Animal models are particularly useful for obtaining specimens from early disease; whereas it is possible to obtain biopsy specimens of synovium at various stages of disease, cartilage and subjacent bone specimens are available only at autopsy or from joints with advanced disease, undergoing replacement. Hence the use of, for example, the anterior cruciate ligament transection (Pond–Nuki) model in dogs. The assumption is that the animal disease mimics human OA; this may be difficult to validate. However, the information gained is useful: early OA in dogs is characterised by a thickening of the articular cartilage as a result of stimulation of matrix synthesis. This is associated with significant synovial inflammation and supports the concept of a reversible, repair, phase of OA.

Other aspects of joint breakdown can be studied. A model of neurogenic arthritis (Charcot joint) can be produced by deafferentation of a limb, but only if the anterior cruciate ligament is transected as well. Thus deafferentation seems to be an accelerator of joint injury, but not sufficient by itself. This seems to fit in with reports of rapid development of onset of joint damage in previously normal joints in patients with diabetic neuropathy after trivial injury (Brandt, 1991).

MODELS OF CARTILAGE REPAIR

There are several clinical and experimental circumstances in which, to some extent, cartilage repair takes place. Immobilised and injured joints may lose over 50% of their matrix proteoglycan (Brandt, 1991), and a model of matrix loss involving intra-articular chymopapain in the rabbit knee shows dramatic release of keratan sulphate, which is subsequently replaced. In this model, markers of bone-specific collagen cross-links were also released, suggesting a link between cartilage changes and underlying bone changes.

Cartilage defects in experimental models heal in a specific pattern: initial filling in of the defect with granulation tissue is followed by replacement with fibrocartilage. This matures to hyaline cartilage, which itself then degenerates to fibrous tissue without much proteoglycan. The process can be followed histologically by staining for matrix components (safranin O or Alcian blue), by immunostaining of the cells for expression of specific phenotype, or by *in situ* hybridisation to detect specific gene expression. Of particular use is staining for the ubiquitous marker of chondrocytes and neural crest-derived cells, S-100. This way, it can be seen that loss of S-100 immunostaining immediately precedes degeneration of the hyaline matrix to the mechanically inferior fibrous tissue (Wolff et al, 1992). Similarly, in experimental models, abrasion chondroplasty as an attempt to repair osteoarthritic lesions led to unsatisfactory fibrous tissue.

EFFECTS OF ANTI-INFLAMMATORY DRUGS ON CARTILAGE DEGRADATION

Brandt (1991) and others have shown that in the Pond–Nuki (cruciate-deficient dog) model of OA, the slowly progressive, compensated, cartilage destruction typically seen changes dramatically when aspirin is administered in therapeutic doses. It becomes rapidly progressive, with complete destruction of the cartilage in a few months. *In vitro*, aspirin inhibits proteoglycan synthesis in a dose-dependent fashion, and to a much greater extent in osteoarthritic than in normal cartilage. This implies a difference in cellular metabolism in the osteoarthritic cartilage. This effect on proteoglycan synthesis was shown by several other (but not all) non-steroidal anti-inflammatory drugs (NSAIDs). This is an issue of great interest and relevance to the clinician, with several NSAIDs said to offer 'chondroprotection', and with definite effects on fracture healing and development of heterotopic ossification.

CONCLUSIONS

Despite the orthopaedic surgeon's radiographically led concentration on the bone changes of the arthritic diseases, it must not be forgotten that most arthritides start with cartilage changes, and even the osteophyte starts as a 'chondrophyte'. If we are to progress from an ability to replace worn-out joints to a time when we can prevent such wear, we need to address the early stages of cartilage change. Much is known, but much more needs to be known to piece together the roles of enzymes, enzyme inhibitors, growth factors and cytokines, chemokines, prostaglandins, hormones and the various cell lines found in normal and arthritic joints.

REFERENCES AND FURTHER READING

Aigner T, Reichenberger E, Bertling W, Kirsch T, Stöß H, von der Mark K. Type X collagen expression in osteoarthritic and rheumatoid articular cartilage. *Virchows Arch B Cell Pathol* 1993; **63**: 205–211.

Brandt KD. Animal models: insights into osteoarthritis (OA) provided by the cruciate-deficient dog. *Br J Rheumatol* 1991; **30**(Suppl 1): 5–9.

Brennan FM, Field M, Chu A, Feldman M, Maini RN. Cytokine expression in rheumatoid arthritis. *Br J Rheumatol* 1991; **30**(Suppl 1): 76–80.

Brown MF, Hazleman BL, Dingle JT, Dandy DJ, Murley AHG. Production of cartilage degrading activity by human synovial tissue. *Ann Rheum Dis* 1987; **46**: 319–323.

Cawston TE. Metalloproteinase inhibitors – crystal-gazing for a future therapy? *Br J Rheumatol* 1991; **30**: 242–244.

Dandy DJ. *Arthroscopic Management of the Knee*, 2nd edn. London: Churchill Livingstone, 1987.

Dieppe P. Osteoarthritis: clinical and research perspective. *Br J Rheumatol* 1991; **30**(Suppl 1): 1–4.

Dingle JT, Saklatvala J, Hembry RM, Tyler J, Fell HB, Jubb RW. A cartilage catabolic factor from synovium. *Biochem J* 1979; **184**: 177–180.

Eyre DR. The collagens of articular cartilage. *Semin Arthritis Rheum* 1991; **21**(Suppl 2): 2–11.

Fell HB, Jubb RW. The effect of synovial tissue on the breakdown of articular cartilage in organ culture. *Arthritis Rheum* 1977; **20**: 1359–1371.

Guthrie D. *A History of Medicine*, 2nd edn. Edinburgh: Thomas Nelson and Sons, 1958.

Hardingham TE, Fosang AJ, Dudhia J. Aggrecan, the chondroitin sulfate/keratan sulfate proteoglycan of cartilage. In: Kuettner KE, Schleyerbach R, Peyron JG, Hascall VC (eds) *Articular Cartilage and Osteoarthritis*. New York: Raven Press, 1992: 5–20.

Kalden JR, Winkler T, Krapf F. Are retroviruses involved in the aetiology of rheumatic diseases? *Br J Rheumatol* 1991; **30**(Suppl 1): 63–69.

Kuettner KE, Aydelotte MB, Thonar EJ-MA. Articular cartilage matrix and structure: a minireview. *J Rheumatol* 1991; **18**(Suppl 27): 46–48.

Larbre J-P, Moore AR, Da Silva JAP, Iwamura H, Ioanou Y, Willoughby DA. Direct degradation of articular cartilage by rheumatoid synovial fluid: contribution of proteolytic enzymes. *J Rheumatol* 1994; **21**: 1796–1801.

Lohmander LS. Articular cartilage and osteoarthrosis. The role of molecular markers to monitor breakdown, repair and disease. *J Anat* 1994; **184**: 477–492.

Malemud CJ. Markers of osteoarthritis and cartilage research in animal models. *Curr Opin Rheumatol* 1993; **5**: 494–502.

Mohamed-Ali H, Scholz P, Merker H-J. Inhibition of the effects of rheumatoid synovial fluid cells on chondrogenesis and cartilage breakdown *in vitro*: possible therapeutic conclusions. *Virchows Arch B Cell Pathol* 1993; **64**: 45–56.

Murphy G, Docherty AJP, Hembry RM, Reynolds JJ. Metalloproteinases and tissue damage. *Br J Rheumatol* 1991; **30**(Suppl 1): 25–31.

Nuki G. *The Aetiopathogenesis of Osteoarthrosis*. Tunbridge Wells: Pitman Medical Publishing, 1980.

Panayi GS. The pathogenesis of rheumatoid arthritis: from molecules to the whole patient. *Br J Rheumatol* 1993; **32**: 533–536.

Rich AM, Pearlstein E, Weissman G, Hoffstein ST. Cartilage proteoglycans inhibit fibronectin-mediated adhesion. *Nature* 1981; **293**: 224–226.

Roitt IM. *Essential Immunology*, 6th edn. Oxford: Blackwell Scientific Publications, 1988.

Salter DM. Tenascin is increased in cartilage and synovium from arthritic knees. *Br J Rheumatol* 1993; **32**: 780–786.

Shinmei M, Ito K, Matsuyama S, Machida A, Miyazaki K. Joint fluid carboxy-terminal type II procollagen peptide as a marker of cartilage collagen biosynthesis. *Osteoarthritis and Cartilage* 1993; **1**: 121–128.

Shiozawa S, Yoshihari R, Kuroki Y, Fujita T, Shiozawa K, Imura S. Pathogenic importance of fibronectin in the superficial region of articular cartilage as a local factor for the induction of pannus extension on rheumatoid articular cartilage. *Ann Rheum Dis* 1992; **51**: 869–873.

Sigerist HE. *A History of Medicine. Vol. 1. Primitive and Archaic Medicine*. New York: Oxford University Press, 1951.

Sledge CB. Biology of the joint. In: Kelly WN, Harris ED, Ruddy S, Sledge CB (eds) *Textbook of Rheumatology*, Vol 1, 4th edn. Philadelphia: WB Saunders, 1993: p. 9.

Stockwell RA. *Biology of Cartilage Cells*. Cambridge: Cambridge University Press, 1979.

Swann AC, Seedhom BB. The stiffness of normal articular cartilage and the predominant acting stress levels: implications for the aetiology of osteoarthritis. *Br J Rheumatol* 1993; **32**: 16–25.

Trippel SB. Growth factor actions on articular cartilage. *J Rheumatol* 1995; **22**(Suppl 43): 129–132.

Unsworth A, Seedhom BB. Biomechanics of articulations and derangements in disease. In: Maddison PJ, Isenberg DA, Woo P, Glass DN, (eds) *Oxford Textbook of Rheumatology*, Vol. 1. Oxford: Oxford University Press, 1993: 276–282.

Urban JPG. The chondrocyte: a cell under pressure. *Br J Rheumatol* 1994; **33**: 901–908.

Wolff DA, Stevenson S, Goldberg VM. S-100 protein immunostaining identifies cells expressing a chondrocytic phenotype during articular cartilage repair. *J Orthop Res* 1992; **10**: 49–57.

Wollheim FA. Rheumatoid arthritis – the clinical picture. In: Maddison PJ, Isenberg DA, Woo P, Glass DN (eds) *Oxford Textbook of Rheumatology*, Vol. 2. Oxford: Oxford University Press, 1993: 639–661.

12

Metabolic Bone Disease

Karim Meeran and Stephen Bloom

INTRODUCTION

Metabolic bone disease is an important cause of bone weakness and hence fractures. It is thus essential that orthopaedic surgeons have a working knowledge of bone metabolism. Although the majority of fractures occur in people without metabolic bone disease, it is important that potential metabolic causes of a fracture are considered and excluded.

The mammalian skeleton serves two completely separate roles. For its role as a structural framework, the skeleton is strong, relatively lightweight, mobile, able to protect vital organs and capable of orderly growth and remodelling. At the same time the skeleton is the reservoir for most of the body's calcium, phosphorus and magnesium. Thus the skeleton has an important metabolic role in calcium homoeostasis, and release of stored calcium will occur in response to a raised concentration of parathyroid hormone (PTH). Activated vitamin D can also mobilise calcium and phosphate from bone cells *in vitro*. To understand the metabolic role of bone, it is first important to have an understanding of the importance of extracellular ionised (free) calcium to the normal functioning of neurones and muscles.

Calcium metabolism

The adult human contains about 25 000 mmol of calcium, 99% of which resides in the skeleton. Calcium is an important intracellular and extracellular cation. Changes in intracellular concentrations are extremely important in the control of cell depolarisation in nerve and muscle. The resting intracellular calcium concentration is in the region of $10 \, \text{nmol} \, \text{l}^{-1}$ ($0.00001 \, \text{mmol} \, \text{l}^{-1}$), whereas the extracellular concentration is tightly controlled to remain

between 2.2 and $2.5 \, \text{mmol} \, \text{l}^{-1}$. Cellular depolarisation of nerve or muscle occurs when calcium is allowed into the cell. The huge gradient in calcium levels is maintained by the active transport of calcium out of nerve and muscle cells.

Only about 40% of the extracellular calcium is free or ionised. A further 40–50% is protein bound, mostly to albumin, with about 10% being complexed to phosphate and bicarbonate. The two most important factors maintaining homoeostasis of extracellular calcium concentrations are the circulating levels of PTH and of activated vitamin D. Both of these serve to raise plasma calcium concentration. PTH also causes a fall in plasma phosphate concentration, whereas vitamin D causes both calcium and phosphate levels to rise simultaneously. Because the extracellular free (ionised) calcium is essential for survival, in particular for normal neuronal and muscle function, homoeostasis of plasma calcium takes priority over bone consistency when calcium is in short supply. Chronic calcium or vitamin D deficiency may therefore result in a significant loss of calcium from bone.

In the presence of a low plasma calcium (or a high plasma phosphate) concentration, PTH levels will rise. This will in turn serve to mobilise calcium from bone, to increase renal reabsorption of calcium (and increase renal phosphate loss) and to increase absorption of calcium from the gut. In addition, PTH serves to activate the renal enzyme 1α-hydroxylase which will in turn activate vitamin D. Once calcium levels have risen to within the normal range, PTH levels will also normalise.

Abnormal calcium homoeostasis occurs with abnormalities in either PTH or vitamin D levels. Metabolic bone disease can occur either due to a deficiency of calcium and vitamin D (rickets in children or osteomalacia in adults) or due to hyperparathyroidism, which results in loss of bone mineral to increase plasma calcium levels. A benign tumour of the parathyroids, for example, which secretes an excess of PTH causes primary hyperparathyroidism, which will result in a slow loss of calcium from bone into the blood. Increased glomerular filtration of calcium then occurs, resulting in increased renal excretion of calcium. An excess of activated vitamin D tends not to produce bone disease, although it does cause a rise in intestinal calcium absorption, plasma calcium concentration and urinary calcium excretion. Activated vitamin D is required for normal mineralisation of osteoid. A deficiency of activated vitamin D can therefore cause rickets in children and osteomalacia in adults.

Renal failure affects calcium metabolism for two reasons. Phosphate cannot be excreted by the kidney and its concentration in the plasma therefore rises. Because calcium and phosphate have a relatively low solubility product, calcium phosphate precipitates, resulting in a fall in ionised (free) plasma calcium concentration. The low ionised calcium and the high phosphate levels stimulate PTH secretion (secondary hyperparathyroidism). In addition to this, the kidney is the site of 1α hydroxylation of vitamin D. In renal failure, this hydroxylation is impaired, resulting in a deficiency of activated vitamin D. 'Renal osteodystrophy' thus results from a combination of secondary hyperparathyroidism with vitamin D deficiency. The clinical presentation of the bone disease depends on the relative severity of each of these.

For clarity, a summary of the clinical effects of PTH and of activated vitamin D is given in *Table 12.1*.

DISORDERS OF THE PARATHYROID GLANDS

Primary hyperparathyroidism

Autonomous secretion of PTH results in hypercalcaemia. Most commonly this occurs with a parathyroid adenoma, which may be single or multiple. Parathyroid hyperplasia occurs in about 20% of cases. The chronically high PTH level results in a raised plasma calcium concentration at the expense of bone, which slowly loses calcium. Although renal tubular calcium resorption is increased, the high plasma calcium level results in a large rise in the amount of filtered calcium, most of which cannot be reabsorbed. The result is an increased urinary calcium concentration which may eventually lead to renal stone formation. The most common biochemical finding is of a raised plasma calcium level with a non-suppressed PTH level. PTH activates renal 1α-hydroxylase. Patients with primary hyperparathyroidism therefore tend to have a low to normal 25-hydroxyvitamin D plasma concentration and a high to normal 1,25-dihydroxyvitamin D plasma concentration.

The apparent rate of complications from primary hyperparathyroidism appears to be falling because routine biochemical screening of plasma calcium allows earlier diagnosis of the condition. Thus the prevalence of nephrolithiasis amongst patients with known primary hyperparathyroidism appears to be falling, from 50% 20 years ago to about 20% more recently (Browder et al, 1983).

Bone manifestations are similarly becoming less pre-

Table 12.1   Clinical effects of PTH and activated vitamin D.

	Effect of PTH	*Effect of active vitamin D*
Plasma calcium	Increase	Increase
Plasma phosphate	Decrease	Increase
Glomerular calcium filtration	Increased (as plasma calcium concentration higher)	Increased
Tubular calcium resorption	Increased	Unchanged
Net calcium excretion	Slightly increased	Increased
Tubular phosphate excretion	Increased ++	Increased
Bone mass	Decreased	Unchanged★
Calcium absorption from intestine	Increased	Increased

★Although excessive vitamin D can mobilise calcium and phosphate from bone cells *in vitro*, bone mass is decreased in vitamin D deficiency because of a combination of impaired mineralisation of osteoid and of secondary hyperparathyroidism.

valent and less severe. Previously the hallmark of primary hyperparathyroidism was osteitis fibrosa cystica. Hand radiography may reveal subperiosteal bone resorption on the radial aspect of the second and third phalanges. When severe, bone cysts may be seen, most commonly in the third metacarpal. These cystic defects can become filled with fibrous tissue. If the fibrous tissue is highly vascular, haemorrhage may occur and pigments may accumulate. These changes cause a reddish-brown hue to the tissue, accounting for the term 'brown tumour'. More recently simple osteopenia, resembling osteoporosis (see below), has been a more common finding.

Other features of hypercalcaemia are non-specific. The mnemonic bones, stones, moans and abdominal groans (referring respectively to fractures, nephrolithiasis, psychiatric features, and pancreatitis, peptic ulceration and constipation) is well known to medical students. Because early in the disease patients may present with only one of these, the diagnosis can easily be missed for a number of years.

The treatment of primary hyperparathyroidism depends on the severity of the clinical presentation. When found incidentally in patients with no symptoms or complications, whose calcium level is less than 2.75 mmol l^{-1}, no treatment may be required. If any symptoms occur, renal impairment supervenes or the calcium level rises to above 2.75 mmol l^{-1}, the ideal treatment is to remove the parathyroid adenoma if one is present, or to perform total parathyroidectomy in patients with parathyroid hyperplasia. The emergency management of hypercalcaemia is given below.

Before arranging parathyroidectomy in a patient with hypercalcaemia with a non-suppressed PTH level, it is important to bear in mind the following differential diagnoses lest a patient has an unnecessary neck exploration.

Familial (benign) hypocalciuric hypercalcaemia

In this condition there is an inherited abnormality in a calcium receptor. Thus all tissues that detect calcium in their normal functioning have an altered set point for calcium handling. There is excessive resorption of calcium from the renal tubules, resulting in a low urinary calcium concentration. Thus renal stones are not a complication. In addition, patients have no bony abnormalities at any stage of life. The plasma calcium and PTH levels are typically raised, but because no organ

that matters senses the raised calcium concentration, no important complications arise, apart from a possible unnecessary neck exploration. The diagnosis is difficult to distinguish from primary hyperparathyroidism without measuring the urinary calcium concentration and taking a family history. The correct management is to do nothing and to warn the patient to avoid parathyroidectomy.

Drug therapy

Lithium can cause plasma PTH levels to rise and hence cause hypercalcaemia. This hypercalcaemia usually resolves when the lithium is discontinued, but confusingly there is a higher prevalence of parathyroid adenomas amongst patients who have been on lithium therapy.

Multiple endocrine neoplasia (MEN)

There are two types of MEN that produce primary hyperparathyroidism, both of which are caused by an autosomal dominant genetic mutation. (1) Patients with MEN type 1 are at risk of parathyroid adenomas, pancreatic neoplasia and pituitary tumours. Once a parathyroid adenoma is found, total parathyroidectomy is generally recommended because of the significant risk of further parathyroid adenomas. (2) Patients with MEN type 2a are at risk of parathyroid **hyperplasia**, medullary thyroid carcinoma and phaeochromocytoma. It is very important to exclude the latter possibility before neck exploration.

Secondary hyperparathyroidism

An appropriately raised PTH level in the face of a low calcium concentration also causes chronic loss of bone. This occurs most commonly with renal failure and vitamin D deficiency.

Tertiary hyperparathyroidism

After a period of chronic secondary hyperparathyroidism, where appropriate parathyroid gland hyperplasia may have occurred, a parathyroid gland may become autonomous. This is most often clinically apparent after resolution of renal impairment, with either dialysis or renal transplantation. The treatment is removal of the offending parathyroid gland.

Management of severe hypercalcaemia

Hypercalcaemia is a medical emergency. Urgent treatment is required if any of the following are found:

- Calcium concentration greater than $3.5\,\mathrm{mmol\,l^{-1}}$
- Clouding of consciousness or confusion
- Hypotension
- Severe abdominal pain
- Severe dehydration causing pre-renal failure

Any drugs known to cause hypercalcaemia should be discontinued. Steroids should be given if the patient is known to have sarcoidosis. If primary hyperparathyroidism is confirmed, a parathyroidectomy should be arranged. A rigorous search for the cause of the hypercalcaemia must be carried out. While awaiting definitive treatment, the following measures should be used:

a) Rehydrate the patient with intravenous normal (0.9%) saline. Aim for about 4–6 litres in 24 hours.

b) If the patient does not pass urine for 4 hours, a urinary catheter must be passed and insertion of a central venous line to monitor central venous pressure (CVP) must be considered.

c) Once the patient is rehydrated, continue normal saline infusion but add frusemide 120 mg every 4 hours to increase renal calcium excretion. Continue monitoring CVP carefully to prevent either fluid overload or dehydration.

d) Monitor electrolytes, especially potassium and magnesium, which may fall rapidly with rehydration and frusemide. Replace potassium ($20{-}40\,\mathrm{mmol\,l^{-1}}$) and magnesium (up to $2\,\mathrm{mmol\,l^{-1}}$) intravenously. If hypercalcaemia persists despite adequate rehydration, the following additional measures can be considered.

e) Salmon calcitonin 400 IU every 8 hours. This has a rapid onset of action (within hours) but its effect lasts only 2–3 days because calcitonin receptors undergo tachyphylaxis and downregulation.

f) Disodium pamidronate is a bisphosphonate which binds to hydroxyapatite in bone and inhibits osteoclast activity. This leads to a reduction in calcium resorption from bone and thereby causes a fall in plasma calcium concentration. Administer 30–60 mg intravenously over 4–6 hours. Calcium levels begin to fall after 48 hours and remain suppressed for up to 14 days.

Hypoparathyroidism

This condition does not cause any bone abnormality but is included for completeness. Hypoparathyroidism can be either congenital (as in Di George syndrome with parathyroid and thymic aplasia) or acquired. Acquired hypoparathyroidism is most commonly due to inadvertent damage to the parathyroid glands at the time of thyroid surgery. Very much less common are metastatic infiltration of the parathyroids, and an autoimmune hypoparathyroidism associated with a polyendocrinopathy, also known as polyglandular autoimmune syndrome type 1 or, by some authors, autoimmune polyendocrinopathy–candidiasis–ectodermal dystrophy (Ahonen et al, 1990). In this condition, candidiasis and hypoparathyroidism are the first features, both usually occurring by the age of 5 years.

Pseudohypoparathyroidism

In this condition there is a PTH receptor defect which results in reduced biological activity of PTH. The calcium level is low and the phosphate level high, giving the initial appearance of primary hypoparathyroidism. However, the PTH level is raised, hence the term pseudohypoparathyroidism. There are at least two abnormalities known to cause pseudohypoparathyroidism. In type I, the abnormality is known to reside in a G protein which normally couples the PTH receptor to adenylate cyclase (*Figure 12.1*).

Of orthopaedic interest is the fact that the phenotype of type 1 pseudohypoparathyroidism, in addition to the features of chronic hypocalcaemia, includes Albright's hereditary osteodystrophy, features of which include short stature, a round face, and short fourth and fifth metacarpals and metatarsals (*Figure 12.2*).

In type 2 disease, the G protein is normal so that adenosine 5′-cyclic monophosphate (cAMP) levels rise normally in response to exogenous PTH. However, there is a defect in the renal tubular response to cAMP.

Pseudopseudohypoparathyroidism

Occasionally orthopaedic surgeons will see patients with the typical phenotype of Albright's hereditary osteodystrophy and confidently make the diagnosis of pseudohypoparathyroidism on account of the patient's appearance alone and without seeing the calcium results. Although

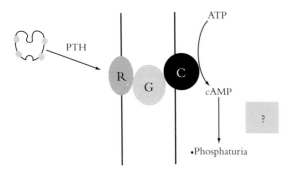

Figure 12.1 Effect of PTH on its receptor in the kidney. Stimulation of the PTH receptor (R) activates adenylate cyclase through the well-known G-protein mechanism. This causes a rise in intracellular cAMP concentration, which in turn has the effect of increasing urinary phosphate through an unknown mechanism. In type 1 pseudohypoparathyroidism, there is a defect in the G-protein, resulting in a failure of the effect of PTH. In type 2 disease, the defect occurs in the unknown pathway beyond the effect of cAMP. Thus patients with type 2 pseudohypoparathyroidism have an increase in urinary cAMP levels but not of urinary phosphate levels when they are given PTH.

these patients have the phenotypic appearance of Albright's hereditary osteodystrophy, there is no demonstrable metabolic abnormality, and the serum calcium level is normal. In this case, the diagnosis given is termed pseudopseudohypoparathyroidism.

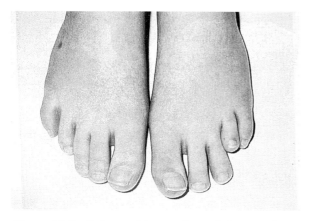

Figure 12.2 Patients with type 1 pseudohypoparathyroidism also have a short fourth and fifth metacarpal, which may be asymmetrical. This is part of Albright's hereditary osteodystrophy.

PAGET'S DISEASE OF THE BONE

Paget's disease of the bone is not a true metabolic bone disease because, however widespread the disease is, it does not affect all bones. Although it is most often asymptomatic, increased bone turnover can cause pain and deformity, and increase the risk of fracture. This, together with the metabolic consequences of Paget's disease, justifies its consideration here.

The incidence and prevalence of Paget's disease is difficult to quantify because only 1% of patients with the condition will have symptoms. Several attempts to estimate the prevalence have been made, including postmortem studies, radiological surveys and reviews of biochemical screening, in particular looking for raised bone-specific alkaline phosphatase. The prevalence of Paget's disease is very low in people under the age of 40 years. The prevalence rises after this age, ranging from about 3% of people over 40 years old to more than 10% in those aged over 80 years. Paget's disease is rare in Japan, China and the Nordic countries, and much more common in Europe and North America. This significant variation in prevalence by geographical area makes an infectious aetiology likely. Some studies have associated Paget's disease with pet ownership (Holdaway et al, 1990). Ultrastructural features of a measles-like virus in Paget's osteoclasts, most commonly seen within the nucleus but occasionally within the cytoplasm, have been identified (Rebel et al, 1980). It is important to note that the finding of this viral-type inclusion on an ultrastructural level is non-specific and may represent an unrelated affliction. No infectious agent has yet been identified and the cause of Paget's disease at present remains unknown.

The bone in Paget's disease has a highly disorganised architecture. All three phases of bone turnover are increased. Initially there is an osteolytic phase, with intense resorption of existing bone. This is followed by accelerated deposition of spicules of lamellar bone in a disorganised fashion, followed by an osteoblastic stage where bone formation is dominant. Any single bone may have all phases visible simultaneously.

Patients with Paget's disease have an increased plasma level of bone-specific alkaline phosphatase, reflecting the increased bone turnover characteristic of the condition. Most multichannel analysers measure total alkaline phosphatase concentration as part of a screen of liver function. If this is raised but other tests of liver function, including hepatic enzymes, bilirubin, albumin and a coagulation screen, are normal, it is likely that the raised alkaline phosphatase level is of bony origin. Hydroxyproline is a marker of bone resorption. It responds more rapidly than alkaline phosphatase to inhibitors of bone resorption and is the first marker of relapse when treatment is withdrawn. Other biochemical findings, including calcium and phosphate levels, are usually normal. If a patient with Paget's disease develops hypercalcaemia, it is important to exclude coincident malignancy and hyperparathyroidism, before attributing the hypercalcaemia to immobility.

The typical radiological findings of a patient with Paget's disease reveal areas of focal bone resorption and formation in a disordered trabecular pattern, seen as areas of lysis and sclerosis. Overall bone size appears enlarged and the cortices are thickened. The sclerosis may be so extensive that it may be confused with metastatic disease from prostate, breast, lung, thyroid or pancreas associated with sclerotic bony metastases. Classically, Paget's disease presents with involvement from one end of the bone to the other. It is also important to remember that Paget's disease and malignancy may coexist.

Clinical features

The majority of pagetic lesions are not painful, although pain may result from the pagetic bone or from complications that arise because of the abnormal bone. The skull is commonly involved and hypertrophy of the bone may cause pressure on the cranial nerves. Blindness or sensorineural deafness may result. Paget's disease can also cause a conductive deafness and difficulty maintaining balance if it involves the temporal bone, owing to involvement of the ossicles and labyrinth. Protrusion of bone through the foramen magnum and pressure on the spinal cord are more severe potential complications.

Fractures are the most common complication of Paget's disease. Characteristically they lie perpendicular to the cortex. Fractures in pagetic bone can heal as efficiently as those in normal bone, whereas the callus underlying the break undergoes the changes of Paget's disease itself. Non-union has been reported to be as high as 40% (Dove, 1980). The long bone deformity and shortening that occurs place abnormal stresses on major joints, and accelerate degenerative change.

The prevalence of malignant change within pagetic bone is about 1% of symptomatic cases, although prevalences as high as 10% have been reported. Osteosarcoma is rare and, for this reason, of all patients with osteosarcoma, about half will have Paget's disease.

High-output cardiac failure is a well recognised but rare complication of Paget's disease. Cardiac output is increased in these patients and this is related to a large increase in bone blood flow. Pathological arteriovenous shunts do not occur and it is unlikely that Paget's disease itself causes high-output cardiac failure in the presence of a normal heart. However, Paget's disease may precipitate cardiac failure when there is an underlying cardiac lesion.

Treatment

Most cases require no treatment. Medical treatment is directed at controlling the pain or reducing the bone turnover. Simple analgesics rather than anti-inflammatory analgesics are useful in controlling pain.

Calcitonin produces a rapid fall in calcium and bone-specific alkaline phosphatase levels in patients with Paget's disease, although no such effect is seen in healthy volunteers. Disease activity should be monitored by measuring alkaline phosphatase levels during treatment with calcitonin. Calcitonin is likely to work by suppressing osteoclast function in these patients. Calcitonin needs to be given by injection and relieves bone pain. It is also effective at relieving some of the nerve compression syndromes such as nerve deafness. Side-effects include nausea, vomiting, flushing and diarrhoea.

Bisphosphonates are synthetic analogues of inorganic phosphate where $-P-C-P-$ (phosphate–carbon–phosphate) bonds are substituted for $-P-O-P-$ (phosphate–oxygen–phosphate) bonds. These bonds are resistant to degradation by osteoclasts. The bisphosphonates bind to the surface of calcium phosphate mineral and thereby inhibit the effect of osteoclasts on the bone. Prolonged (up to several months) remission can be maintained after a single infusion, although relapse may occur after 6 weeks. Various infusion schedules have been described to achieve remission with the different bisphosphonates. Most commonly, a single infusion is repeated every 6 weeks until biochemical markers indicate remission. Bisphosphonates are also used in the treatment of hypercalcaemia and osteoporosis.

OSTEOPOROSIS

Despite its inert appearance, bone is metabolically extremely active with a very high turnover. Osteoporosis is defined as a loss of bone mass. Osteoporotic bone is normal in quality but reduced in quantity. Bone mass is a balance between bone formation and bone resorption, and these two processes are normally tightly coupled (*Figure 12.3*). Loss of bone mass can therefore occur secondarily to either increased bone resorption or decreased bone formation.

Osteoporosis must be distinguished from osteomalacia (see below), where bone is weakened because of decreased mineralisation and is not normal in quality (*Figure 12.4*). The distinction between osteoporosis and osteomalacia can be established with certainty only by bone biopsy and inspection of appropriately stained, undecalcified, histological sections.

Before the advent of accurate methods of quantifying bone mass, osteoporosis was defined as being present only after a fracture had occurred. There are many people with a reduced bone mass who never sustain a fracture. Reduced bone mass is a risk factor for fractures, however, and for this reason the term 'osteopenia' has been coined. Osteopenia can be reliably observed radiologically only after 30% bone mass has been lost. To the radiologist,

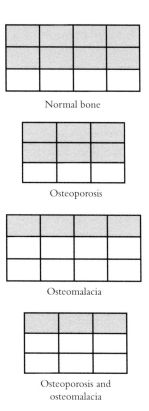

Normal bone

Osteoporosis

Osteomalacia

Osteoporosis and
osteomalacia

Figure 12.4   Schematic representation of bone mass and mineral–osteoid relationships. Each large block represents a hypothetical bone segment. The shaded areas represent mineralised osteoid and the clear areas poorly mineralised or non-mineralised osteoid. In osteoporosis, the bone segments comprise fewer bone units. Thus, in osteoporosis, the bone mass is decreased although mineral : osteoid ratio is normal. In osteomalacia, however, the bone mass may be normal but the mineral : osteoid ratio is decreased.

osteoporosis represents increased radiolucency of bones, particularly of the vertebrae.

Estimates of bone mineral content (BMC) or bone mineral density (BMD) can be made more reliably by the use of quantitative computed tomography, dual-energy X-ray absorptiometry (DEXA), or single- or dual-photon absorbtiometry (SPA or DPA).

DEXA is the most precise measurement of BMC or BMD, and involves only very low levels of ionising radiation. For postmenopausal women, it is now recommended that osteopenia is defined as BMD or BMC between 1 and 2.5 standard deviations below the mean for young adults, and that osteoporosis is defined as values greater than 2.5 standard deviations below the mean; severe or established osteoporosis is osteoporosis in the

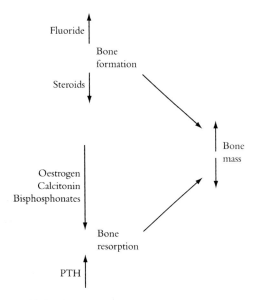

Figure 12.3   Bone mass is a balance between bone formation and bone resorption.

presence of one or more fragility fractures (World Health Organisation, 1994).

Factors influencing bone mass

Bone mass at any time depends on the peak bone mass attained and subsequent bone loss. Factors affecting peak bone mass and rate of bone loss are discussed below.

Peak bone mass

Peak bone mass is the main determinant of osteoporosis in the elderly. The range of bone densities in young adults (at least 20% on either side of the mean) is large relative to the mean rate of bone loss (1% per annum). To a large extent, peak bone mass is genetically determined. A low peak bone mass may be attributed to a low value at birth or failure to achieve optimum bone density during growth. Osteoporosis is positively correlated with a positive family history and being of Caucasian or Asian ethnicity. Black individuals have a higher peak bone mass and a lower age-adjusted fracture rate.

Age

The rate of bone formation declines with age but the rate of resorption does not. Thus, as coupling between bone formation and bone resorption declines, osteoporosis sets in. Any cause of such uncoupling will produce osteoporosis. Age-related bone loss may be seen as normal, but is labelled as pathological either when a fracture occurs or when a treatable secondary cause can be found (see *Table 12.2*).

Table 12.2 Associations of osteoporosis.

Gonadal failure (menopause is the commonest association)

Immobilisation, weightlessness, inactivity
Nutritional disorders including life-long low calcium intake, vegetarian dieting, malabsorption, alcohol abuse, smoking

Excessive exposure to glucocorticoids, either as medication or from Cushing's syndrome

Hyperthyroidism
Hyperparathyroidism
Pregnancy
Drugs including anticonvulsants, loop diuretics (not thiazides) and phenothiazines
Acromegaly

Gonadal failure

Bone loss is more rapid in postmenopausal women. Ovarian failure (either premature or physiological) is the commonest treatable cause of osteoporosis. Oestrogens in hormone replacement therapy (HRT) will prevent bone loss in women who have had a natural or surgically induced menopause. Further details about HRT are given in the treatment section below.

Hypogonadism in the male also causes osteoporosis. This can be prevented with testosterone replacement. However, anabolic steroids will not improve bone mass when given to adults with idiopathic osteoporosis who do not have gonadal failure.

Lifestyle factors

Exercise is known to increase bone mass in normal subjects. Decreased stress on the skeleton leads to loss of bone. This is well demonstrated by the effects of immobilisation, bed rest, paralysis and weightlessness in astronauts.

Although exercise is known to have a beneficial effect on bone mass, excessive exercise in young women can lead to amenorrhoea and mimic the effect of menopause on bone. Menstrual cycle disturbances are associated with significant vertebral bone loss regardless of the level of exercise (Prior et al, 1990).

Nutritional factors

Calcium absorption from the gut is known to be decreased in the elderly. Calcium and vitamin D supplementation in the elderly has been shown to reduce fracture rates (Chapuy et al, 1992). A large proportion of the world's population has borderline calcium deficiency and, rather than try to target people with reduced bone density (by scanning, etc.), it is cheaper to treat the entire population with calcium supplementation.

Steroid-induced osteoporosis

Osteoporosis was one of the features described by Harvey Cushing in 1932 when describing what has become his syndrome. Osteoporotic fractures, especially vertebral compression fractures, were reported with the use of steroids, as they were first used therapeutically. Osteocalcin is a peptide secreted into the plasma by osteoblasts.

Corticosteroid therapy reduces osteoblastic activity as measured by estimation of plasma osteocalcin levels (Meeran et al, 1995). Minimising exposure to steroids is the best way to avoid steroid-induced osteoporosis. Calcium supplementation and activated vitamin D therapy have also been used.

Hyperthyroidism

Thyroid hormones act directly on bone to increase bone resorption *in vitro* (Mundy et al, 1976) and this leads to an increase in plasma calcium concentration. The rise in plasma calcium levels in turn results in increased glomerular filtration of calcium and hence in hypercalciuria. Hyperthyroidism therefore causes a negative calcium balance, hypercalcaemia and hyperphosphataemia, with bone loss leading to fractures. Florid bone disease is no longer seen because of the prompt diagnosis and treatment of overt hyperthyroidism.

The only abnormal investigation in patients with osteoporosis is measurement of bone density. The results of all blood tests, including plasma calcium, urinary calcium, alkaline phosphatase and plasma phosphate levels, are normal.

Treatment of osteoporosis

Postmenopausal women benefit from oestrogen replacement (*Figure 12.5*) (Christiansen et al, 1981). A minimum dose of 0.625 mg conjugated equine oestrogen is required to prevent postmenopausal bone loss (*Figure 12.6*).

The efficacy of oestrogen at preventing fractures in epidemiological studies reveals that vertebral fracture rates are reduced by 90% over 5 years, whereas hip fracture rates are reduced by less than 50%. Fracture rates in other bones are not reduced.

Endometrial carcinoma, breast carcinoma, hypertension and risk of thromboembolic disease have all been cited as potential reasons for women to consider avoiding oestrogen replacement (HRT). Although a past history of breast or endometrial malignancy is a contraindication to HRT, it has now been shown that HRT (unlike the oral contraceptive pill) does not increase blood pressure or cause thromboembolism. Unlike oral contraceptives, therefore, HRT should not be discontinued before surgery. In addition, because of the significant decrease in the cardiovascular mortality rate resulting from oestrogen replacement therapy, its use is associated with a

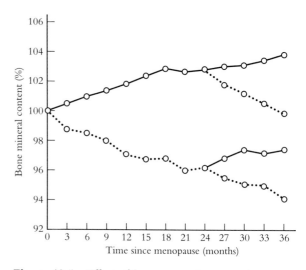

Figure 12.5 Effect of hormone replacement therapy on bone mineral content over 3 years. Bone mass increases in subjects on HRT (—) and decreases in those on placebo (– – –). The effects are reversible even after 2 years, suggesting that continued HRT is beneficial.

significant fall in age-adjusted all-cause mortality. A 15% reduction in stroke incidence and a 20% reduction in ischaemic heart disease have been reported (Meade and Berra, 1992).

Calcium and vitamin D treatment has been shown to reduce the incidence of fractures in the elderly (Chapuy et al, 1992). All causes of osteoporosis must be investigated and any medication that may be responsible (including drugs such as diuretics or corticosteroids) reduced to the minimum dose possible. Although fluoride has been shown to increase apparent bone density, this is not associated with any reduction in fracture rate. In fact, the fracture rate is increased, probably because bone containing a high proportion of fluoride is weaker.

Early remobilisation of a patient is an excellent way to prevent immobilisation osteoporosis.

Bisphosphonates (see section on treatment of Paget's disease) are potent antiosteoclast agents. Etidronate is now licensed for use in established vertebral osteoporosis.

OSTEOMALACIA AND RICKETS

Activated vitamin D is required for normal mineralisation of bone. The mineralisation lag time is defined as the time

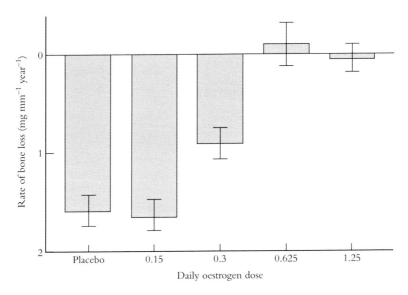

Figure 12.6   Dose–response of bone mass changes with conjugated equine oestrogen.

interval between the deposition of an individual moiety of bone matrix and its mineralisation (Baylink et al, 1970). This time is increased in both osteomalacia and rickets. Lack of activated vitamin D produced a defect of mineralisation so that osteoid is formed but remains unmineralised. In addition to this defect of mineralisation, secondary hyperparathyroidism occurs due to the hypocalcaemia of vitamin D deficiency. This results in further loss of mineral from bone.

Causes

Any causes of activated vitamin D deficiency will cause osteomalacia and rickets. Nutritional vitamin D deficiency is the most important treatable cause. Vitamin D is a fat-soluble vitamin, and bile salts are needed for its efficient absorption.

Any cause of fat malabsorption can result in vitamin D deficiency. This includes chronic pancreatitis, liver disease and bowel resection where the enterohepatic circulation may be interrupted. Where a blind loop of small bowel exists, there may be breakdown of bile salts by bacteria within the loop. The liver is the site of 25-hydroxylation of vitamin D, an early step in vitamin D activation, so that liver failure can cause a deficiency of 25-hydroxycholecalciferol. In addition, coeliac disease and gastrectomy have been associated with osteomalacia.

The rate-limiting step of vitamin D activation is 1α hydroxylation in the kidney, forming 1,25-dihydroxy-

cholecalciferol (1,25-$(OH)_2D_3$). Chronic renal failure can therefore also result in deficiency of activated vitamin D. In addition, a congenital lack of the enzyme 1α-hydroxylase causes 'vitamin D-dependent rickets'.

Finally, vitamin D deficiency can also be caused by rapid degradation of vitamin D. This occurs in 'anticonvulsant rickets'. It is believed that anticonvulsants cause induction of certain hepatic enzymes that result in rapid degradation of vitamin D. The causes of osteomalacia and rickets are summarised in *Table 12.3*.

Table 12.3   Causes of osteomalacia and rickets.

Vitamin D deficiency
   Nutritional
   Lack of sunlight

Malabsorption
   Coeliac disease
   Chronic pancreatitis
   Gastrectomy
   Blind loops of small bowel
   Bowel resection
   Liver disease (also causes 25-hydroxylase deficiency)

1α-Hydroxylase deficiency
   Congenital vitamin D-dependent rickets
   Chronic renal failure

Rapid breakdown of vitamin D
   Anticonvulsant therapy

Clinical features

When defective mineralisation begins in childhood, rickets results. The main difference between osteomalacia and rickets is the presence of the growth plate. In rickets, in addition to increased osteoid, there is failure of calcification and resorption of mature cartilage cells on the metaphyseal side of the growth plate, producing a widened and irregular radiological appearance. Infants may present with features of hypocalcaemia such as tetany and convulsions. Older children may present with skeletal deformity. The costochondral junctions may be enlarged, producing a 'rickety rosary'. If this persists untreated into adulthood, severe deformity and gross radiological deformity will result. Short stature, kyphosis, coxa vara and protrusio acetabuli may occur. Protrusio acetabuli can ultimately compress the pelvic inlet to a triradiate shape and narrow the pubic arch, so that childbirth is possible only by caesarean section.

Bone pain and tenderness are characteristic features of osteomalacia. The pain is dull and poorly localised but is clearly felt in the bones rather than in the joints. Muscle weakness, especially of the proximal limb girdles, often occurs in osteomalacia. Clinical examination reveals mild atrophy, reduced tone but increased deep tendon reflexes. These findings imply a combination of upper and lower neurone features together with those of a myopathy. Specific symptoms include difficulty rising from a chair or climbing stairs. A striking finding is a waddling gait, which occurs as a result of a combination of the pain and the weakness. If the glutei cannot keep the pelvis horizontal on walking, the upper body swings over the leading leg in order to keep the centre of gravity over the leading leg. The combination of trunk oscillation and short steps results in the classical waddling gait of osteomalacia.

Investigations reveal a raised plasma alkaline phosphatase concentration with a low to normal calcium and phosphate concentration. Radiography reveals cupping of the metaphysis and irregularity of the epiphyseal plate in rickets. In osteomalacia, the pseudofracture, or Looser's zone, is a characteristic feature.

Treatment

Osteomalacia should be treated with oral vitamin D. An initial dose of 50 000 units vitamin D daily should be given for 1 week, followed by a maintenance dose of 400 units daily. For patients with chronic renal failure or a deficiency of 1α-hydroxylase, activated vitamin D is now available orally as 1,25-$(OH)_2D_3$. Hypercalcaemia is a danger with activated vitamin D, so calcium concentrations should be monitored regularly. Because the half-life of activated vitamin D is very short, hypercalcaemia can be rapidly controlled by discontinuing the drug.

BONE IN MALIGNANT DISEASE

Hypercalcaemia is a well-known complication of malignancy. The mechanism of hypercalcaemia includes a 'humoral' hypercalcaemia where circulating hormones induce hypercalcaemia, and the hypercalcaemia due to localised osteolysis resulting from bone metastases. Humoral hypercalcaemia is often associated with a low plasma phosphate concentration, and it has long been presumed that the circulating factor is PTH. However, although 'ectopic PTH' secretion has been described with squamous cell carcinoma of the lung, in many other instances the PTH level has been found to be very low. It appears that, in several of these cases, the circulating factor is a factor related to PTH known as PTH-related protein (PTHrp). This is a peptide with 60% sequence homology to PTH over the first 13 amino acids. The PTH-like bioactivity is contained within the first 34 amino acids.

The function of PTHrp is not known but may be important in the change in calcium homeostasis during pregnancy, enabling the foetus to obtain calcium from the mother. PTHrp concentrations have recently been shown to be raised during pregnancy (Bertelloni et al, 1994) in the presence of a raised plasma calcium concentration. PTHrp binds to the PTH receptor in bone and in the renal tubule, producing hypercalcaemia. PTHrp has been found to be secreted into breast milk. Plasma PTHrp levels are raised in several malignancies, including squamous cell carcinoma of the bronchus, breast cancer and renal cell carcinoma.

A number of cytokines have been shown to contribute to hypercalcaemia in patients with multiple myeloma. These have been given the generic term 'osteoclast-activating factor'. They are now known include IL-1, tumour necrosis factor (TNF) α and TNF-β.

Bone involvement in multiple myeloma classically produces extensive bone destruction with pain and susceptibility to fracture. Skeletal radiography reveals osteoporosis, lytic lesions and fractures. Characteristic skeletal lesions are punched-out lytic areas which are sharply circumscribed. The vertebrae, skull, thoracic cage and pelvis are the most common sites of involvement. Pathological fractures are common and should suggest the possibility of multiple myeloma. In contrast to patients with metastatic carcinoma, the vertebral pedicles are rarely involved in myeloma.

The kidney is the normal site of action of 1α-hydroxylase. This enzyme is normally tightly regulated by PTH. Occasionally, renal cell carcinomas can produce 1α-hydroxylase that is not regulated. This is a further mechanism by which hypercalcaemia can occur. In this case, the plasma phosphate concentration will not be low because the mechanism of hypercalcaemia is through an excess of activated vitamin D.

REFERENCES

Ahonen P, Myllarniemi S, Sipila I, Perheentupa J. Clinical variation of autoimmune polyendocrinopathy–candidiasis–ectodermal dystrophy (APECED) in a series of 68 patients. *N Engl J Med* 1990; **322**: 1829–1836.

Baylink D, Stauffer M, Wergedal J, Rich C. Formation, mineralization, and resorption of bone in vitamin D-deficient rats. *J Clin Invest* 1970; **49**: 1122–1134.

Bertelloni S, Baroncelli GI, Pelletti A, Battini R, Saggese G. Parathyroid hormone-related protein in healthy pregnant women. *Calcif Tissue Int* 1994; **54**: 195–197.

Browder W, Rakinic J, Schlecter R, Krementz ET. Primary hyperparathyroidism in the seventies. A decade of change? *Am J Surg* 1983; **146**: 360–365.

Chapuy MC, Arlot ME, Duboeuf F et al. Vitamin D₃ and calcium to prevent hip fractures in the elderly women. *N Engl J Med* 1992; **327**: 1637–1642.

Christiansen C, Christensen MS, Transbol I. Bone mass in postmenopausal women after withdrawal of oestrogen/gestagen replacement therapy. *Lancet* 1981; **i**: 459–461.

Dove J. Complete fractures of the femur in Paget's disease of bone. *J Bone Joint Surg [Br]* 1980; **62B**: 12–17.

Holdaway IM, Ibbertson HK, Wattie D, Scragg R, Graham P. Previous pet ownership and Paget's disease. *Bone Miner* 1990; **8**: 53–58.

Meade TW, Berra A. Hormone replacement therapy and cardiovascular disease. *Br Med Bull* 1992; **48**: 276–308.

Meeran K, Hattersley A, Burrin J, Shiner R, Ibbertson K. Oral and inhaled corticosteroids reduce bone formation as shown by plasma osteocalcin levels. *Am J Respir Crit Care Med* 1995; **151**: 333–336.

Mundy GR, Shapiro JL, Bandelin JG, Canalis EM, Raisz LG. Direct stimulation of bone resorption by thyroid hormones. *J Clin Invest* 1976; **58**: 529–534.

Prior JC, Vigna YM, Schechter MT, Burgess AE. Spinal bone loss and ovulatory disturbances. *N Engl J Med* 1990; **323**: 1221–1227 (published erratum appears in *N Engl J Med* 1993;p **328**(23): 1724).

Rebel A, Basle M, Pouplard A, Malkani K, Filmon R, Lepatezour A. Bone tissue in Paget's disease of bone. Ultrastructure and immunocytology. *Arthritis Rheum* 1980; **23**: 1104–1114.

World Health Organisation. Assessment of fracture risk and its application to screening for postmenopausal osteoporosis. *WHO Technical Report Series 843*. Geneva: World Health Organisation, 1994.

13

Osteonecrosis

Jean WM Gardeniers

INTRODUCTION

One of the first, if not the first, descriptions of osteonecrosis appeared in the medical literature in 1794, when James Russell (1755–1836), who was the first Professor of Clinical Surgery at the University of Edinburgh, published his book *Necrosis of Bone*. In the nineteenth century osteonecrosis was predominantly of septic origin and characterised by Russell as the formation of sequestra in the long bones of the skeleton. The distinction between septic and aseptic necrosis was not recognised until much later, by Axhausen and Koenig in 1888.

For more than a century we have known that osteonecrosis of the femoral head has a vascular pathogenesis. For this reason, the process was called aseptic, or avascular, necrosis. Today, osteonecrosis of aseptic origin has become more and more important in orthopaedics, manifest in all the large joints, but with the highest incidence in the femoral head. In 1978, Jones wrote that osteonecrosis of the femoral head had become an increasingly significant problem in the twentieth century, particularly in connection with deep diving, high-altitude operations, alcohol and corticosteroid treatment of recipients of organ transplants.

The precise aetiology of both traumatic and non-traumatic osteonecrosis is still uncertain. Traditional concepts have been challenged frequently by many authors. Glimcher et al (1978) challenged the concept of 'creeping substitution' which, until then, had been a widely accepted mechanism of bone reconstruction following osteonecrosis. Several groups recognised a new preradiological stage in the evolution of the disease, and introduced a new guideline for early diagnosis and treatment of the disease (Arlet and Ficat, 1968). New treatments have also been developed by Judet, Meyers, Hori, Ganz and Sugioka, with the objective of revascularising and/or preserving the femoral head (Sugioka et al, 1992).

Many questions concerning the aetiology, pathogenesis and treatment of idiopathic osteonecrosis of the femoral head (IONF) still remain unanswered. This was, and still is, the stimulus for many scientists and clinicians to start experimental and clinical studies to investigate the histomorphological and mechanical behaviour of normal, avascular and revascularising cancellous bone and to investigate and follow up different treatment modalities. For a detailed review of the literature relating to osteonecrosis the reader is referred to the references by Gardeniers (1988) and Monticelli (1982).

DEFINITION

Bone is an organ that comprises vascular, fat, marrow, cartilage and bone tissues. Living bone is composed of osteogenic cells and the extracellular bone substance. Bone substance is inert and consists of collagenous and non-collagenous proteins and minerals.

Necrosis of bone infers death and lysis of the cells of all tissues within the organ, except the cartilage. Following cell necrosis, the extracellular matrices of all tissues, except bone, undergo lysis as well. In general, necrosis of bone can be caused by either infectious or non-infectious factors. The difference between these two causes is shown not only in the aetiology but also in the reactions of the surrounding tissues. In septic necrosis, caused by an infection with microorganisms, the process is well demarcated by the surrounding tissues, which try to dispose of it. The reactions of the surrounding tissues in non-infectious, aseptic, avascular or, synonymously called, osteonecrosis are completely different. All tissue reactions are organised in such a way that healing of the necrotic part becomes the main goal.

Osteonecrosis of bone implies death of bone, following a circulation disturbance in the bone. Only in trauma is the aetiology of this vascular injury well understood. In all other types of osteonecrosis the aetiology is not yet clear. Idiopathic osteonecrosis includes all types of aseptic necrosis associated with various pathological conditions or treatments, as well as those not associated with any disease entity (Kenzora and Glimcher, 1985).

EPIDEMIOLOGICAL FACTORS

Incidence

In 1962 Mankin described five bilateral cases of IONF. Some 10 years later, Marcus et al (1973) presented a series of 53 bilateral cases. This higher number may be due to an increased incidence in general or to better diagnostic acumen. The incidence may be higher as a result of more frequent alcoholism, steroid use and hyperlipidaemia. A diagnostic factor may be that necrosis, in some femoral heads, has been masked by degenerative changes. One study concluded that 68% of degenerative hips were based on underlying avascular necrosis.

Several authors, however, have confirmed the increase of IONF in large series over prolonged periods. In one study it was found that 70% more cases were seen in the period from 1975 to 1980, than in 1970–1975, although their criteria for the diagnosis of IONF did not change between 1970 and 1980. Hence, there was a real increase in the incidence of IONF between 1950 and 1981. This is still true today due to the increasing number of transplant recipients.

Sex distribution

The male prevalence for IONF is invariably reported as a mean of 81.4%, although the prevalence varies in different studies. In the literature the male : female ratio varies from 8:1 to 2.6:1. The percentages given for male prevalence in the literature do not show large variations.

Age

The age distribution is wide, from 14 to 83 years. The vast majority of patients, however, are younger than 50 years. Comparison of the average age shows that the incidence has increased, and that the average age has decreased. This is in agreement with other reports. The average age of females exceeds that of males by almost 10 years.

Site affected

In the literature, 34–72% of cases were reported to be bilateral. The majority of authors found a percentage of 50–60% for bilateral involvement, including Merle d'Aubigné et al (1965) who reported a value of (50%). Jaffe (1972) reported that these variations are probably due to variations in the time at which the diagnosis was made, and the period of observation. Another study reported a slightly increased prevalence for the right hip (58.6%).

General health

It is not unusual for other diseases to be associated with IONF. Some researchers found that only 4.7% of all patients with IONF were otherwise healthy. It was also reported that in 89% of the cases IONF occurred concurrently with systemic disorders: 72.8% were associated with alcohol, steroid use or hyperuricaemia, and 23% with multiple coexistent disorders.

AETIOLOGY

The conditions that are directly associated with osteonecrosis of bone can be divided into two groups: the certain and the probable causative factors.

The certain causes are major trauma to the blood vessels of the femoral head, emboli obstructing these blood vessels, systemic diseases with sludging in the blood vessels, severe obstruction of the blood vessels by arterial disease, and radiation causing direct cell death in bone marrow. The list of probable causative factors contains conditions statistically associated with IONF. These aetiological associations are as follows.

Corticosteroids

An association between high dosages or length of treatment with corticosteroids and the incidence of avascular necrosis has been reported, but there is no agreement about how strong this association is. The relationship between corticosteroid treatment and IONF is beyond doubt, but the mechanisms involved, and whether they have a vascular or mechanical cause, or both, are not known.

In many experimental studies the role of steroids has been examined (Jones, 1985). Studies have shown that steroid treatment produces marked lipaemia in humans and animals. Long-term administration of steroids is associated with systemic fat embolism and increased fat in the liver in animal studies. Wang showed that large fat cells develop in bone marrow of rabbits. Nishimura showed that steroids lead to the proliferation of foamy cells in the walls of the vein intima, producing venous stasis. Both authors reported that these effects of steroids lead to increased intraosseous pressure and subsequent collapse of the sinusoidal vessels in the femoral head. Subsequently, marrow oedema and fatty necrosis appeared, and finally focal osteonecrosis occurred.

The main feature is that there are often multiple foci of osteonecrosis in the skeleton. Many authors have reported different values for the indicence of IONF, ranging from 14.6% to 37% (mean 27.0%) (eg. Merle d'Aubigné et al, 1965 (36%)). The higher values include patients undergoing renal dialysis, renal transplants or with lupus erythematosus; the lower figures do not include these patients. In approximately 24% of all recipients of renal transplants osteonecrosis developed somewhere in the skeleton.

Alcoholism

The reports by different authors present a great variation in the incidence of IONF in patients taking large quantities of alcohol. It is, of course, difficult to define the precise characteristics that qualify an invididual to be an alcoholic. Authors, patients and family have their own subjective opinion about these qualifications and this affects the percentages quoted. The lowest value is 10.2%, the highest 74%.

The relationship between the consumption of large quantities of alcohol and the incidence of IONF is beyond any doubt, but the extent or absence of osteonecrosis in many alcoholics suggests that there are other factors to be considered.

Hyperlipaemia

Between 1965 and 1994 Jones published many articles about hyperlipaemia as a causative factor for osteonecrosis (Jones, 1978, 1985). He suggests three pathological mechanisms, all combined with hyperlipaemia: a fatty liver, destabilisation and coalescence of endogenous plasma lipoproteins and disruption of bone marrow or adipose tissue depots. His clinical and experimental data explain the relationship between fat embolism and osteonecrosis, and suggest 13 clinical conditions to be associated with this relationship.

Jacobs (1978) also found fat embolism or disorders in fat metabolism in 89% of all patients with non-traumatic osteonecrosis. Calandriello observed an increase in blood lipid levels in 26% of patients with osteonecrosis, triglycerides in 78.9% and cholesterol in 44.7%.

Hyperuricaemia

The incidence of IONF in patients with hyperuricaemia, as reported by different authors, varies from 16.2% to 53%. In patients with hyperuricaemia IONF is more common in men (80.6%) than in women (19.4%).

However, some other conditions associated with hyperuricaemia are predisposing factors for IONF, such as alcoholism and corticosteroid treatment. None the less, a direct link between hyperuricaemia and avascular necrosis is feasible only if uric acid crystals are found in the affected bone tissue.

Liver disease

This is difficult to define, because various conditions associated with liver disease predispose to or are associated with IONF, for example alcoholism and corticosteroid treatment. It is not always possible to decide which condition developed first. In the literature, only Calandriello has mentioned an incidence of IONF of 14.3% in patients in whom liver disease was an important factor; two-thirds of these patients also had other disorders with a relevant association with IONF, such as alcoholism and corticosteroid treatment.

Loads and minor injuries

Type of work has no correlation with IONF, and mechanical load at work alone cannot explain the predominance of IONF in men. Minor injuries are always mentioned in the literature, but the incidence of IONF in patients who had minor injuries ranges from 5%

up to 36%. It may be that minor injury is the inductive factor, producing symptoms in a patient with previously asymptomatic IONF. The relevance of any injury in the development of IONF should always be considered.

Congenital dysplasia of the hip

This is seldom considered as a predisposing factor (Merle d'Aubigné et al, 1965) and doubt has been cast on its possible relevance for IONF. The incidence of IONF in patients with congenital dysplasia of the hip joint varies from 5% to 52% (Merle d'Aubigné et al, 1965; Kerboul, 1974).

Pancreatitis

In one article, pancreatitis has been suggested as a factor associated with IONF (Jones, 1985). Alcoholism, hyper-lipaemia and pancreatitis constitute a triad. The real effect of pancreatitis is not yet well understood, but fat necrosis was found in 10.4% of the pancreatitic cases. Lipolytic enzymes may cause lysis of the fat cells in the bone. One author found no cases of acute pancreatitis, but observed an increase in the level of amylase which, however, was not statistically significant.

Obesity and diabetes

Obese patients are common in series of osteonecrosis of the knee joint. Jacobs had six obese and three diabetic patients among 23 cases of osteonecrosis not associated with alcohol or corticosteroids. Hyperglycaemia (12.3% of cases), however, has no significance as far as the aetiology of IONF is concerned.

Other predisposing and risk factors

These are, according to the literature, deep and superficial phlebitis (4.1%), thromboembolic disease, artherosclerosis (up to 42.8%), polycythaemia (up to 25%) and gastric uclers (10.9%).

All the above-mentioned factors, in particular those related to diseases of the blood and liver, may interact in a complex way to produce IONF. Many authors also suggest the involvement of environmental or social factors. However, the femoral head is so commonly affected that local factors must be involved. One of the local factors is the inadequacy of the blood supply to the femoral head.

Vascularity of the femoral head

A major risk factor to the circulation of the femoral head is the scarcity or absence of anastomoses between the terminal arterioles. These end arterioles branch off at right angles from the major rami, which enter the femoral head through areas of rigid bone. Two principal groups of arterioles supply the whole of the femoral head: the lateral and medial epiphyseal arterioles and the superior and inferior metaphyseal arterioles. Functionally, however, the largest and therefore the most precarious area is that dependent only on the lateral epiphyseal arterioles. These arterioles vary in number from two to six and follow the line of the former epiphyseal growth plate (Trueta and Harrison, 1953; Trueta, 1963; Crock, 1980).

Mechanical factors

Another local factor, mechanical stress on the femoral head, provides a possible explanation for the major involvement of the anterosuperior weight-bearing seg-ment in IONF. According to Frost's (1964) theory, the resistance of necrotic bone to mechanical stress is reduced. It is assumed that the weakening starts with a small fatigue fracture in the subchondral bone, which is not followed by adequate repair. By confluence of more microfractures, a segmental collapse eventually results. However, this mechanical factor is only an additional one in IONF, related in most cases to subsequent events such as collapse and fragmentation.

PATHOGENESIS

The effects of ischaemia are seen in both marrow and bone structure. Haematopoietic marrow is the most vulnerable structure and is therefore the first to show effects. These appear within 24 hours of the interruption of blood flow and consist of loss of cell outline, homo-geneity of the cytoplasm, reduced basophilia, pycnosis of nuclei and, finally, cellular dissolution leading to the appearance of lacunae, which become larger and coalesce. The haematopoietic marrow is completely dissolved within 5–6 days.

Fatty marrow appears to be more resistant. As late as 3 days from the onset of ischaemia, the general architecture of the cells begins to change, with disappearance of the nuclei, interruption of the septa and conglutination of more cells into optically empty vacuoles. Last to be dissolved is the collagen matrix of the marrow.

Early endothelial lesions in the vessels appear within the first 48 hours. The sinusoids and capillaries are destroyed more quickly than larger vessels such as the venules and arterioles. In the trabecular bone, the first elements to be affected are the osteoblasts. Within the first 48 hours regressive changes appear, such as loss of natural basophilia in the cytoplasm, nuclear pycnosis, karyolysis and, at a later stage, cellular disintegration. Ischaemic lesions of the osteocytes appear much later. Many of these cells seem substantially intact in the histological sections, even weeks or months after the ischaemic damage (up to 4–5 months: Catto, 1965). This is undoubtedly misleading because, from the first week of ischaemia, osteocytes show morphological and functional changes, involving the principal organelles, mitochondria and endoplasmic reticulum. Deductions based on light microscopy of histological sections are not reliable in evaluating the viability of osteocytes. Within 1 week of ischaemia, haematopoietic marrow cells and the reticuloendothelium show necrosis, whereas approximately 50% of fat cells, osteoblasts and osteoclasts remain morphologically intact. Osteocytes appear to be undamaged. Some 2 weeks after the onset of ischaemia only the osteocytes appear to be morphologically intact, but there is absence of functional activity.

Peculiar to bone is the fact that the bony framework, organic matrix and mineral component are not affected by the enzymes released by necrotic cells. The mineral part of bone protects the matrix, and the mineral part, the apatite, is protected from phagocytic recognition by the bone lining cells and the extracellular barrier, the lamina limitans or α2HS glycoproteins (Chambers, 1980). The bony framework therefore remains unchanged.

The process of revascularisation originates in the unaffected medullary spaces at the edge of the ischaemic area and from the synovial membrane. New capillaries and cells invade the marrow spaces between the dead trabeculae (Atsumi et al, 1984; Kenzora and Glimcher, 1985; Atsumi and Kuroki, 1992). A dense network of vessels develops, partly newly formed by mesenchymal differentiation and partly formed by subsequent branch-

ing of pre-existing vessels. The extent of penetration depends on the size of the necrotic area and the reduced intensity of the revascularisation with time. The latter is probably due to loss of an additional chemotactic signal. This process is not yet completely understood, but it is known that lipopolysaccharide, prostaglandins, parathyroid hormone and an osteoclast-activating factor play significant roles (Chambers, 1980).

A second source of revascularisation is the synovial membrane. An intense proliferation of vessels starts at the 'circulus vasculosus' and the vessels enter at the point where the synovial membrane reflects at the osteochondral junction.

Around the newly formed vessels, primordial mesenchymal cells and monocytes appear in the first few days. These cells multiply actively and are very immature. Phagocytosis of necrotic marrow is heralded by the appearance of histiocytes. Progressive differentiation of the primordial cells into fibroblasts becomes more and more evident until it gives rise to areas of marked fibrosis. Differentiation into lipocytes can also occur, but differentiation into haematopoietic marrow is extremely doubtful in humans.

Differentiation into osteoclasts, osteoblasts and osteocytes takes place in another phase of the repair process: osteogenesis and resorption. Osteogenesis, by means of metaplasia, sometimes takes place in the newly formed connective tissue when this is well vascularised, but the common mechanism is apposition of new bone on the dead trabeculae. These dead trabeculae are an excellent framework, and support by necrotic bone therefore plays an important role in osteogenesis. Necrotic bone remains unchanged for a long period of time (for up to 6 months from the onset of ischaemia in laboratory animals; Favenesi et al, 1984a,b; Gardeniers et al, 1989), and is able to act as a continuous stimulus for the osteopathic front. Some of the primordial cells polarise themselves towards the surfaces of dead trabeculae and differentiate into osteoblasts and osteocytes. They coat the dead trabeculae with osteoid, which often mineralises into bone.

In humans, lamellar bone is preponderant and woven bone is often absent. Trabeculae with appositional bone are thicker than normal because they consist of a mixture of newly formed bone with a necrotic centre. In humans, this increased bone mass becomes manifest on radiographs as a small area of high density 4–6 months after the onset of ischaemia. Increased radiodensity is therefore not characteristic of early osteonecrosis, but is a manifestation of the repair process.

For reasons presently unknown, osteoapposition eventually becomes exhausted. Osteoapposition rarely extends more than 4–5 mm into the necrotic area before the undifferentiated cells become fibroblasts. When this osteoblastic front disappears, areas of aggressive medullary fibrosis are formed and they penetrate the bone. Also, new vascular penetration proceeds. Periosteocytic osteolysis starts along the edge of the necrotic bone where the osteocytes assume osteoclastic activity and form a shallow niche in the necrotic bone. These local bone changes lead to a phagocytic recognition of the apatite. The protective bone lining cells and the extracellular barrier disappear. Mononuclear phagocytes migrate to the bone, also attracted by an additional chemotactic signal. Osteoclasts are formed via fusion of these cells, and resorption commences. This resorption often penetrates deeper into the necrotic area than the osteogenetic front (Chambers, 1980; Kenzora and Glimcher, 1985).

This predominance of resorption over osteogenesis undermines the mechanical strength of the necrotic bone (Glimcher and Kenzora, 1979). The old and strong but dead trabeculae are being removed and replaced by young, weak, but living, bone. The total strength of the bony structure is diminished and this leads to fracture as a result of normal mechanical loading. Fracture of the necrotic bone, collapse and fragmentation are therefore the result of normal weight-bearing and motion. The presence of the fracture is a stimulus for further ingrowth of vessels, but this vascular penetration again stimulates resorption rather than osteogenesis. For this reason, the repair process in humans is not sufficient to achieve complete reossification of the whole necrotic area, and fracture, collapse and fragmentation are the result of the revascularisation process (Favenesi et al, 1984a,b, 1988; Gardeniers et al, 1989).

NATURAL HISTORY OF IDIOPATHIC OSTEONECROSIS OF THE FEMORAL HEAD

The natural history of osteonecrosis has been described extensively by many authors (Marcus et al, 1973; Springfield and Enneking, 1978; Hungerford, 1979; Enneking, 1979, 1986; Ficat, 1983; Steinberg et al, 1984, 1995;

ARCO, 1992; Mont and Hungerford, 1995). Depending on the specific researcher and based on clinical, radiological and histological findings, five to seven stages of osteonecrosis have been recognised.

Early staging systems were based on standard radiographic examinations, and Arlet and Ficat (1968) were among the first to create a workable system. They were also the first to recognise that the early onset of osteonecrosis lies in the preradiological stage. They referred to this stage as 'the silent hip' in osteonecrosis. In their stage 1, the radiograph does not show any abnormality and the diagnosis is confirmed by biopsy. Many authors did not agree with a preradiological stage because nearly all bone imaging was based on plain radiography and tomography.

In 1973, Marcus et al described a staging system based on radiographic changes and clinical symptoms and signs. This six-stage system never became widely accepted because the relationship between symptoms, radiographic findings and treatment was not completely proven, especially in the situation where the patient had initial symptoms and the radiographs showed a normal image.

In 1985, Bluemm and colleagues, Hungerford, Jergesen, Kittrup and Mitchell wrote the first reports about magnetic resonance imaging (MRI) of osteonecrosis. The marrow cavity of bone and, of course, the femoral head emit a strong MR signal. This is very useful in the diagnosis of osteonecrosis because the first effects of ischaemia occur in the bone marrow. Necrosis of the marrow, degradation of marrow lipids and their replacement by water-equivalent tissue, and the growth of vascularised mesenchymal tissue produce changes that can be detected by MRI.

In 1990, Hungerford and Lennox modified the staging system of Ficat and Arlet and added a stage 0, in which the plain radiograph is normal and only the MRI shows a double-line sign (T1-weighted image) or a band of low intensity (T2-weighted image). The double-line sign was consistent with the process of osteonecrosis and became the pathognomonic image on MRI in the early stage of osteonecrosis (Hungerford, 1990; Steinberg et al, 1995).

Steinberg et al (1995) also proposed a seven-stage system, which is also based on that of Ficat and Arlet. They divided the third stage in a stage IIIA and IIIB, without or with collapse of the femoral dome. As Mont and Hungerford wrote in their recent article in 1995, the major contribution of Steinberg's classification to the Ficat and Arlet system is the addition of quantification of involvement of the femoral head, which includes the extent of the necrotic area and is predictive of the final outcome of the disease and applied treatment.

The Japanese Investigation Committee for Adult Idiopathic Avascular Necrosis of the Femoral Head was founded in 1984. The Japanese recognised the increasing problem of osteonecrosis in their country and saw the need for a single, uniform, classification. The Committee also modified the Ficat and Arlet system. They recognised the importance of the radiographic location of the osteonecrosis in accordance with the weight-bearing part of the femoral head and acetabulum. The first report of this Committee (Ono, 1989) shows the sub-classification in medial, central and lateral lesions and the importance of progression of the disease according to this subclassification. Many authors (Ohzono et al, 1991; Sugioka et al, 1992) have shown the importance of the location of the lesion with respect to prognosis and different treatment modalities.

In 1990, in Ischia, Italy, at the General Assembly of ARCO (the international 'Association de Recherche sur la Circulation Osseuse') it was accepted by the members that **one uniform and international classification of osteonecrosis** was needed. The use of different classifications, however good, could lead only to confusion and disagreement. The International Committee on Terminology and Classification was formed. The members (J. Gardeniers, chair, J. Arlet, B. Mazieres, P. Acquaviva, M. Steinberg, Y. Sugioka, B. Stulberg and R. Burkhardt) had their first meeting in Nijmegen, The Netherlands, and proposed to ARCO the first concept of '**one uniform classification**', based on the Ficat–Arlet system, the Japanese staging system and subclassification, and the Steinberg system of staging and subclassification. This system was finalised in 1994, but is not yet accepted universally. The system consists of five stages and incorporates the subclassification advocated by Steinberg and the Japanese Investigation Committee. The ARCO classification is a good compromise between the original systems predominating in Europe, the USA and Japan.

Within ARCO it was agreed that the definition of necrosis of bone had to be: 'Bone is an organ that consists of mineralized and non-mineralized tissues. Bone necrosis is a disease which causes death of bone and is therefore called "osteonecrosis"'. ARCO agreed on this definition because the many terms used for necrosis of bone are at least confusing. The list is long − avascular necrosis, aseptic necrosis, infarction of bone, Chandler's disease − and these terms are frequently used at random.

The goal has to be to make the diagnosis of 'true osteonecrosis' as early as possible in the course of the disease. The diagnostic criteria available at present are: anamnesis, physical examination, radiography, scintigraphy, MRI, functional bone investigation and histology.

DIAGNOSTIC CRITERIA

Anamnesis and physical examination

The patient in the early stages of the disease will complain of pain in the hip region, often located in the groin but sometimes also in the trochanteric region or buttocks. Later in the course of the disease the pain will radiate to the mid-thigh and knee. The pain starts vaguely with many free intervals but becomes more and more intense and is felt deep in the groin. As more of the femoral head is affected, the pain will become more steady, and when finally the femoral dome fails mechanically (seen as a crescent sign or collapse on radiograph) the pain becomes intense and severe. At this stage the pain is disabling and the patient needs external support. In the end stage of the disease, the patient has the same complaints as somebody with severe osteoarthritis. The investigator must interview the patient carefully to try to record all the risk factors of osteonecrosis such as alcohol intake, medication especially corticosteroids, tablets or ointments, associated diseases and professional risk factors.

Anyone with hip pain, negative radiography and associated risk factors needs to be examined carefully and followed with sequential re-examination.

In the early onset of the disease, the findings on physical examination are often very subtle. The range of motion might be normal but painful at the extremes, especially on maximal abduction, external and internal rotations. When the disease progresses, these findings become more pronounced and all movements are painful and become gradually more and more limited.

When the femoral dome starts to fail mechanically, the figure-of-four sign becomes positive. This test is a manoeuvre in which the examinator flexes the hip 90°, abducts, and at the same time externally rotates the hip with gradual force by placing the heel on the contralateral knee. The anterosuperior segment is forced into acetabulum and pressure is put on the subchondral fracture. The patient experiences intense pain. This sign is pathognomonic for fracture and collapse in osteonecrosis.

Special attention is needed for the contralateral hip, because of the high incidence of bilateral involvement of up to 80%. Often, the diagnosis of osteonecrosis in the contralateral hip is made as a result of a high degree of clinical suspicion.

This high degree of clinical suspicion is also present in patients with vague pains in the hip region accompanied with negative radiographic findings but who have one or more risk factors for osteonecrosis, such as alcoholism, corticosteroid use, systemic lupus erythematosus, sickle cell anaemia, Gaucher's disease, trauma, coagulation disorders, exposure to radiation, and risky professional activities such as deep diving or high-altitude occupations. All the previously mentioned epidemiological and aetiological factors can be involved and should be taken into consideration.

Radiography

The problem with radiography is that when the signs of osteonecrosis are visible the disease has already progressed beyond the initial stage. Radiography should, however, always be performed in a plain anteroposterior view and a lateral or true lateral view. The true lateral view has been described extensively by Sugioka et al (1992) and is taken with the leg in 90° flexion, 45° abduction and neutral rotation. It projects the femoral head in a perpendicular view to the anteroposterior projection and clearly shows the site of the affected area.

The first signs visible on a plain radiograph are subtle changes in radiodensity often not noticed at the time of the first examination. Local osteoporosis, osteosclerotic or early cystic changes are often seen retrospectively in the anterosuperior segment. When the disease progresses, these changes become more and more pronounced and eventually, especially on the lateral or true lateral views, the crescent sign, the subchondral fracture line, is seen. Finally, in the later phase of the disease, radiographs show the picture of collapse and the start of advanced osteoarthritis with flattening of the femoral dome, irregularity of the femoral articular surface, joint space narrowing and finally complete joint destruction.

Tomography can be helpful as it may show the first osteosclerotic or osteolytic changes in the early phase, and it might be helpful in estimating the extent of the lesion.

Scintigraphy

Scintigraphy has the same problem as radiography: it is not reliable in the early phase. The osteonecrotic area is avascular in the early phase. Around this avascular area lies a reactive zone from which the vascularity tries to invade the infarction.

On a ^{99m}Tc scan, this is visible as 'cold in hot'. However, this image is not observed frequently because it represents only one short phase in the disease. More often, a plain low uptake or a plain high uptake is seen, and these signs are not pathognomonic. Increased uptake is seen in many conditions such as osteoarthritis, bacterial arthritis, tumours, post-trauma and reflex dystrophy. However, scintigraphy should always be considered because it shows involvement of the hip and will therefore focus the attention of the examiner on the hip joint.

Magnetic resonance imaging

MRI is a non-invasive method and can be used to visualise early changes in the bone. It is both sensitive and more specific than other non-invasive diagnostic measures, and gives an image of the existing process in the bone. The marrow cavity in the femoral head emits a strong MRI signal. The first effects of ischaemia occur in the bone marrow; oedema, necrosis, degradation of marrow lipids and their replacement by water-equivalent tissue and the ingrowth of vascularised mesenchymal tissue produce changes that can be detected by MRI.

Classical T1-weighted images in a frontal and axial plane with sections of 5 mm, taken every 2.5 mm, are basic recommendations (*Figure 13.1*). The early finding in osteonecrosis is a 'band-like image of low intensity' on the classical T1-weighted image. As an addition, a T2-weighted image is made which shows the so-called 'double-line sign'. The high-intensity signal in the double line represents the revascularisation front surrounding the ischaemic area. The 'band-like image of low intensity' on T1 and the 'double-line sign' on T2 are pathognomonic for osteonecrosis.

MRI is also useful to estimate the extent of the involved area (Steinberg et al, 1995). View perpendicular to the femoral neck axis are the most useful images to determine the position and to calculate the extent of the lesion.

The Japanese Investigation Committee and several Japanese authors (Atsumi et al, 1984; Ono, 1984–1989;

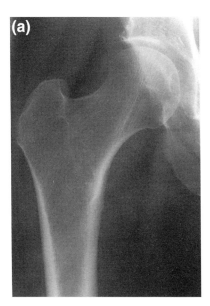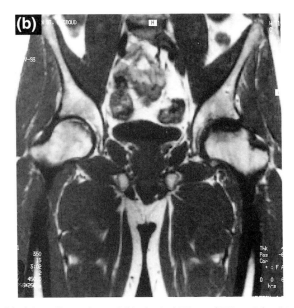

Figure 13.1   Early changes in osteonecrosis as shown by (a) plain radiography and (b) classical T1- and T2-weighted MRI.

Ohzono et al, 1991; Atsumi and Kuroki, 1992; Sugioka et al, 1992) have indicated the importance of localisation of the involved area with respect to the weight-bearing part of the femoral dome and acetabulum. In the early stages, MRI will show the localisation clearly. MRI is also important in the sequential evaluation of asymptomatic lesions in the femoral head and, furthermore, the effects of operative treatment modalities can be assessed more objectively.

Functional bone investigation

Functional bone investigation is an invasive technique first described by Arlet, Ficat and Hungerford (Arlet and Ficat, 1968; Hungerford, 1979; Ficat, 1981, 1982, 1983). It consists of measurement of intraosseous pressure, intraosseous venography and core biopsy, the latter as a diagnosticum and also as a therapeutic method. The great value of this method has been that it distinguished the 'preradiological stage of osteonecrosis' in the days before MRI. This stage is now recognised as the probable onset of the disease.

The technique is invasive and therefore should not be used routinely to stage the disease. It is not pathognomonic for osteonecrosis because the derived data are also positive in other circulatory bone diseases. It remains, however, of great value in the research of osteonecrosis

and other bone disorders in which the great advantage is obtaining bone for histological examination.

Histology

Histological examination should be done at every possible opportunity, but not as a standard diagnostic method. Biopsy remains the 'golden standard', although it is invasive. However, it is often also a curative procedure.

The biopsy often shows non-conclusive data in the very early phase. Oedema, foci of cellular necrosis and red blood cells outside the vessels can also be seen in other bone diseases. However, when diffuse marrow necrosis covering an area of more then one square centimetre and empty lacunae become visible, the diagnosis of osteonecrosis can be made.

THE ARCO INTERNATIONAL CLASSIFICATION

'Staging of osteonecrosis' is a method of defining the development of the disease (*Figure 13.2*). It has to include the very onset of the disease, stage 0, and extend till the final end, the complete joint destruction; this covers the full spectrum of the disease. 'Staging' is also a guideline for

Stage	0	1	2	3	4
Findings	All present techniques normal or non-diagnostic	X-ray and CT are normal; at least one of the below mentioned is positive	No crescent sign. X-ray abnormal: sclerosis, osteolysis, focal porosis	Crescent sign on the X-ray and/or flattening of articular surface of femoral head	Osteoarthritis: joint space narrowing, acetabular changes, joint destruction
Techniques	X-ray, CT, scintigraphy MRI	Scintigraphy, MRI ★Quantitate on MRI	X-ray, CT, scintigraphy, MRI ★Quantitate on MRI and X-ray	X-ray, CT only ★Quantitate on X-ray	X-ray only
Subclassification	No	Location (see figure) 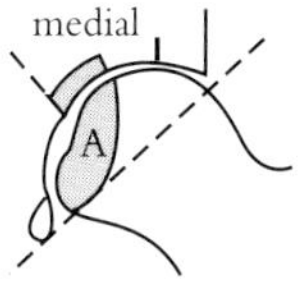	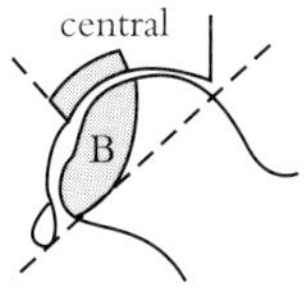	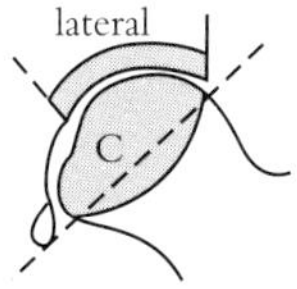	No
Quantitation	No	Quantitation / % Area involvement: minimal A<15%, moderate B 15–30%, extensive C>30%	Length of crescent: A<15%, B 15–30%, C>30%	% Surface collapse and dome depression: 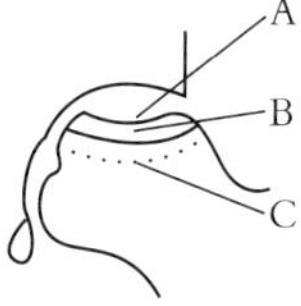 A <15% <2mm, B 15–30% 2–4mm, C >30% >4mm	No

Figure 13.2 ARCO international classification of osteonecrosis. From *ARCO News* 1993; **5**(2): 82.

treatment of the patient with osteonecrosis. It is clear that the success of the treatment of osteonecrosis of the femoral head is related to the stage at which treatment is started. If treatment is initiated early, the biological and mechanical capacities of the bone might be restored.

Stage 0

All present diagnostic techniques are normal or non-diagnostic. Future diagnostic techniques will at some point enable a diagnosis to be made in stage '0'.

Stage 1

Plain radiographic and computed tomography (CT) findings are normal. At least one of the following techniques is positive: scintigraphy and/or MRI. An open biopsy will confirm the diagnosis (*Figure 13.3*). This stage is subdivided into three categories according to the **location** and **extension** of the lesion under the weight-bearing dome of the acetabulum. These three

subcategories are **medial, central** and **lateral** (see *Figure 13.2*). For further study and follow-up on the results of different forms of treatment and the development of the disease, **quantitation** is added. This quantitation is a calculation of the area of femoral head involvement (according to Steinberg et al, 1995):

- Minimal – less than 15%
- Moderate – 15–30%
- Extensive – more than 30%

Stage 2

Radiography shows areas of abnormality: a mottled aspect, sclerosis, osteolysis and focal porosis (*Figure 13.4*). There is **no** subchondral fracture, known as the **crescent sign**. The femoral head remains spherical on anteroposterior and lateral views on radiography and CT. Again, scintigraphy and MRI are positive. Subclassification is important, as described in stage 1.

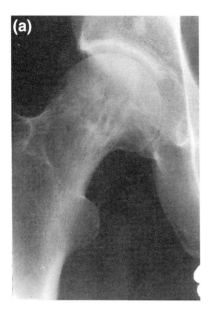
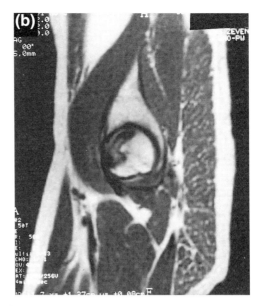

Figure 13.3   Stage 1 osteonecrosis: (a) radiograph and (b) positive T1-weighted MRI.

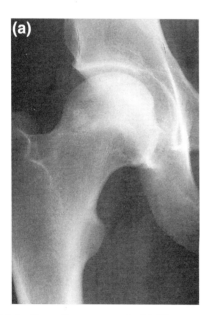
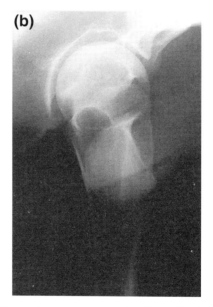

Figure 13.4   Stage 2 osteonecrosis. (a) The anteroposterior radiograph shows a clear sclerotic rim in the anterosuperior segment. (b) The axial radiograph shows no crescent sign.

Stage 3

A **crescent sign** is visible on the radiograph, especially in lateral or axial views. The femoral head fails mechanically and axial radiographs show a fine radiolucent subchondral fracture line. Progressive flattening of the femoral dome will occur. The spherical configuration starts to deterio-

rate and finally the dome will collapse. Late radiographs show the articular surface of the femoral head to be flattened, but there is no evidence of joint-line narrowing or acetabular involvement (*Figure 13.5*). CT laminograms might be helpful if there is no evidence of collapse on the plain radiographs.

Subclassification and quantitation is added, but quanti-

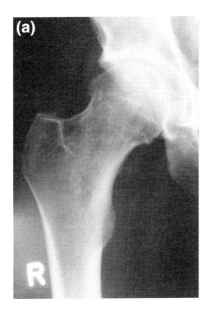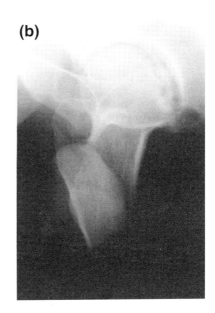

Figure 13.5   Stage 3 osteonecrosis. (a) Slight flattening of the femoral dome on the anteroposterior view. (b) The axial view clearly shows the crescent sign, the subchondral fracture.

tation can also be done by calculation of the amount of flattening of the femoral dome according to Steinberg et al (1995). First, it is determined whether the crescent sign appears more prominently in the anteroposterior or lateral view. After selection of the most prominent view, the length of the crescent is expressed as a percentage of the length of the entire articular surface:

- Minimal – less than 15% involvement or a depression of less than 2 mm
- Moderate – 15–30% involvement or a depression of 2–4 mm
- Extensive – more than 30% involvement or a depression of more than 4 mm

Stage 4: progression to osteoarthritis

Radiographically the femoral articular surface is flattened and the joint space starts narrowing (*Figure 13.6*). This is associated with progressive changes on the acetabular side of the joint and with signs of osteoarthritis with areas of sclerosis, cysts and marginal osteophytes. Later, radiographic examinations show advanced degenerative changes and finally complete joint destruction is seen. Subclassification and quantitation are not needed any more.

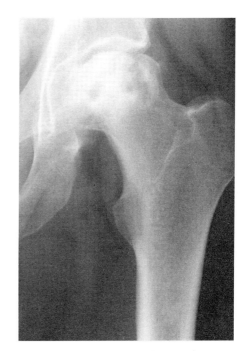

Figure 13.6   Stage 4 osteonecrosis: secondary osteoarthritis.

The Committee suggests strongly that the minimum requirements for reporting results on clinical and scientific work must include the following:

1. Staging according to this 'international classification', in which the classification is considered to be a minimum requirement.
2. A clinical quantitation by means of any hip score rating (e.g. the Harris hip score).
3. Radiographical and MRI quantitation to be reported separately from the clinical quantitation.
4. Therapeutic results on survival of the femoral head.

A more detailed or more specified subdivision of any stage and all other diagnostic techniques or examinations can be added freely but separately. Steinberg et al (1995) have divided stage 3 into stages III and IV, and stage 4 into stages V and VI. The ARCO Committee has tried to keep the system as compact as possible, with only four stages, while allowing for any subclassification needed (e.g. stage 3A = crescent sign without collapse and stage 3B is with collapse, but both represent the same mechanical failure of the femoral head).

The above-mentioned requirements are a **minimum** for meaningful comparison of all the different reports on osteonecrosis.

Biopsy should be performed at every possible opportunity. It remains a 'golden standard', although it is an invasive method; it can, however, be curative in the early stage of the disease. A descriptive histological classification of the disease is not yet available but is urgently needed.

TREATMENT OF OSTEONECROSIS

In this section the different methods of treatment are discussed. Some are of only historical importance, but they are reviewed because of the underlying principles, which appear to be rational. It is important to recognise that the indication for all surgical interventions has to be based on accurate assessment of the individual case, including the patient's age, the previously mentioned risk factors, the stage of the disease, the extent of articular damage, whether the condition is monolateral or bilateral, the results of laboratory tests and the histological findings of a possible biopsy.

The first operations that were thought to have positive results for osteonecrosis were denervation of the hip joint, coxolysis and cervicocephalic perforations. Denervation,

chiefly an anterior denervation (resection of the articular branches of the obturator nerve), was used in the past. The aim was pain relief, correction of any contracture caused by the adductor muscles, and production of active hyperaemia. The results, however, were poor. The later addition of posterior denervation of the quadratus femoris muscle produced no improvement. Total or subtotal capsulectomy was a further attempt to improve the denervation, but progression of the disease was not affected (Parrini and De Bastiani, 1982).

Coxolysis was devised by Voss in 1952 and subsequently modified by several authors. The operation produced a 'hanging hip' by sectioning muscles in order to diminish the intra-articular pressure. It included transverse section of the fascia lata and detachment of the greater trochanter and the abductor muscles. Tenotomy of the rectus femoris and iliopsoas muscles was sometimes added. The results were poor, because the assumption that the procedure would result in arrest of the necrotic process did not become true. There was no effect on vascular insufficiency and of weight-bearing on the necrotic area (Parrini and De Bastiani, 1982).

In the early stages of osteonecrosis – on the stages with no or very minor symptoms, featuring only a positive MRI or very subtle radiographic signs and an intact joint congruity – the prevention of a subchondral fracture and the subsequent start and stimulation of spontaneous repair of the infarct are the goals of the treatment.

The spectrum of different treatments starts with 'observation and non-weight-bearing'. In children with Perthes' disease the necrotic bone usually heals in this way, but in adults with post-traumatic osteonecrosis of the femoral head (ONF) this happens only occasionally, and in IONF rarely.

Cervicocephalic perforation through the femoral neck into the necrotic area (Beck's operation) is based on the assumption that this would induce hyperaemia and therefore produce revascularisation by ingrowth of blood vessels from the surrounding healthy bone. At the same time, increased intraosseous pressure and oedema in the marrow spaces is relieved by decompression. Arlet and Ficat (1968), and Hungerford (1979), propose core decompression and non-weight-bearing. Spontaneous revascularisation is assumed to take place through the cored tunnel. Intramedullary venous pressure is reduced by means of perforation of the medullary canal.

If raised intramedullary pressure is indeed the origin of the ischaemia, it is extremely important to make the diagnosis at the earliest possible moment. In the mid-1980s many authors reported the results of coring to be favourable. They operated on the unaffected hips in patients with symptomatic ONF on the contralateral side.

Today, MRI permits a more accurate diagnosis in the early pre-collapse hips and a more accurate assessment of this and other treatment techniques, which are designed to prevent progression of the disease (Steinberg et al, 1984, 1995; Bluemm et al, 1985; Mont and Hungerford, 1995).

Some authors have combined simple perforation with the introduction of cortical or cancellous bone grafts. The function of the grafts is to provide mechanical support and to promote local bone regeneration (Phemister, 1949).

The cortical graft is intended to fix the subchondral layer of bone and introduce osteogenic material into the necrotic area (Marcus et al, 1973; Springfield and Enneking, 1978) (*Figure 13.7*). The viability of the grafts and the osteogenic activity was improved by using tensor fascia lata muscle pedicled grafts of the iliac crest in hip fusion. Judet and Meyers proved that muscle pedicled grafts from the greater trochanter were superior to Phemister's cortical strut grafts for the treatment of

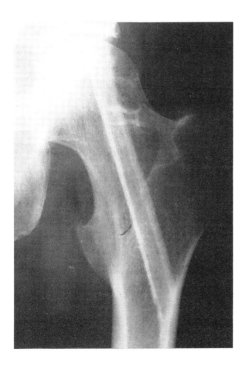

Figure 13.7   Cortical fibular graft supporting the antero-superior segment.

fractures and non-union of femoral neck fractures and the treatment of the silent phase of osteonecrosis. Judet and Chacha used free vascularised fibula grafts for the treatment of osteonecrosis, with good results. The procedure requires microvascular technique and is therefore time consuming; donor site morbidity can also be a problem. The authors recommend the operation only for stage 1 and 2 osteonecrosis in young patients, in whom the only alternative would be arthrodesis or total hip replacement.

Another alternative is the diversion of arterial and/or venous blood flow to the bone to try to revascularise the avascular segment. Many authors have described different methods with little success. In 1973 and 1978, Ganz and Buechle combined this technique with a flexion osteotomy in six patients.

Based on the assumption that the biological effects of osteotomy alone are rather slow, a cancellous bone graft can be added to accelerate the process.

The operations described above are suitable only in stage 1 and 2 IONF, where there is no subchondral fracture. Sugioka described an extracapsular intertrochanteric femoral osteotomy to rotate the infarct away from the weight-bearing zone. The operation prevents refracture of already repaired parts of the necrotic area, thus preventing reinfarction, and brings unaffected and healing bone under the acetabular roof in the weight-bearing area. Sugioka suggests his technique for patients with stages 1, 2 and 3 disease with a central or lateral location of the necrotic area.

When IONF reaches stage 3, the pain is a true sign of the occurrence of a subchondral fracture. In stage 4, the pain increases due to the onset of osteoarthritis. The femoral dome changes its shape and the joint is not congruent any more. In stages 3 and 4 of IONF, the above-mentioned operations are, in general, not possible any more. A cortical bone graft is considered to be inadequate as a method of immobilising the fracture and preventing further collapse. Except in some cases, Sugioka's osteotomy is still possible when a major part of the femoral head remains intact. The infarct is often more extended than is visible on radiographs, and rotational osteotomies must be planned on the basis of serial radiographs and MRI. The infarct must be completely rotated away from the weight-bearing zone, or further collapse will not be prevented (Sugioka, 1992) (*Figure 13.8*).

In experimental studies, starting back in the 1970s, it has been shown that osteogenesis and revascularisation

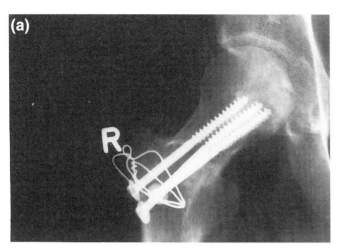
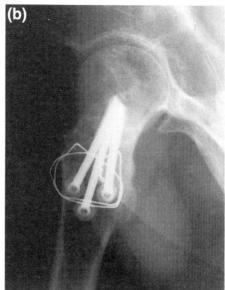

Figure 13.8   Sugioka's intertrochanteric osteotomy. The osteonecrotic segment is rotated from the weight-bearing to the non-weight-bearing part of the femoral head. (a) Anteroposterior view. (b) True lateral view.

are enhanced by electrostimulation. This technique has been used clinically in the treatment of pseudoarthrosis and delayed union of fractures.

Several authors have tried to treat osteonecrosis with electrostimulation with no effect at all, or at least doubtful effects. In 1983, Eftekhar and co-workers described the positive effects of pulsed electromagnetic fields on clinical and radiographic symptoms in the majority (approximately 70%) of treated patients. Steinberg et al (1984) used a combination of core biopsy and bone grafting with or without electrostimulation. They reported no clear difference between the two groups. At present, the use of electrostimulation in osteonecrosis is doubtful and needs further investigation.

Recently, the first results of a new therapy for osteonecrosis in stages 1 and 2 has been presented to the 43rd Annual Orthopaedic Research Society Meeting in San Francisco and the Fifth European Orthopaedic Research Meeting in Barcelona (Gardeniers et al, 1997). The technique of impacted grafting of the femoral head seemed to be successful in the first small group of patients and in an animal model. The anterosuperior segment is removed completely and all osteonecrotic bone is excised. The cavity is then filled with autograft and fresh frozen allograft bone chips from the bone bank. These chips are impacted solidly in the cavity. The first results

seem very promising (Gardeniers et al, 1997) (*Figure 13.9*).

Hemiarthroplasty or total arthroplasty is the operation of choice when the femoral head shows signs of collapse (*Figure 13.10*). Hemiarthroplasty has been suggested in the past, but long-term pain relief is not guaranteed. Hemiarthroplasty can damage the acetabular side of the joint after several years, causing the femoral prosthesis to protrude gradually into the pelvis.

For young patients a resurfacing arthroplasty is not always a satisfactory solution because of long life expectancy and an active lifestyle. Long-term problems such as low-grade infection and loosening of the prosthesis can be expected. Tharies' hip resurfacing, ICLH-prosthesis, double cup arthroplasty according to Wagner and other double cup arthroplasties have shown to be unreliable in IONF. In IONF, the mechanical support provided by the cancellous bone of the femoral head is not adequate. Loosening of the femoral component is the main long-term problem.

In stage 4 IONF, the joint is deformed. The only operation suitable for such a degenerated hip joint is total joint replacement. The opposition of the patient to arthrodesis of the hip joint is well known and easy to understand. Arthrodesis of the hip joint has a higher failure rate in IONF and, even after extensive excision of

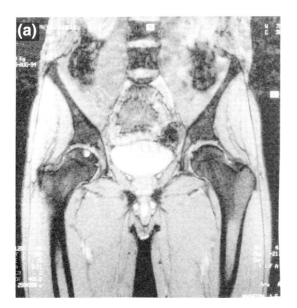
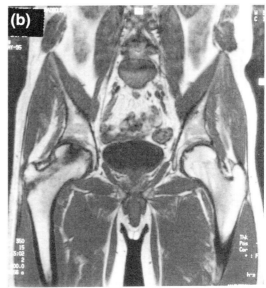

Figure 13.9 (a) Preoperative and (b) postoperative MRI of a patient with stage 2 osteonecrosis treated with impacted grafting.

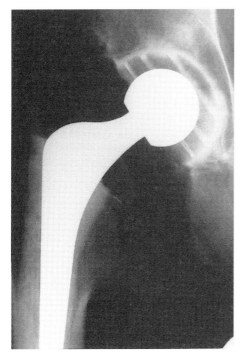

Figure 13.10 Total hip arthroplasty (cemented Exeter hip arthroplasty).

the necrosis and bone grafting, a higher failure of consolidation is seen.

Finally, there is the occasional patient in whom the resection angulation osteotomy (Girdlestone–Milch osteotomy) offers a rational treatment, but only if total joint replacement is undesirable or where the infarct penetrates deeply into the proximal femur (seldom in IONF, but more frequent in ONF due to sickle cell disease). Non-cemented hemiarthroplasties with a double articulating femoral component (e.g. Osteonics universal head prosthesis) might offer an alternative in younger patients, but non-cemented prostheses have not yet proven to be a better alternative for the cemented prosthesis.

CONCLUSIONS

IONF has become an increasingly significant disease in the twentieth century, evident in the deep-diving industry, high-altitude operations, alcohol consumption, and corticosteroid treatment of recipients of organ transplants. There was, and is, a real increase in the incidence of IONF and a higher number of bilateral cases. The male prevalence of IONF is invariably reported, and the average age has decreased in the past 20 years.

The precise aetiology of IONF is still unknown. It is a problem of inadequate blood supply to the bone relative to metabolic need. Many factors play a role in the aetiology, such as treatment with corticosteroids, alcoholism and, in particular, factors related to disease of the liver and blood. They work in a complex way to produce IONF. However, the femoral head is so often involved that local anatomical and mechanical factors must play an important role.

The anatomical factor is the precarious blood supply of the anterosuperior segment of the femoral head. This is the area in the femoral head that is most affected in IONF and is completely dependent on the lateral epiphyseal endarterioles. Vascular damage or occlusion does cause interruption of the blood flow to the anterosuperior segment, but it has been suggested by several authors that extravascular intraosseous elements can also cause ischaemia by increasing the pressure in the intertrabecular spaces. Because bone acts as a closed compartment, this rise in intraosseous pressure produces a decrease in medullary blood flow.

Mechanical stresses on the femoral head are the factors that finally lead to the collapse and fragmentation of the anterosuperior segment. Weakening of the bone starts with a small fatigue fracture in the subchondral plate which is not followed by adequate repair. The effects of ischaemia can be seen both in the marrow tissues and in the bone cells, but the marrow tissues are affected first. Peculiar to bone is the fact that the bony framework itself is not affected by the ischaemia. Changes can be seen only once the process of repair has started and the osteogenic cells arrive. Primarily, the avital trabeculae act as a frame-work for new bone apposition and therefore play a major role in the osteogenesis. But, for reasons presently unknown, this osteoapposition rarely extends more than 4–5 mm into the necrotic area, when the osteoblasts disappear and are replaced by fibroblasts, forming exten-sive areas of medullary fibrosis. Osteoresorption by osteoclasts starts. This resorption often penetrates deeper into the necrotic area than the osteogenetic front. The predominance of resorption over osteogenesis under-mines the mechanical strength of the necrotic bone. Fracture of the necrotic bone, and finally collapse and fragmentation, are the result of normal weight-bearing and motion.

It can be concluded that the treatment of avascular necrosis must be based on two principles: revascularisa-tion (and revitalisation) of the necrotic bone, and pre-vention of the collapse. These requirements are analogous to those for reconstruction of an old building: the supporting structure must be renewed, but at the same time the building must be upheld. Evidently, in bone, this procedure can be conducted successfully only when

enough is known about the effects of the revascularisation process, on both the remodelling process and the bone strength. It is also evident that these processes are not well documented in the literature. In particular, little is known about the velocity of the remodelling process and the relationship between remodelling and bone strength.

REFERENCES

ARCO (Association de Recherche sur la Circulation Osseuse. Committee on Terminology and Classification. *ARCO News* 1992; **4**: 41–46.

Arlet J, Ficat P. Diagnostic de l'ostéo-nécrose fémoro-capitale primitive au stade I. *Rev Chir Orthop* 1968; **54**(7): 637–648.

Atsumi T, Kuroki Y. Role of impairment of blood supply of the femoral head in the pathogenesis of idiopathic osteonecrosis. *Clin Orthop* 1992; **277**: 22–30.

Atsumi T, Kuroki Y, Saito S, Ohgiya H, Sugimori H, Yoshida M. On the revascularization in both idiopathic and traumatic necrosis of the femoral head. In: *The Hip. Clinical Studies and Basic Research*. Paris: Elsevier, 1984: 177–180.

Bluemm RG, Falke THM, Ziedses des Plantes BG Jr, Steiner RM. Early Legg–Perthes disease (ischemic necrosis of the femoral head) demonstrated by magnetic resonance imaging. *Skeletal Radiol* 1985; **14**: 95–98.

Bucholz RW, Ogden JA. Patterns of ischemic necrosis of the proximal femur in non-operatively treated congenital hip dis-ease. In: *The Hip (Proceedings of the Sixth Meeting of the Hip Society, 1978)*. St Louis: CV Mosby, 1978: 43–63.

Catto M. A histological study of avascular necrosis of the femoral head after transcervical fracture. *J Bone Joint Surg [Br]* 1965a; **47B**: 749–776.

Catto M. The histological appearances of late segmental collapse of the femoral head after transcervical fracture. *J Bone Joint Surg [Br]* 1965b; **47B**: 777–791.

Chambers TJ. The cellular basis of bone resorption. *Clin Orthop* 1980; **151**: 283–293.

Crock HV. An atlas of the supply of the head and neck of the femur in man. *Clin Orthop* 1980; **152**: 17–27.

D'Ambrosia RD, Shoji H, Riggins RS, Stadalnik RC, DeNardo GL. Scintigraphy in the diagnosis of osteonecrosis. *Clin Orthop* 1978; **130**: 139–142.

Eftekhar NS, Schink-Ascani MM, Mitchell SN, Bassett CAL. Osteonecrosis of the femoral head treated by pulsed electro-magnetic fields (PEMFs): a preliminary report. In: *The Hip (Proceedings of the 11th Meeting of the Hip Society, 1983)*. St Louis: CV Mosby, 1983; 306–330.

Enneking WF. The choice of surgical procedures in idiopathic aseptic necrosis. In: *The Hip (Proceedings of the Seventh Meeting of the Hip Society, 1979)*. St Louis: CV Mosby, 1979; 238–243.

Enneking WF (ed.) *Clinical Musculoskeletal Pathology*. Gainesville, Florida: 1986.

Favenesi JA, et al. *Mechanical Properties of Normal and Avascular Bone.*

Biomat adn Biomech van der Perre G, Aubert AE (eds). Amsterdam: Elsevier Science, 1984a; 121–126.

Favenesi JA, et al. Mechanical properties of normal and avascular cancellous bone. *Transactions of the 30th Annual Meeting of ORS* 1984b; **9**: 198.

Ficat RP. Early diagnosis of osteonecrosis by functional bone investigation. *Prog Orthop Surg* 1981; **5**: 17–28.

Ficat RP. Idiopathic osteonecrosis of the femoral head: forage-biopsy. *Ital J Orthop Traumatol* (Suppl) 1982; **VIII**: 123–130.

Ficat RP. Treatment of avascular necrosis of the femoral head. In *The Hip (Proceedings of the Eleventh Meeting of the Hip Society, 1983)*. St Louis: CV Mosby, 1983; 279–305.

Gardeniers JWM. Behaviour of normal, avascular and revascularizing cancellous bone. Thesis, Catholic University of Nijmegen, The Netherlands, 1988.

Gardeniers JWM, et al. Behaviour of normal, avascular and revascularizing cancellous bone in the femoral head. *Transactions of the 35th Annual Meeting of the ORS* 1989; **14**: 73.

Gardeniers JWM. The ARCO perspective for reaching one uniform staging system of osteonecrosis. In: Schoutens A, et al (eds) *Bone Circulation and Vascularization in Normal and Pathological Conditions*. 375–380. New York: Plenum Press, 1993.

Gardeniers J, Yamano K, Buma P, Slooff T. Impaction grafting for osteonecrosis in the femoral head. *Transactions of the 43rd Annual Meeting of the ORS*, Vol. 22, section 1. San Fransisco, 1997: 134.

Gardeniers JWM. Impaction grafting for osteonecrosis in the femoral head. *Transactions of the 7th Annual Meeting of the EORS, Barcelona.* 1997; **7**: 82.

Glimcher MJ, Kenzora JE. The biology of osteonecrosis of the human femoral head and its clinical implications: III. Discussion of the etiology and genesis of the pathological sequelae; comments and treatment. *Clin Orthop* 1979; **140**: 272–312.

Hungerford DS. Bone marrow pressure, venography, and core decompression in ischemic necrosis of the femoral head. In: *The Hip (Proceedings of the Seventh Meeting of the Hip Society, 1979)*. St Louis: CV Mosby, 1979; 218–237.

Jones JP. Editorial comment. Osteonecrosis. *Clin Orthop* 1978; **130**: 2–4.

Jones JP. Fat embolism and osteonecrosis. *Clin Orthop* 1985; **16**: 595–634.

Kenzora JE, Glimcher MJ. Pathogenesis of idiopathic osteonecrosis: the ubiquitous crescent sign. *Orthop Clin North Am* 1985; **16**(4): 681–696.

Kerboul M, Thomine J, Postel M, et al. The conservative surgical treatment of idiopathic aseptic necrosis of the femoral head. *J Bone Joint Surg* 1974; **56**(2): 299–296.

Marcus ND, Enneking WF, Massam RA. The silent hip in idiopathic aseptic necrosis. *J Bone Joint Surg [Am]* 1973; **55A**: 1351–1366.

Merle d'Aubigné R, et al. Idiopathic necrosis of the femoral head in adults. *J Bone Joint Surg [Am]* 1965; **47B**: 612–633.

Meyers MH. The treatment of osteonecrosis of the hip with fresh osteochondral allografts and with the muscle pedicle graft technique. *Clin Orthop* 1978; **130**: 202–209.

Meyers MH. Avascular necrosis of the femoral head – diagnostic techniques, reliability and relevance. In: *The Hip (Proceedings of the 11th Meeting of the Hip Society, 1983)*. St Louis: CV Mosby, 1983; 263–278.

Mont MA, Hungerford DS. Non traumatic avascular necrosis of the femoral head. *J Bone Joint Surg [Am]* 1995; **77A**(3): 459–474.

Monticelli G, et al. Idiopathic osteonecrosis of the femoral head. Proceedings of the LXVII Congress of the Italian Society of Orthopaedics and Traumatology, Turin, 20–23 October 1982. *Ital J Orthop Traumatol* 1982; **VIII**(Suppl): 9–66.

Ohzono KM, et al. Natural history of non-traumatic avascular necrosis of the femoral head. *J Bone Joint Surg [Am]* 1995; **77B**: 68–72.

Ono K. *Annual Report of the Investigation Committee for Adult Idiopathic Avascular Necrosis of the Femoral Head.* Tokyo: Ministry of Health and Welfare, 1989.

Phemister DB. Treatment of the necrotic head of the femur in adults. *J Bone Joint Surg [Am]* 1949; **31A**: 55–66.

Schoutens A, Arlet J, Gardeniers JWM, Hughes SPF. *Bone Circulation and Vascularization in Normal and Pathological Conditions.* New York: Plenum Press, 1993.

Springfield DS, Enneking WF. Role of bone grafting in idiopathic aseptic necrosis of the femoral head. In: *The Hip (Proceedings of the Third Meeting of the Hip Society, 1975)*. St Louis: CV Mosby, 1975: 3–18.

Springfield DS, Enneking WJ. Surgery for aseptic necrosis of the femoral head. *Clin Orthop* 1978; **130**: 175–185.

Steinberg ME, Brighton CT, Hayken GD, Tooze SE, Steinberg DR. Early results in the treatment of avascular necrosis of the femoral head with electrical stimulation. *Orthop Clin North Am* 1984; **15**: 163–175.

Steinberg ME, Hayken GD, Steinberg DR. A quantitative system for staging avascular necrosis. *J Bone Joint Surg [Br]* 1995; **77B**(1): 34–41.

Stulberg BN, Davis AW, Bauer TW, Levine M, Easley K. Osteonecrosis of the femoral head. A prospective randomized treatment protocol. *Clin Orthop* 1991; **268**: 140–151.

Stulberg BN, Gardeniers JWM. Methodologic problems in staging and evaluating osteonecrosis. In: Schoutens A, et al (eds) *Bone Circulation and Vascularization in Normal and Pathological Conditions.* New York: Plenum Press, 1993: 373–374.

Sugioka Y, Hotokebuchi T, Tsutsui H. Transtrochanteric anterior rotational osteotomy for idiopathic and steroid-induced necrosis of the femoral head. Indications and long-term results. *Clin Orthop* 1992; **277**: 111–120.

Trueta J. The role of vessels in osteogenesis. *J Bone Joint Surg [Br]* 1963; **45B**: 402–418.

Trueta J, Harrison MHM. The normal vascular anatomy of the femoral head in adult man. *J Bone Joint Surg [Br]* 1953; **35B**(3): 442–461.

Section III

Biomechanics

14

Basic Biomechanics

Edward RC Draper

INTRODUCTION

A good orthopaedic surgeon will have a 'good feel' for many of the biomechanical problems that face him or her. The role of biomechanics is not to replace these important attributes but to supplement them, both by allowing more detailed investigations and by being less subjective.

Biomechanics can be considered to be the application of engineering mechanics to the body, in that it helps in the measurement and analysis of the forces and movements of the body. However, it is probably better to consider the study of biomechanics as the interplay between the biological systems and the mechanical environment, in which case the practitioner of biomechanics must consider far more than just the mechanics of the body. This chapter will not attempt to delve into the details of this interplay; instead it will concentrate on the techniques borrowed from the more traditional engineering field.

Engineering mechanics is the physical science concerned with how forces can affect physical bodies. It is the oldest of all the physical sciences: the Ancient Egyptians have left obvious signs of many of its principles in their building of the pyramids prior to 2000 BC. The fundamentals of the subject, as we know it today, were properly established about three centuries ago by Sir Isaac Newton (1642–1727) in his laws of mechanics and of motion.

BASIC QUANTITIES: MASS, LENGTH AND TIME

Fundamental to any science is the concept of quantification, either through measurement or through calculation.

For any measurement of any parameter to be understood without confusion it will need to be quoted in specific units that are relevant to that parameter and understood by the reader.

The Imperial or English system, which includes units such as inches and ounces, and is still in use in many parts of the world, was derived from measuring systems used by the Babylonians to the Norman French. It is a complicated system in that several different units are often used to describe the same parameter over a large range of sizes; length goes from the inch, to the foot, to the yard, to the mile. It is further complicated by the fact that each of these units is related to the next by a factor that is rarely ten. This requires not only knowledge each of the units but also the factors by which they relate to the other units describing the same parameter. There are 12 inches to the foot, 3 feet to the yard and 1760 yards to the mile.

In 1960 a revised version of the metric system was adopted. This modern metric system was named Le Système International d'Unités and is abbreviated to the SI units. At the heart of this system are four base units: length in metres, mass in kilograms, time in seconds and temperature in kelvin. There is also a supplementary unit for plane angles, the radian. From these units all other mechanical engineering units can be derived, which means that most SI units are derived units.

The SI system is further simplified by being based on the decimal system, and each base unit being defined in a way that is independently reproducible.

Most of the derived SI units are expressed in terms of how they are derived. For instance, the SI units for volume is the cubic metre (m^3), and for density it is kilograms per cubic metre ($kg\,m^{-3}$). There are, however, some derived units that have been given special names after famous scientists and mathematicians (*Table 14.1*).

Table 14.1   Common SI units used in biomechanics.

Quantity	SI unit	
Mass	kg	
Length	m	
Time	s	
Area	m^2	
Volume	m^3	
Velocity	$m\,s^{-1}$	
Acceleration	$m\,s^{-2}$	
Force	newton (N)	$(kg\,m\,s^{-2})$
Work, energy	joule (J)	(N m)
Power	watt (W)	$(N\,m\,s^{-1})$
Pressure	pascal	$(N\,m^{-2})$
Torque	N m	
Stress	$N\,m^{-2}$	

In biomechanics there are five of these special units: the newton (N), which is the unit of force (equivalent to $kg\,m\,s^{-2}$); the pascal (P), which is the unit of pressure and stress (equivalent to $N\,m^{-2}$); the joule (J), which is the unit of energy and work (equivalent to N m); the watt (W), which is the unit of power (equivalent to $J\,s^{-1}$); and the degree Celsius (°C), a unit of temperature (equivalent to $K - 273.15$).

To accommodate the vast range of sizes that can be covered, a system of prefixes has been incorporated into the SI system (*Table 14.2*). Each prefix has a precise meaning and can be applied to any of the SI units. It then indicates that the parameter is being quoted in some multiple of a thousand times that unit. For instance, the millisecond (ms) is used to represent one thousandth of a second, and the meganewton (MN) is one million newtons.

Table 14.2   Prefixes used with SI units.

Prefix	Symbol	Exponent or power of ten
tera	T	10^{12}
giga	G	10^{9}
mega	M	10^{6}
kilo	k	10^{3}
milli	m	10^{-3}
micro	μ	10^{-6}
nano	n	10^{-9}
pico	p	10^{-12}
femto	f	10^{-15}

In summary: (1) SI units should be used at all times; (2) they are based on mass, length, time and temperature; (3) all other units can be derived from these; and (4) prefixes are used to indicate a multiple of a thousand times the unit.

SCALAR AND VECTOR QUANTITIES

When considering some parameters (e.g. force) it is important to know the direction in which the measurement was taken, whereas others (e.g. volume) should remain the same whichever direction the measurement is taken.

Whether or not a parameter has this dependence on direction is of fundamental importance. Consequently parameters are divided into two groups: those that do and those that do not exhibit this dependence. Those in which direction is either not appropriate or is meaningless are referred to as scalar quantities, whereas those that require both the magnitude and direction to be quoted before the quantity can be fully understood are known as vector quantities.

To understand the importance of direction to vector quantities it is best to consider some examples. Imagine there is someone trying to get through a door. What they do not know is that the door slides and moves to one side. If that person were to pull or push then they would not open it, not because the force was too small but because it was being applied in the wrong direction. Force is a vector. Applying the same level of force but in the correct direction will cause the door to open.

Imagine being in a car that is travelling due west, then no matter how long the car is driven its latitude would never change; it would never go further north or further south no matter how fast or for how long the car is driven. However, if you drive the same car at the same speed but in a different direction say north-west, then you would travel as many miles north as you drive west.

Speed, therefore, is a scalar quantity, but there is another vector quantity that is similar to speed but which takes direction into account. It is given the name velocity. Both are measured in metres per second, but velocity needs to have its direction stated.

The difference between these two types of quantity becomes even more important when we consider how they add or subtract.

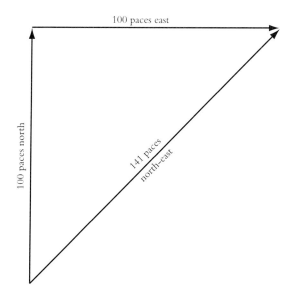

Figure 14.1 Resultant distance after walking north and then east.

If one cubic metre is added to another, we will have two cubic metres of water. However, *Figure 14.1* illustrates that if we take 100 paces north then 100 paces east we will not be 200 paces from our starting position. The total distance walked will be 200 paces but we will be just over 141 paces away from the start and to the north-east. Combining the effect of two or more vectors, and breaking down a vector into its components, will be described in detail in the next section.

In summary: (1) there are two groups of parameters, scalar and vector; (2) scalar quantities require no description of direction; (3) vectors do; (4) scalar quantities can be added using simple mathematics; (5) the additive effect of two vectors is not necessarily the same as the sum of two magnitudes.

VECTORS: ADDITION AND RESOLUTION

One only has to watch a professional sportsperson throw a ball to see that the segments of an individual limb, although joined, can be travelling in quite different directions and at quite different speeds. If one considers the individual forces acting upon the structures of the

body it will be rare, if ever, that only one force will act upon it at any one time. Consequently, it is fundamental to the study of biomechanics to be able to add vectors together and to break them down, or resolve them, into their components.

Figure 14.1 illustrated a simple addition of vectors, but it is rare that one vector will begin at the point at which the other finishes. Often vectors act at roughly the same point simultaneously, making it more difficult to see how to examine their combined effect.

To illustrate this, consider the typical forces on the patella at a flexion angle of 120°, limiting the analysis to the plane in which the leg lies, the sagittal plane, and ignoring friction. It should be pointed out that in this analysis it is assumed that the forces are in equilibrium and therefore there is no movement. The angles of the tendons are taken from a tracing of a lateral radiograph of the knee (Williams and Lissner, 1962). *Figure 14.2* shows the three forces acting on the patella: the overall force due to the action of the quadriceps, *M*; the force within the patellar tendon, (because there is no friction this is also *M*); and the compressive force that acts between the patella and the femur, *P*.

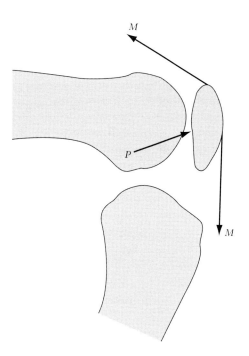

Figure 14.2 Forces on the patella with the knee flexed at 120°.

(a)

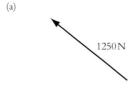

1250 N

(b)

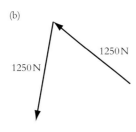

1250 N

1250 N

(c)

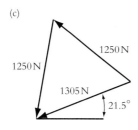

1250 N

1250 N

1305 N

21.5°

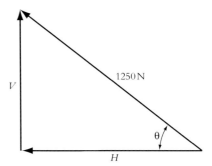

V

1250 N

θ

H

Figure 14.4   Horizontal and vertical components of the quadriceps force on the patella.

Figure 14.3   Graphic vector addition of forces on the patella: (a) the quadriceps force on the patella; (b) the forces of the quadriceps and the patella tendon; (c) the resultant forces of the quadriceps and the patella tendon.

If the muscle force, *M*, is taken to be 1250 N, the force *P* can be calculated. We begin by drawing an arrow (see *Figure 14.3a*) in the same direction as the action of the quadriceps and whose length is equal or proportional to the magnitude of this force. Then, at the end of this arrow, we draw a second arrow (see *Figure 14.3b*), which represents the force applied by patellar tendon. Finally, in *Figure 14.3c* the combined force, *F*, is drawn from the starting point of the first arrow to the end of the second arrow. The patella is not moving; consequently this force, *F*, is resisted by the equal and opposite compressive force, *P*, shown in *Figure 14.3c*. *P* can be measured from this arrow. It has a magnitude of 1305 N and lies at an angle of 21.5° to the horizontal.

This example shows how two vectors can be added to produce a resultant vector. This technique can be used to define the effect of any number of vectors. In general, therefore, if a series of vector parameters acts together,

they can be combined and considered as one resulting vector.

As two vectors can be combined to form one resultant, it should be possible to break one vector down into its components. In the previous example, an analysis of the forces on the patella in sagittal plane, each of the forces could have been broken down into two components, the horizontal and vertical components. If it had been a full three-dimensional analysis, the third, lateral, component could also have been calculated.

If we consider the action of the quadriceps alone, *M*, it can be broken down into its horizontal, *H*, and vertical, *V*, components; this is shown in *Figure 14.4*. Because *H* and *V* lie at right angles, it is also possible to calculate them arithmetically:

$$H = M \cos(\theta) \qquad (1)$$

$$V = M \sin(\theta) \qquad (2)$$

where θ is the angle from the horizontal that the force *M* acts.

By breaking down the forces in this way into their horizontal and vertical components, we can calculate the force between the femur and patella using equations. *Figure 14.5* shows both the magnitude and the angles of the forces. The quadriceps force of 1250 N acts at 37° above the horizontal and towards the left; the patella tendon also exerts a force of 1250 N but at an angle of 80° below the horizontal and towards the left; the patello-femoral force is unknown, and so is given the symbol F, and lies at an angle of ϕ° below the horizontal and towards the right.

Considering all the horizontal components of these forces, they must cancel each other out. This is known as

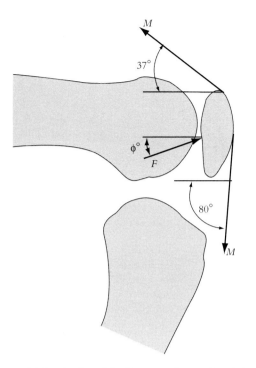

Figure 14.5   Angles of the forces on the patella relative to the horizontal.

resolving the forces horizontally. We can write the equation:

$$F \cos\phi = 1250 \cos37° + 1250 \cos80° \qquad (3)$$

In other words, the horizontal components of force to the right must equal the horizontal components of force to the left. The only horizontal component to the right is that of the patellofemoral force, $F\cos\phi$. This is matched by the components of force to the left, that of the quadriceps force, $1250\cos37°$, and the patellar tendon $1250\cos80°$. From this we can calculate that:

$$F \cos\phi = 1215 \text{ N} \qquad (4)$$

Now resolving vertically:

$$F \sin\phi + 1250 \sin37° = 1250 \sin80° \qquad (5)$$

That is to say, the upwards components of force, that of the quadriceps and the patellofemoral forces, must balance the downward force, that of the patellar tendon.

We can calculate from equation 5 that:

$$F \sin\phi = 479 \text{ N} \qquad (6)$$

Dividing equation 4 by equation 6 we get:

$$\frac{F \sin\phi}{F \cos\phi} = \frac{479}{1215} \qquad (7)$$

From this, the tangent of the angle may be calculated:

$$\tan\phi = 0.394 \qquad (8)$$

Therefore:

$$\phi = 21.5° \qquad (9)$$

Substituting this into equation 6:

$$F \sin21.5° = 479 \qquad (10)$$

From which, we find the magnitude of F:

$$F = \frac{479}{\sin 21.5°} = \frac{479}{0.367} = 1305 \text{ N} \qquad (11)$$

By resolving these forces into their horizontal and vertical components it has been possible to perform the same analysis as in the previous graphical technique. Of the two, this second technique is more suited for more general and computer analysis, and is consequently more widely adopted, except for the simplest of cases.

In summary: (1) the effect of two or more vectors can be added together to produce one resultant vector; (2) the resultant vector can be discovered graphically; (3) any vector can be broken down into its components; (4) in two-dimensional analysis a vector is broken down into two components, and in three dimensions it is resolved into three components; (5) by breaking vectors down into their components, their effects can be analysed arithmetically.

LINEAR AND ANGULAR LOADS: FORCES AND MOMENTS

A force is a load that acts in a particular direction; its action is linear. Like velocity and acceleration, it has a counterpart, which is angular, called a moment. *Figure 14.6* illustrates a moment being applied to a bolt: a force is applied at a distance from the nut; the spanner acts to transmit it. The applied moment could be increased by increasing the force, or by applying the same force to a longer spanner, that is using a longer lever arm.

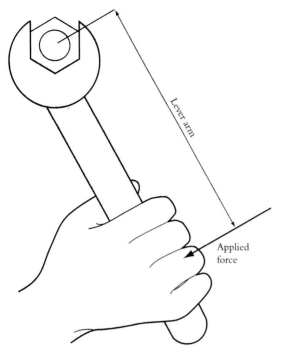

Figure 14.6   Moment applied to a bolt.

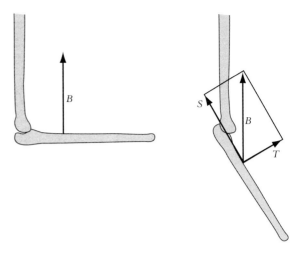

Figure 14.7   Two components of the force applied by the biceps.

In fact, the magnitude of the moment is the applied force, *F*, multiplied by the length of the spanner, *l*

$$M = F \times l \qquad (12)$$

where M is the magnitude of the moment. The unit for a moment is therefore the newton metre.

The concept of the moment is fundamental to biomechanics because, with a few exceptions, the joints of the body rotate. Muscles apply linear forces at a distance from the joint. Consequently, the joint moments are dependent both on the tension within the muscle and on the lever arm at which it acts.

This is important because the lever arm of a muscle will invariably alter as the joint flexes and extends. For instance, consider the action of the biceps brachii on the elbow at flexion angles 30° and 90°, as shown in *Figure 14.7*. It can be seen that the distance from the joint to the arrow representing the force B is greater at 90° than at 30°. This means that the lever arm is greater. Consequently, for the biceps to apply the same moment they have to be under greater tension at 30° than at 90° of flexion.

Rather than trying to define the distance to a vector, Williams and Lissner (1962) considered the force applied

by the biceps in two components: *S*, the component that acts in the direction of the ulna and radius and tends to stabilise the elbow by compressing it; and *T*, the component that acts at 90° to the ulna and radius and causes the elbow to flex.

As the elbow flexes so the component *S* decreases and the component *T* increases. From *Figure 14.7* it can be seen that *S* and *T* can be calculated:

$$S = M \cos\theta \qquad (13)$$

$$T = M \sin\theta \qquad (14)$$

where *M* is the force applied by biceps and *θ* is the angle of elbow flexion.

Component *S* acts straight towards the elbow and therefore contributes nothing to the flexion moment, whereas *T* acts a set distance, *L*, from the elbow and therefore applies an elbow moment equal to *T* × *L*:

$$\tau_{elbow} = TL = ML \cos\theta \qquad (15)$$

where τ_{elbow} is the elbow moment due to the biceps.

From *Figure 14.7*, and equations 13 and 14, it can be seen that the stabilising component, *S*, begins high and falls slowly to nothing at 90° (cos90° = 0). However, the rotating component, *T*, starts low and builds to a maximum at 90° (sin90° = 0). This means, from equation 15, that the biceps have to work harder at the ends of movement to apply the same moment than at 90°

Moments, like forces, are vector quantities: they act about an axis and have direction, that is they act within a plane. They can be represented with arrows, using the same technique as for angular velocity, that is the arrow points along the axis about which the moment acts. Consequently, in the example given of the flexion moment applied to the elbow by the biceps brachii, the moment can be represented by an arrow at $90°$ to the plane of the elbow. In this way the effect of moments acting in different planes can be calculated, although this is beyond the scope of this chapter.

In summary: (1) a force is a linear load and a moment is its angular equivalent; (2) the magnitude of a vector is dependent on the force multiplied by the lever arm; (3) the muscles of the body apply forces that act at a distance from the joints they flex, and consequently apply a moment; (4) the moment arms of the musculature vary throughout the movement of the joint; (5) a moment is a vector.

STATICS

In *Figure 14.2*, we were able to calculate the patellofemoral contact forces resulting from the action of the quadriceps. We did this because we knew that all the forces were perfectly balanced. This required that the overall resultant force on the patella was zero. That, in turn, meant that the patella was not moving; it was stationary.

The branch of engineering mechanics that deals with this state of equilibrium is known as 'statics'. The importance of this state of equilibrium is that all forces and moments must cancel each other out; there must be no overall resultants. There have been many techniques developed in the area of statics based on this aspect of equilibrium.

As an example, consider the calculation of the force at the elbow resulting from a weight carried in the hand. The object applies a force of F_o due to its weight, the forearm also applies a force due to its weight, F_{FA}, both of which are opposed by the biceps brachii.

If we use the simplified model given in *Figure 14.8*, in which there are only four forces – the force at the elbow, the force due to the biceps, the weight of the forearm and the weight of the object in the hand – then we can calculate the elbow force quite easily.

Because the elbow is in equilibrium there can be no

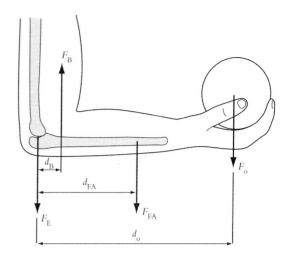

Figure 14.8 Forces on the elbow when carrying an object in the hand.

resultant force or moment. There are no horizontal forces, so let us consider the vertical forces.

Taking moments about the elbow:

$$F_B.d_B = F_{FA}.d_{FA} + F_o.d_o \qquad (16)$$

where F_B is the biceps force, d_B is the moment arm of the biceps, F_{FA} is the force due to the mass of the forearm, d_{FA} is the moment arm of the F_{FA}, F_o is the force due to the weight of the object, and d_o is the moment arm of F_o.

If we take typical values (d_B of 50 mm, F_{FA} of 20 N, d_{FA} of 130 mm, F_o of 10 N, d_o of 300 mm), then we can calculate F_B:

$$F_B = \frac{20\,\text{N} \times 130\,\text{mm} + 10\,\text{N} \times 300\,\text{mm}}{50\,\text{mm}} = 112\,\text{N}$$

$$(17)$$

If we now consider the linear forces in the vertical direction, that is if we resolve vertically:

$$F_E + F_{FA} + F_o = F_B \qquad (18)$$

From this we can calculate the elbow force:

$$F_E = F_B - F_{FA} - F_o = 112\,\text{N} - 20\,\text{N} - 10\,\text{N} = 82\,\text{N}$$

$$(19)$$

According to this model the force required by the biceps is about 11 times greater than that at the hand, and the force at the elbow is about eight times greater.

In fact, this model ignores many important forces, such as the wrist and finger flexors, which will be active; these groups originate above the elbow and consequently will increase the elbow forces.

However, this example does illustrate several points: (a) because the model is in equilibrium, we can write a series of equations that helps us to calculate the forces inside the body; (b) muscles, in general, work at a mechanical disadvantage and have to apply greater forces than those applied externally; this results in even greater forces at the joints upon which they act.

Using a static analysis of a joint to investigate the internal forces is further complicated by antagonistic activity. If, in the above model, the triceps brachii are considered, then there are too many unknown quantities and these equations cannot be solved. The model is then said to be 'statically indeterminate'. Because of the large number of muscles within the body, most joints of the body are statically indeterminate most of the time. There are methods to allow analysis in these situations but they are beyond the scope of this chapter.

In summary: (1) for a system to be in equilibrium the resultant forces and moments must be zero; (2) equations can be written considering the forces and the moments in the different directions; these help to calculate the unknown loads; (3) muscular and joint forces tend to be far greater than external loads; (4) the large number of muscles that act on each joint makes it difficult to analyse the internal loads.

LINEAR AND ANGULAR MOTION

To describe how an object has moved in three-dimensional space, it is necessary to include six components for a full description, because not only are there three linear components of motion (up and down, left and right, and forward and back; see *Figure 14.9*), there are also three angular movements (in nautical and aeronautical terms these are roll, pitch and yaw; see *Figure 14.9b*).

If we want to describe the position of an object in space relative to a fixed point, we can say how far forward, up and to the left it is. This is usually represented by distances parallel to an *x*, *y* and *z* axis (the direction in which these lie will be defined by the researcher). If it were then to move without rotating, the displacement could be described in terms of its *x*, *y* and *z* components (i.e. linear displacement is a vector).

If we want to describe how an object is rotated relative to a fixed axis, we can describe the angle of roll, pitch and

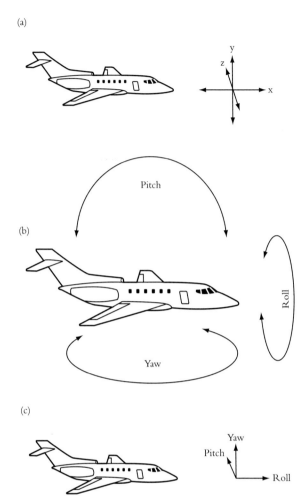

Figure 14.9 Six components of motion: (a) three components of linear motion; (b) three angular components of motion; (c) representation of angular velocities by arrows.

yaw. However, this requires an understanding of what these angles are. Imagine that the aeroplane shown in *Figure 14.9* has a line passing through it from front to back, and is free to rotate about this line. This line is its axis of rotation. The movement allowed around this axis is roll, and it is possible to measure its angle. If we then imagine the same for a line passing from left to right, we get pitch; with a line running up and down we get yaw.

These angles can be related to the *x*, *y* and *z* axes by measuring the angles about each of these axes. Angles measured in this way are conventionally given the symbols: θ_x, θ_y and θ_z, where the subscripts indicate about which axis the movement occurs.

Velocity and acceleration

During normal walking the human foot spends part of its time on the ground and is stationary. It is then brought forward, first speeding up and then slowing down, before being placed back on the floor. In addition, the foot needs to be raised and lowered, and moved out to the side and back in. Consequently, from instant to instant the direction in which it travels is quite complex, but, if we know all three components of velocity, the resultant velocity can be calculated.

This is fairly clear when considering linear velocity; what is more obscure is how to describe complex angular motions. Angular velocity, the rate of change of angle, is also a vector (Shames, 1970), but it is at first difficult to see how it can be drawn as an arrow and represented as a vector. The convention is to draw an arrow along the axis about which it is spinning, with its length representing the magnitude of the angular velocity. Roll would therefore be represented by an arrow pointing forward, pitch as a side-facing arrow and yaw as an arrow pointing up; this is illustrated in *Figure 14.9c*. In this way any angular velocity of an object can be broken down into its three components.

Acceleration of an object is the rate of change of its velocity. An object can experience both linear and angular accelerations, and both of these are vectors. It is quite clear, if an object was travelling at $6\,\mathrm{m}^{-1}$ and is now travelling at $8\,\mathrm{m\,s}^{-1}$, that it has accelerated. However, it is possible for an object to remain at the same speed but to change directions, such as a ball being swung around on the end of a string; in this instance, the object is also accelerating.

This is explained in *Figure 14.10a*, in which a ball on the end of a string is travelling at the same speed, S. After a short time, t, it has turned through an angle, θ; it can be seen in *Figure 14.10b* that there has been a change in velocity, V. Consequently, the ball has been accelerating at a rate of V/t towards the centre of the circle.

In summary: (1) the position of an object can be represented by x, y and z, and θ_x, θ_y and θ_z; (2) linear and angular velocities and accelerations are vectors; (3) angular velocity can be represented by an arrow; (4) velocities and accelerations can be broken down into their components; (5) an object that is travelling at the same speed but changing direction is accelerating.

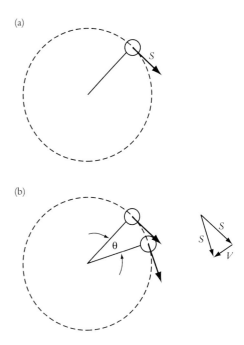

Figure 14.10 (a) Ball travelling in a circle with constant speed. (b) Same ball a short time later.

WORK, ENERGY AND POWER

Imagine having to push a car: you apply a force until it moves and as it moves you have to do work. The heavier the car, the harder the work; equally the further the car has to be pushed, the greater the work. In fact, work is calculated by multiplying the force by the distance moved in the direction of the applied force. Turning a stiff handle also requires work. This time, work is the moment multiplied by the angle. Work is measured in joules.

In biomechanics this is confused by the fact that a muscle may be active and expending energy, while not moving the joint upon which it acts. Because the joint does not move, no external work is done.

For example, Courtney et al (1995) examined the work required to break a series of proximal femora. They simulated a fall on to the greater trochanter by resting it on to a load cell and applying a force to the femoral head, in such a way as to mimic the bending moment that can be expected at the neck. By measuring the applied load and the distance through which it travelled, they showed that a sample from older donors (mean age 74 ± 7.4 years) had an average work to fracture of 5.5 ± 3.0 joules, whereas a sample from younger donors (mean age 33 ± 12.8 years) required a mean of 18.0 ± 8.3 joules of work to break the neck of their femora, a significant difference ($P < 0.001$).

In this example, when the femoral necks broke, the work expended was lost. This, however, is not always the case; in some instances the work can be stored.

Energy is defined as the ability to do work; consequently, it is also measured in joules. For instance, when winding up the spring of a clockwork toy, the work is stored in the form of energy in the coiled spring, which is later released as the toy performs.

In engineering mechanics it is useful to consider energy in one of two forms: kinetic and potential energy. A moving object has energy by virtue of its movement; this is known as kinetic energy and it is dependent on the mass and the square of the speed of the object.

An object at rest can store energy; for instance, the weights of a grandfather clock store energy because they are raised up, or coiling up a spring can store energy. This form of stored energy is referred to as potential energy.

During locomotion the human body utilises these energy stores to improve efficiency, as will be discussed below. Kinetic energy is stored in the moving limb segments, and potential energy is stored in the raising of limb segments and the stretch of tendons and ligaments.

Power is the rate at which work is done; in other words, the rate at which energy is used. It is measured in joules per second.

In summary: (1) if a force or a moment is required to move an object, work has to be expended; (2) work is the force multiplied by the distanced moved, or the moment times the angle; (3) energy is the ability to do work; (4) both work and energy are measured in joules; (5) power is the rate of work and is measured in joules per second.

TENSION COMPRESSION, SHEAR, TORSION AND BENDING

Figure 14.11a shows a tibia whose distal end has a force being applied along its axis. This leads to either tension

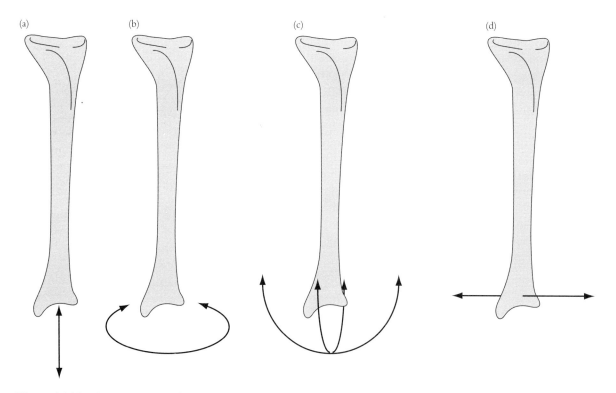

Figure 14.11   Forces acting on the tibia: (a) tension – compression force; (b) torsion; (c) bending moments; (d) bending moment and shear.

(distraction) or compression, depending on the direction of the load. If there is no other load, that is if no muscles attached are active, then the force will be transmitted along the whole length of the bone, and the level of tension or compression will be the same over the whole bone.

If a moment is applied to the end of the bone about its axis, as in *Figure 14.11b*, that is the bone is twisted, then the bone is in torsion. Again, the same torsion will be the same along the whole tibia if no other loads are applied.

If we now try to apply a moment to the distal end but at 90° to its axis, as in *Figure 14.11c*, then it will bend. This type of load is known as a bending moment. As the figure shows, there are two bending moments: one in the sagittal plane and one the coronal plane.

However, if we apply a force to the distal end of the tibia while restraining the proximal end, as in *Figure 14.11d*, then loading is a little more complex. The tibia will bend; it experiences a bending moment which increases further away from the applied force as the lever arm increases, but it also experiences a type of loading known as shear.

To explain the concept of shear, place a large book on a table top, put a hand on to the book and push the uppermost cover as shown in *Figure 14.12*. The resulting movement is known as shear. In shear, each page tends to slip relative to the next.

The tibia in *Figure 14.11d* will experience this type of load – shear – along its whole length which, unlike the bending moment, will not change along its length.

In fact, most types of loading result in tension–compression and shear. Consider the tibia in *Figure 14.11c*, which experiences bending. As it bends, the fibres on the convex side stretch and on the concave side squash; that is, there are regions that experience tension and those that experience compression. In fact, between adjacent layers of fibres going from the tensile face to the compressive face there is also shear. In pure compression and pure tension there are also both compression, tension and shear, although the nature of these loads is beyond the scope of this chapter.

In summary: (1) there are four types of loading that a long bone can experience: tension–compression, shear, torsion and bending; (2) tension–compression and shear are linear loads; (3) torsion and bending are angular loads; (4) a bone in bending will have layers of fibres in tension, layers of fibres under compression, and shear in between each of these adjacent layers; (5) in general, although the external loads can be simple, the internal loads can be highly complex.

LOADS AND DEFORMATIONS WITHIN A MATERIAL OR TISSUE

We have looked so far at how objects behave if they are considered to be rigid. However, no material or tissue is completely rigid; in fact, loads are transmitted within a solid by deformation of the solid.

Let us consider the form in which loads appear within an object. *Figure 14.13* shows a tibia under a compressive force, *F*. The loading within the diaphysis will depend on the magnitude of this force and the cross-sectional area of the cortex. A larger force will lead to greater loads within the bone, and a large cross-sectional area will reduce the loads.

This internal loading is known as 'stress'; it is given the symbol, σ, and is calculated by dividing the applied force by the cross-sectional area.

$$\sigma = \frac{F}{A} \qquad (20)$$

where F is the applied force, and A is the cross-sectional area.

Stress, consequently, has the same units as pressure (N m^{-2}).

Any loading or stress on a material will result in the material deforming. This can be illustrated by again

(a)

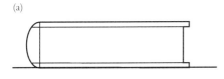

(b)

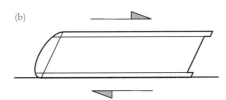

Figure 14.12   Effect of shear on a book.

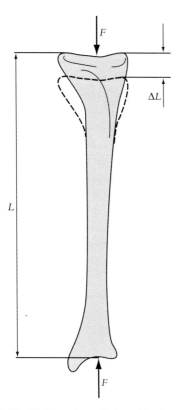

Figure 14.13 Deformation of the tibia due to a compressive force.

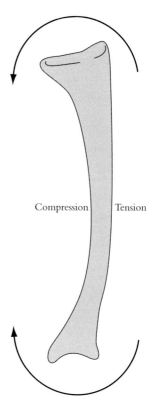

Figure 14.14 Stresses within the tibia in bending.

considering the tibia under a compressive load, but this time considering how it will deform.

Figure 14.13 shows that the tibia will shorten by a small amount, ΔL. It is best to consider this change of length relative to the original length of tibia. This relative change in length is referred to as strain, ε. That is:

$$\varepsilon = \frac{\Delta L}{L} \qquad (21)$$

where L is the original length of the tibia.

As strain is a relative change in length it has no units.

It is important to realise that, although these terms have been defined in terms of a whole object, the tibia, they can both vary throughout the material or tissue. For instance, if the tibia experiences the bending moment illustrated in *Figure 14.14*, then the medial surface will be in tension and the lateral surface will be in compression. This means that the medial stresses will be tensile and lateral stresses will be compressive. The bone will be stretched, experiencing tensile strains, on the lateral

border, and will be squashed on the medial border, experiencing compressive strains.

Stiffness, strength and energy to fracture

The stiffness of a tissue will be defined by how much it deforms under load. In engineering mechanics this is known as Young's modulus, or E. If two tissues are considered, bone and cartilage, bone will deform less than cartilage under a given load. Bone is stiffer and has a higher Young's modulus.

The Young's modulus of a material is measured by dividing the applied stress by the resulting strain:

$$E = \frac{\sigma}{\varepsilon} \qquad (22)$$

where σ is the applied stress and ε is the resulting strain.

For Young's modulus to have any meaning the relationship between stress and strain needs to be roughly linear. Unfortunately, the stress–strain curves for different tissues tend to be a little more complicated.

Figure 14.15 shows typical stress–strain curves for

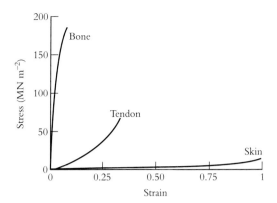

Figure 14.15 Typical stress–strain curve demonstrating the material properties.

bone, tendon and skin. Although bone and tendon do have initial regions which are linear, the mechanical property of skin is more complex. The highest point on these curves, the point of maximum stress, indicates the maximum load that the tissue can tolerate; in other words, its strength.

As has been explained earlier, work is done if the point at which a load acts is allowed to move. Consequently, these curves can measure the amount of energy absorbed by the tissues; the absorbed energy is equal to the area under the stress–strain curve. The amount of energy a material absorbs before it fails is a measure of its toughness. A material such as glass can be quite strong but not tough, whereas another material, such as some plastics, can be tough but not strong.

Plasticity and elasticity

If you take a rubber band and measure its unloaded length, then stretch and release it, you will find that, as long as you have not exceeded the limits of the rubber band, it will return to its original length. In fact, for a particular load the length of the band will be the same; increase the load and it will be greater, decrease the load and it will be less. A material or tissue that has this ability to return to the same length for a given load is referred to as being 'elastic'.

On the other hand, if you take a piece of modelling clay and pull it slightly, it will change shape and remain in that new shape even after the load has been removed.

Materials that exhibit this property are referred to as being 'plastic'.

Both elastic and plastic materials absorb energy when they are loaded, but only elastic materials release the energy back as the load is removed.

In summary: (1) stress is the load within a material and is calculated by dividing the overall load by the area over which it is acting; (2) strain is the deformation within a material, and is calculated by dividing the change in length by the original length; (3) most biological materials have a non-linear relationship between load (stress) and deformation (strain); (4) the area under the stress–strain curve indicates the energy absorbed when the object was loaded; (5) elastic materials go back to their original shape and release energy as they are unloaded, whereas plastic materials do not.

KINEMATICS

The study of motion, without regard to the loads involved, is known as 'kinematics'. This type of analysis reveals not only how the body segments move in space, but also how they move relative to each other. The movement is measured in terms of both linear and angular displacements, velocities and accelerations.

The bones of the body are considered to be completely rigid. This will be shown later not to be the case. However, the deformations within the bones are much smaller than the movements they make as a whole object; consequently, they are negligible and can be ignored.

If we consider the movements of the tibia during normal walking, its movement is mainly in the sagittal plane. It moves forward rapidly while the leg is swung. The distal end is brought almost to a standstill as the foot lands on the floor. While the leg is swinging, the tibia rotates so that its distal end moves forward. However, when the foot is on the ground it continues to rotate, but this time with its proximal end moving forward. Therefore, there is a complex pattern of linear and angular motions.

Figure 14.16 shows a tibia during the swing phase of walking. The arrows indicating the velocity vectors of each end of the bone are marked for this instant. Of

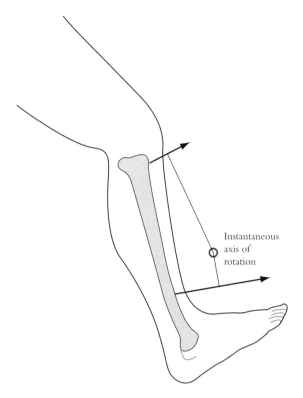

Figure 14.16   Instantaneous axis of rotation of the tibia during walking.

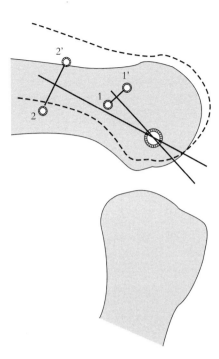

Figure 14.17   Instantaneous axis of rotation of the femur relative to the tibia.

course, these velocities will be different the instant before or after the one shown in this figure.

These vectors are in different directions, yet the tibia is moving as a rigid solid body. This is explained by the fact that the tibia is rotating. The velocity vectors at the rim of a spinning wheel vary, with the vectors being in opposite directions on either side of a diameter.

In fact, at this instant, the tibia is rotating about a single point. This point is outside the body and can be discovered quite easily. If we draw a line at right angles to each of the velocity vectors, they will cross at a point, as shown in *Figure 14.16*. This intersection is the instantaneous centre of rotation. The different linear velocities at each end can now be considered to be one angular velocity about this point. The velocity vector for any point on the tibia can now be calculated because that point must also have the same angular velocity about the same point. However, since the velocity vectors at each end of the tibia will vary from instant to instant, the instantaneous centre of rotation and the angular velocity will also vary.

The analysis of movement using this technique can be extremely useful. For instance, examination of the relative motion of two neighbouring bones, defining the instantaneous centre of rotation of one bone relative to the other, gives a clear indication of the behaviour of the joint.

Analysing the movement of the femur relative to the tibia using this technique allows a good understanding of the function of the knee (Frankel and Burstein, 1970). In this case, the position of the instantaneous centre of rotation is calculated by comparing two radiographs taken at slightly different angles of knee flexion. Because the knee is at rest, velocity vectors cannot be defined; instead the displacement of two (or more) points is considered.

Figure 14.17 shows how two points on the femur have moved. To calculate where the instantaneous centre of rotation lies, a line is first drawn between the two positions of the same point, then another line is drawn half-way along this and at right angles. Where these bisecting lines cross lies the instantaneous centre. Note that it lies well above the surface of the tibia. If the instantaneous centre lay on the surface, it would indicate that the knee joint is a pure rolling joint. As a wheel rolls, its instantaneous centre is always at the point of contact. Since that does not happen, it indicates that the knee joint is sliding as well as rotating.

The majority of synovial joints in the body exhibit this sliding behaviour, that is they allow rotation but the joint surfaces do not just roll on each other but also slip relative to each other.

In summary: (1) analysing the motion of the body without considering forces is known as kinematics; (2) the complex motions of the body segments can be defined in terms of the instantaneous centre of rotations; (3) the position of the instantaneous centre of rotation can be calculated from known linear velocities or known linear displacements at two or more points on the bone; (4) the instantaneous centre of rotation of the knee lies above the surface of the tibia; (5) the majority of synovial joints are sliding joints.

DYNAMICS

If the forces or moments within a system are out of balance, that is there is an overall resultant load, then the system cannot be in equilibrium. In other words, statics is no longer directly applicable. The resultant load will cause the system to accelerate.

If we consider again the leg during normal walking, it goes through cycles of linear and angular accelerations and decelerations. These must be due to forces and joint moments. The study of this movement with reference to the loads that cause them is known as 'dynamics'.

The relationship between force and acceleration is quite simple; it is often referred to as Newton's second law:

$$F = m.a \qquad (23)$$

where F is the resultant force, m is the mass and a is the acceleration.

The acceleration that an object experiences is dependent on the applied force and its mass. The heavier the object, the slower the acceleration; the greater the force, the higher the acceleration.

There is a comparable equation that describes the angular acceleration in response to a moment:

$$M = I.\alpha \qquad (24)$$

where M is the resultant moment, I is the moment of inertia and α is the angular acceleration.

The concept is similar; we can consider the moment to be comparable to the force and the two accelerations also to be comparable. The moment of inertia, therefore, is comparable to mass in some way.

The moment of intertia of an object is dependent not only on the mass but also on how it is distributed. The further away from the centre of rotation the mass is situated, the higher the moment of intertia. A mass strapped to the ankle requires a greater moment at the hip to accelerate it than if the same mass were strapped to the thigh.

The moment of inertia also depends on the axis of rotation. The moment of inertia of the whole leg is less when it is being internally and externally rotated than when the hip is flexed and extended with a straight leg.

Dynamic studies of the body are made difficult by the fact that there is no acceptable way of measuring the forces within the body. Techniques have been developed to measure the loads in implants (Rydell, 1966), but studies of the loads within the body have relied on more indirect techniques.

For instance, in 1967 Paul produced some seminal work in which he estimated the peak forces at the hip from kinematic data for the normal hip coupled with measurements of the external forces. The only external forces on the leg are when the foot is on the ground, so he measured the force vector being applied to the ground (or more precisely the force with which the ground reacts to the foot).

By knowing the magnitude of the force and its direction relative to the leg, he was able to estimate what the external moment was at the hip. He developed a technique to calculate the moments due to the active musculature and showed that the resultant peak force during normal walking was higher than had been expected at between four and seven times body-weight.

In summary: (1) the study of forces, moments and resulting accelerations is known as dynamics; (2) the linear acceleration of an object is dependent on both the applied force and its mass; (3) the angular acceleration of an object is dependent on the resultant moment it experiences and its moment of inertia; (4) the moment of inertia of an object is dependent on its mass and how that mass is distributed; the further away from the axis of rotation the mass is, the greater the moment of inertia;

(5) dynamics studies have been performed to estimate the internal forces and moments on joints.

BIOMECHANICS OF THE MUSCULOSKELETAL SYSTEM

Lower limb

Hip

The hip is a large ball and socket joint, made up of the head of the femur and the acetabulum. It is the most difficult joint to dislocate (Kapandji, 1987); the acetabulum, being hemispherical, cannot hold the head of the femur without the assistance of the labrum acetabulare. It was also shown by the Weber brothers (1836) that the partial vacuum within the joint plays an important role in holding the joint in apposition. If this vacuum is released, the joint becomes less stable. Unlike the shoulder, the direction of the resultant force due to body-weight also tends to assist in stabilising the joint.

Being a ball and socket joint, the hip is able to rotate in all three planes: flexion–extension occurs in the sagittal plane, abduction–adduction in the frontal plane and internal–external rotation in the transverse plane. The full range of motion is greater in flexion–extension (140°) than in the other directions; 75° in abduction–adduction and 90° in internal–external rotation.

The forces on the hip depend on both activity and anatomy. Rydell (1966) used a hip prosthesis that had been strain-gauged to measure the hip joint loads directly. He showed that the load on the hip when standing on one leg was 2.6 times body-weight. This agreed well with that predicted by other researchers who had calculated this load from knowledge of the anatomy, measured external forces and estimated muscular activity.

Full biomechanical models of the major joints of the body are beyond the scope of this chapter. However, a simplified model of the loads on the hip during one-leg standing can give close approximations to the measured hip loads. In this simple model, shown in *Figure 14.18*, only one muscle group is active, the gluteal group, which in this model is assumed to act between the greater trochanter and the pelvis.

In this model, we look at the forces of the body above the hip and including the contralateral limb. As one leg weighs about one-sixth of body-weight, the rest of the body weighs five-sixths of body-weight. The centre of

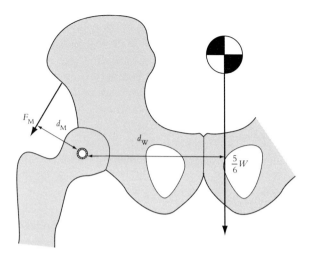

Figure 14.18   Loads on the hip during one-leg standing.

gravity of the rest of the body is in a different position, without the leg that is on the ground; the centre of gravity moves away from the hip in question, and so increases the moment arm. If we now consider moments about the femoral head we find that:

$$F_M d_M = \frac{5}{6} W d_W \tag{25}$$

where F_M is the muscular force, d_M is the moment arm of the muscular force, W is body-weight, and d_W is the moment arm of the weight.

If the person has a mass of 73 kg, then body-weight will be 720 N. If we take d_M to be 60 mm and d_W to be 150 mm, we can calculate F_M:

$$F_M = \frac{5 \times 720 \, N \times 150 \, mm}{6 \times 60 \, mm} = 1500 \, N \tag{26}$$

The muscular force in this simplified model is 1500 N or 2.1 times body-weight.

We now know the magnitudes and the directions of the force due to gravity and the muscle group, from which we can calculate the remaining unknown, the forces on the hip.

From the triangle of forces drawn in *Figure 14.19*, it can be seen that the hip force, F_H, can be measured to be 2042 N, that is nearly three times body-weight. Rydell and others have shown that the load on the hip during walking and running is considerably greater than this: 4.2 times body-weight during slow walking to 7.6 times body-weight during running.

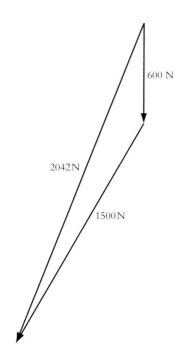

600 N

2042 N

1500 N

Figure 14.19   Triangle of forces at the hip during one-leg standing.

In summary: (1) the hip joint is a naturally stable ball and socket joint; (2) range of movement is 140° flexion–extension, 75° abduction–adduction and 90° internal–external rotation; (3) a force on the hip of 2.6 times body-weight can be expected during one-leg standing; (4) the hip force during slow walking is around 4.2 times body-weight; and (5) the hip force during running is around 7.6 times body-weight.

Knee

Unlike the hip, the knee depends completely on its soft tissue structures for its mechanical stability: the collateral ligaments resist mediolateral bending moments, torsion and to a certain extent mediolateral shear; the cruciate ligaments resist anteroposterior shear forces; and the musculature deals with anteroposterior bending, with compressive forces being passed directly across the joint surfaces.

By far the greatest range of motion of the knee occurs in flexion–extension, about 150°. However, it would be wrong to consider the movement only in this plane (Cochran, 1982); during the last 15° or so of extension there is an external rotation of the knee through 4–5°.

There is also about 10° abduction–adduction at the knee.

Normal daily activities require the knee to be free through a large range of flexion–extension: normal walking requires 70° of flexion; descending stairs requires about 90° of flexion and sitting comfortably on a bus requires more than 90° of flexion. Some 110° of flexion of the knee is recommended as a good goal to allow daily activities to be performed in comfort.

A lateral view of the femoral condyles reveals that they are not circular, but that their radius of curvature changes over their length. The curve of the anterior surface of the condyles is relatively shallow and tightens up posteriorly. The knee therefore cannot have one centre of rotation like a hinge, but the position of the centre of rotation varies with flexion. The path of these instantaneous centres of rotation of the femur relative to the tibia have been mapped out by Frankel et al (1971).

In normal standing, the knees are held in extension with the line of action of body-weight passing slightly anteriorly to the centre of the joint. The requirements for balancing from the musculature are therefore minimal and the knee loads can be estimated from body-weight: one knee experiences half of the body-weight less the weight of the lower leg and foot.

Varus or valgus deformities will cause the line of action of the joint load to move away from its centre, producing an increase in the load in one or other compartment: genu valgum leads to higher loads in the medial compartment, genu varum in the lateral compartment.

The static loads increase to three or five times body-weight in such activities as standing with flexed knees or slow stair-climbing. During normal walking, the knee can experience forces as high as three times body-weight; even during the swing phase of walking, when the foot is off the ground, the active musculature can produce forces up to that of body-weight.

As the femoral condyles and the tibial plateau are not congruent, the medial and lateral menisci have a role to play in distributing the loads over a wider area than would otherwise be possible by enlarging the area of contact. The menisci have to be relatively mobile to remain between the femur and tibia throughout the flexion–extension range. Without the menisci, the contact area is smaller; consequently, for the same joint forces the stresses are higher, which can lead to detrimental effects on the cartilage.

The patella acts both as a simple pulley, changing the

direction of the action of the quadriceps, and more importantly to increase the moment arm of the quadriceps especially towards full extension. At larger flexion angles the patella rides down between the condyles and has less effect. The consequence of this is that the moment arm of the quadriceps varies throughout flexion–extension, ranging from about 60 mm at full extension to about 40 mm at 120° flexion.

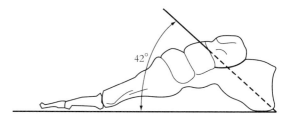

In summary: (1) the stability of the knee is dependent on its ligaments; (2) the largest amount of movement occurs in flexion–extension, range 150°; (3) 110° of flexion of the knee is required for daily activities; (4) knee forces during normal walking are about three times body-weight; and (5) the patella acts to increase the moment arm of the quadriceps.

Ankle and foot

The ankle complex consists of three joints: the tibiotalar, the fibulotalar and the distal tibiofibular joints. The configuration of the ankle is inherently stable, like the hip. It is a saddle joint, allowing mainly dorsiplantar flexion, although a few degrees of inversion–eversion and internal–external rotation are allowed.

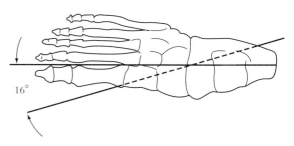

Figure 14.20   Axis of the subtalar joint.

The range of movement at the ankle is normally around 45°, although far larger ranges are not uncommon. This is usually broken down into 10–20° dorsiflexion and 25–35° plantar flexion.

The subtalar joint is located between the talus and the calcaneus; its axis does not lie parallel to the main axes of the body, consequently it allows motions in all three planes, although mainly inversion–eversion with a range of about 25°: 20° inversion and 5° eversion. The axis shown in *Figure 14.20* makes an angle of 42° to the horizontal and an angle of 16° to the midline of the foot.

The transverse tarsal joint, or Chopart's joint, lies anterior to the talus and calcaneus, and allows complex movement between the talus and navicular and between the calcaneus and cuboid. Manter (1941) recorded two motions about two axes. These axes allow for both inversion–eversion and dorsiplantar flexion.

The force on the ankle during normal two-legged standing will be greater than half body-weight because the musculature constantly acts to balance the body in a similar manner to that of the guy ropes holding up a flagpole. This force will be experienced by the ankle in addition to body-weight. Rising up and standing on tiptoe on one leg can result in a force equivalent to four times body-weight at the ankle.

During standing, the weight-bearing of the forefoot is distributed between the metatarsal heads in a ratio of about 2 : 1 between the first metatarsal and each of the others. However, during walking, especially when the foot is pushing off, the second metatarsal transmits more load.

The longitudinal medial arch of the foot is an important shock-absorbing mechanism. Normally the arch fails to collapse because of three components: the bony structures themselves form a fairly stable structure; the anterior and posterior bases to the arch are prevented from moving apart by the plantar fascia; and the intrinsic muscles of the foot aided by tibialis anterior also help to elevate the arch.

In summary: (1) the ankle is a naturally stable saddle joint; (2) movement in the hindfoot can be considered at the subtalar and the transverse tarsal joints; (3) standing up on one's toes can produce ankle forces of four times body-weight; (4) during normal standing the first metatarsal head carries about twice as much load as each of the other heads, whereas during walking the second metatarsal head carries the most load; and (5) the longitudinal medial arch acts as a shock absorber.

Upper limb

Shoulder

The shoulder is possibly the most intricate joint complex of the body, involving four bones (humerus, scapula, clavicle and sternum) and four distinct articulations (glenohumeral, acromioclavicular, sternoclavicular and scapulothoracic joints).

The glenohumeral articulation is a ball and socket joint similar to the hip; however, the socket is quite shallow. Consequently the shoulder is not inherently stable and requires soft tissue structures to prevent dislocation.

The shoulder, like the hip, allows movement in all planes. The glenohumeral joint is not rigidly attached to the trunk; the scapula provides one of the joint surfaces. The scapula is able to move relative to the thorax; its scapulothoracic joint is not a true anatomical joint but a bone–muscle–bone articulation. Shoulder abduction is the result of motion both at the glenohumeral joint and of the scapula; it is generally accepted that after the first 30–60° the ratio of these movements is 2 : 1; that is, for every 15° of shoulder abduction 10° occurs at the glenoid and 5° is due to scapula movement. The total range of movement of glenohumeral motion is, with the arm in external rotation, 120°; the total scapular range is 60°. External rotation of the arm avoids impingement of the greater tuberosity, and consequently allows for a greater range of abduction.

Up to 90° of abduction, the sternoclavicular joint moves about 4° for every 10° of arm movement, and then motion ceases at this joint. The acromioclavicular joint moves through 20–25° during the first 30° of shoulder abduction, after which it ceases to move until the end of the range of this movement.

Full acromioclavicular joint motion is possible only if it relieves the tension in the coracoclavicular ligament; this tension is an important factor in the stability of the shoulder complex. The tension is released by the clavicle rotating about its long axis up to a maximum of 40°.

The forces at any joint come in part from the stabilising muscles around it; the role of the musculature in stabilising the shoulder complex is particularly important. Any raised position of the arm requires a minimum of three forces: the weight of the arm, the force to raise the arm and at least one other force to balance these other two.

It has been shown that, at 90° abduction, the force applied by the deltoid is about eight times that of the weight of the arm. The biomechanical models of the shoulder are by necessity highly complex; they estimate that the force at the shoulder is about 90% of body-weight when the arm is in this position.

In summary: (1) the shoulder complex comprises four separate articulations and is not inherently stable; (2) the shoulder allows movement in all planes; (3) the ratio of movements of the glenoid and of the scapula is 2 : 1; (4) at 90° abduction of the shoulder, the deltoid applies a force about eight times the weight of the arm; and (5) at 90° of abduction, the shoulder load is about 90% of body-weight.

Elbow

The elbow allows two movements: flexion–extension and pronation–supination. It has three separate articulations: the ulnohumeral, radiohumeral and radioulnar joints.

In supination the radius and ulna lie roughly parallel to each other: however, in pronation they cross. This occurs by allowing the radius to undergo internal–external rotation relative to the humerus. Abduction–adduction of the ulna allows it to cross the radius, but internal–external rotation is prevented. At the wrist the movements are reversed: the radius does not rotate, whereas the ulna does.

The distal humerus has two articular surfaces, the trochlea and the capitulum; the trochlea is pulley shaped and the capitulum is spherical.

The trochlea articulates with the trochlear notch of the ulna, and has good congruency throughout flexion. As a result, there is a relatively high area of contact of this joint and the forces are more evenly distributed. Degenerative changes of this articulation are infrequent when there is no specific cause.

The head of the radius makes the other half of the ball and socket joint with the capitulum. Like the glenohumeral joint, this joint has no inherent stability; it relies for this on the ligaments, muscular action and its stable neighbour, the ulna. In particular, the radial head is kept in apposition by the annular ligament, which is located immediately behind the head.

The elbow has a range of flexion–extension of up to 150° and a range of pronation–supination of about 180°.

The simplified model of the elbow, forearm and hand given in *Figure 14.8* revealed an approximation of the forces experienced at the elbow. This model ignores the fact that the wrist, and probably finger flexors, will be active and they are inserted above the elbow, and so will in turn add to the forces at this joint.

Nicol et al (1977) showed that during simple daily living activities, such as eating and dressing, the elbow forces could be about half body-weight. More energetic actions, such as lifting or pulling, could result in elbow forces greater than twice body-weight.

In summary: (1) the elbow comprises three separate articulations; (2) the elbow allows two movements, flexion–extension and pronation–supination; (4) the ulnohumeral joint has good congruency whereas the radiohumeral joint does not; (4) there is about 150° flexion–extension and 180° pronation–supination; and (5) the elbow can experience over twice body-weight.

Axial skeleton

The spine consists of 32 vertebrae: seven cervical, twelve thoracic, five lumbar, five sacral and three coccygeal. Apart from the sacrum and coccyx, these vertebrae are separated by an intervertebral disc and various ligaments. The whole spine therefore behaves like a segmented rod.

The ligaments are normally in tension and the discs in compression, conveying a state of stability to the spine. Excised whole spines can stand unsupported, although they buckle under compressive loads of over 20 N. The stability is greatly improved *in vivo* by the muscles acting as guy ropes. This muscular activity in turn increases the amount of compressive force experienced by the discs.

Motion in the spine occurs between each pair of vertebrae, and an intervertebral disc with its two neighbouring vertebrae is known as a 'spinal motion segment'. These motion segments are capable of limited angular movement in all three planes and limited translational movements in all three directions including compression–distraction (i.e. it has six degrees of freedom).

It is common to consider the motion segment in two portions: anterior and posterior. The anterior portion comprises the two vertebral bodies, the intervertebral disc and the longitudinal ligaments. The intervertebral joints formed by the facets, the transverse and the spinous process, with the corresponding vertebral arches and various ligaments, make up the posterior portion.

In the anterior portion the intervertebral disc carries load yet is flexible; it is composed of an inner and an outer structure. The inner portion is the nucleus pulposus, which is a hydrophilic gelatinous mass that becomes progressively less hydrated with age. This degeneration results in loss of elasticity, energy–storing ability and shock-absorbing capacity, as well as a loss of disc height.

The outer layers of the vertebrae make up the annulus fibrosus, which consists of layers of fibrocartilage in a criss-cross arrangement. The vertebral endplates, which sit immediate above and below the discs, are composed of hyaline cartilage.

In compression, the disc tends to bulge slightly, putting the nucleus into compression but the annulus into tension; in the lumbar spine it has been shown that this tensile stress can be four to five times greater than the applied compressive stresses (Nachemson, 1960; Galante, 1967).

The movement of the motion segment is guided by its posterior portion. This guidance is dependent on the orientation of the facet joints, which varies between levels of the spine. There is also a considerable variation between individuals, although a general pattern can be described.

The two uppermost cervical vertebrae are atypical and their facets are parallel to the transverse plane. The other cervical facets lie at about 45° to the transverse plane, which allows flexion–extension, lateral flexion and rotation. The facet joints of the thoracic spine lie at 60° to the transverse plane and 20° to the frontal plane, allowing these motion segments to move in lateral flexion, rotation and limited flexion–extension. In the lumbar region the facets are oriented at about right angles to the transverse plane and at 45° to the frontal plane (White and Panjabi, 1978), allowing almost all movements except rotation, which is highly restricted. The lumbrosacral joints of facets lie obliquely and allow appreciable rotation (Lumsden and Morris, 1968).

The facet joints carry an appreciable load; the amount of load that is shared between these joints and the intervertebral discs varies with the position of the spine. King et al (1975) showed that the greatest loads on the facet joints occur when the spine is hyperextended, when the loads are about 30% of the total load; they are also high during forward bending coupled with rotation (El-Bohy and King, 1986).

Patients with degenerative changes in the vertebral arches or defective intervertebral joints, such as spondylosis, are at greater risk of forward displacement of the vertebral bodies (Adams and Hutton, 1983; Miller et al, 1983), indicating the importance of these structures in resisting shear forces in the spine. The transverse and spinous processes serve as sites of attachment for the spinal muscles.

The role of the ligaments of the spine contributes to its intrinsic stability. Most of these structures around the spine have high collagen content and are therefore relatively inelastic. However, the ligamentum flavum, which runs between adjacent vertebral arches, has a large proportion of elastin. Its elasticity allows it to elongate during flexion, but not to fold back in extension. In the neutral position it has been shown to be in tension and therefore prestresses the intervertebral disc (Rolander, 1966; Nachemson and Evans, 1968).

In summary: (1) the spine can be considered to consist of a series of motion segments; (2) the spine is commonly considered as being in two portions, anterior and posterior; (3) the anterior portion, with the intervertebral disc, allows flexion–extension, twist and shear, which are guided by the structures in the posterior portion; (4) the range and type of motion allowed at a motion segment varies with the spinal level; and (5) the ligamentum flavum, unlike the other spinal ligaments, is relatively elastic and prestresses the intervertebral disc in the neutral position.

REFERENCES

Adams MA, Hutton WC. (1983) The mechanical function of the lumbar apophyseal joints. *Spine* 1983; **8**: 327.

Cochran GvB. *A Primer of Orthopaedic Biomechanics*. Edinburgh: Churchill Livingstone, 1982.

Courtney AC, Wachtel EF, Myers ER, Hayes WC. Age-related reductions in the strength of the femur tested in a fall-loading configuration. *J Bone Joint Surg* 1995; **77A(3)**: 387–395.

El-Bohy AA, King AI. Intervertebral disc and facet contact pressure in axial torsion. In: Lantz SA, King AI (eds) *Advances in Bioengineering*. American Society of Mechanical Engineers, New York: 1986: 26–27.

Huang TC. *Engineering Mechanics*. Addison-Wesley, 1967.

Frankel VH, Burstein AH. *Orthopaedic Biomechanics*. Philadelphia: Lea and Febiger, 1970.

Frankel VH, Burstein AH, Brooks DB. Biomechanics of internal derangement of the knee. Pathomechanics as determined by the analysis of instant centres of motion. *J Bone Joint Surg [Am]* 1971; **53A**: 945–962.

Galante JO. Tensile properties of the human lumbar annulus fibrosus. *Acta Orthop Scand Suppl* 1967; **100**: 1–91.

Kapandji IA. *The Physiology of the Joints*. Singapore: Churchill Livingstone, 1987.

King AI, Prasad P, Ewing CL. Mechanism of spinal injury due to caudocephalad acceleration. *Orthop Clin North Am* 1975; **6**: 19.

Lumsden RM, Morris JM. An *in vivo* study of axial rotation and immobilisation at the lumbrosacral joint. *J Bone Joint Surg [Am]* 1968; **50A**: 1591.

Manter JT. Movements of the subtalar and transverse tarsal joints. *Anat Rec* 1971; **80**: 397.

Miller JAA, Haderspeck KA, Schultz AB. Posterior element loads in lumbar motion segments. *Spine* 1983; **8**: 331.

Nachemson A. Lumbar intradiscal pressure. *Acta Orthop Scand Suppl* 1960; **43**: 1–140.

Nachemson AL, Evans JH. Some mechanical properties of the third human lumbar interlaminar ligament (ligamentum flavum). *J Biomech* 1968; **1**: 211.

Nicol AC, Berne N, Paul JP. A biomechanical analysis of elbow joint function. In: Joint replacement in the upper limb. London: Institution of Mechanical Engineers, 1977; 45–51.

Paul JP. Forces transmitted by joints in the human body. *Proc Instn Mech Eng* 1967; **Part 3J, 181**: 8–15.

Rolander SD. Motion of the lumbar spine with special reference to the stabilizing effect of posterior fusion. An experimental study on autopsy specimens. *Acta Orthop Scand Suppl* 1966; **90**: 1–144.

Rydell NW. Forces acting on the femoral head prosthesis. A study of strain gauge supplied prosthesis in living persons. *Act Orthop Scand Suppl* 1966; **88**: 1–132.

Shames, IH. *Engineering Mechanics*. Prentice-Hall, London, 1970.

Weber W, Weber E. *Mechanik des Menschlichen Gehwekzeuge*. Goltingen: Dietrich, 1836.

White AA, Panjabi MM. *Clinical Biomechanics of the Spine*. Philadelphia: JB Lippincott, 1978.

Williams M, Lissner HR. *Biomechanics of Human Motion*. Philadelphia: WB Saunders, 1962: 102–103.

15

Biomechanics of Bone, Tendon and Ligament

Andrew A Amis

INTRODUCTION

In this chapter the mechanical characteristics of bones, tendons and ligaments will be examined. In each case, this will start with a description of the materials themselves, their constituents and the material properties, and then progress to examine how these properties manifest themselves in the function of the complete structure.

As the text progresses, one aim is to demonstrate that the bones, tendons and ligaments have structures that are adapted remarkably well to withstand the loads imposed on them in use, not just for the structure as a whole, but even at a local level within each structure. The level of sophistication in this respect is way beyond that attainable by normal manufactured engineering components: one needs to think only of the changing cross-section along a long bone, and to compare it with the constant cross-section of a girder in a bridge, to see this.

BIOMECHANICS OF BONE

Bone structure and material

The reader will probably be familiar with the cross-sectional anatomy of the cortical bone from the diaphyseal region, and an appreciation of the micro-structure helps with understanding the mechanical behaviour under load and as the bone fails. In mature bone, the cross-section is primarily made up of lamellar bone arranged into concentric tubular structures known as haversian systems, each of which has a blood vessel passing along the haversian canal on its central axis. This arrangement, with small canaliculae branching out centrifugally from the central canal, means that all parts of the cross-section are relatively close to a vascular supply; this obviously allows nutrition but, by inference, also allows adaptation to changing circumstances such as disuse. The canaliculae of adjacent haversian systems are prevented from communicating with each other by the presence of a boundary wall, the cement line; the assembly within the cement line is known as an osteon. At the endosteal and periosteal walls of the bone, there is usually a layer of lamellar bone that is laid down as a flat surface, and not arranged into haversian systems.

On a smaller scale, the material from which the lamellae are constructed is of two main constituents: collagen fibres and ground substance; the latter consists of inorganic crystals of hydroxyapatite (calcium phosphate) and related species, which are embedded in an amorphous organic material.

Collagen fibres are the main tensile load-bearing material in the body, and small differences in their molecular structure have allowed the identification of a number of collagen species that are tissue specific. They have in common, however, a structure made up of long-chain amino acid molecules, that are arranged into a triple helical pattern to form collagen protofibrils, and these are bundled together to form collagen microfibrils. Thus, the collagen structure is very similar to that of a piece of string. These structures pass along the lamellae within haversian systems, giving tensile strength along their length.

Collagen exhibits a fairly complex mechanical behaviour, of a viscoelastic nature, which means that the deformation and stresses induced in collagen are time dependent and, therefore, depend on the speed with which a load is applied. As the word implies, viscoelasticity consists essentially of time-dependent viscous effects acting on a structure that contains elements that could behave elastically. If a load is applied to an elastic structure, it elongates immediately to a new length that depends on the load applied. If it is affected by some viscous milieu, then the resistance of the viscosity means that it will take some time for the structure to deform, as it must overcome the viscosity, or flow resistance. This phenomenon allows collagen-based structures to withstand a load applied momentarily that would lead to failure if it were applied slowly and for a longer time, and this will be shown later.

It is the inorganic crystals that give bone its rigidity, when compared to other collagen-based structures. The crystalline micro-structure varies both regionally and with age, and this can be related to the strength of the bone. It can be imagined that the crystals will give bone its compressive strength, as they are packed together under load, but also that their presence could interfere with the ability of the collagen fibres to withstand being stretched in tension, leading to bone failing at a lower tensile stress than compressive.

Material properties: bone strength – cortical bone

The material properties of bone vary from person to person, from time to time, from bone to bone, and also vary from position to position within each bone. It follows that although much work has been published on bone strength, and some data will be given in this chapter, it is usually the case that a researcher with a particular interest must do the strength testing in person, in order to obtain specific data. Much of the methodology of bone strength testing has existed for some time, and a particularly important factor is that the specimens must be maintained in a fully hydrated state during storage and preparation. If the bone surface gets hot and dries out when it is being cut into a test specimen, then premature failure will be inevitable. Extensive review articles on cortical bone strength have been written by Swanson (1971) and Reilly and Burstein (1974).

Regional variation of material properties of cortical bone

The majority of bone strength investigators have machined their test specimens from the cortical mid-shaft region, usually because the thick cortex here facilitates this. However, much work relates to the ends of the bones, as joint replacements are located here, and the

strength is different. This has been shown elegantly by Pope and Outwater (1974), who tested mature bovine tibiae. Specimens were taken from every part of the bone, and were in several different orientations in each zone: longitudinal, circumferential and radial, the latter being facilitated by the thick cortices in this species. The fresh bones were machined and tested wet, to preserve the mechanical properties, and a high strain rate was used, to minimise viscoelastic effects. A three-point bending test configuration was used, in which the two ends of the specimen were supported, and the load was applied to bend the specimen at the mid-point. This arrangement causes the greatest bending stress at the midpoint.

The results (*Figure 15.1*) show that the bone had effectively equal fracture strength (approximately 120 MPa) and stiffness in all directions at the ends, and this is known as 'isotropic' behaviour. Conversely, at the mid-shaft region, the bone exhibited marked anisotropy, with much greater tensile fracture strength and elastic modulus in the longitudinal direction: 230 MPa longitudinally, compared with only 35 MPa circumferentially. These results are not surprising when the loads imposed on the bone are considered: the bone is subjected to loads in many directions at the ends, as a result of joint forces, ligament tensions and muscle loads at a range of joint postures. However, the mid-shaft region must act as both a compression strut and resist some bending and torsion loading, which will give predominantly axial stresses, and a robust tubular structure is ideal for this. The microstructure of haversian systems is seen to be well adapted to resisting axial loads in the diaphysis.

Effects of different loading patterns

Axial loads. The predominant load acting on the shaft of a long bone will be axial compression. This arises primarily because of the tensions in the muscles, which are usually arranged alongside the bones, and which combine to give compressive forces much larger than the external loads acting on the body, such as the foot–floor reaction force. This is illustrated by work on joint forces, in which it has been shown that the tibiofemoral joint is subjected to three or four times body-weight when walking, for example (Morrison, 1968). In this situation, the bone is acting as a compression strut, and it may fail either by compressive yielding of the bone material or by buckling, when the structure becomes suddenly unstable. The transverse forces are relatively

(a)

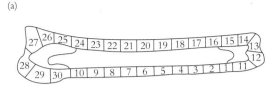

(b)

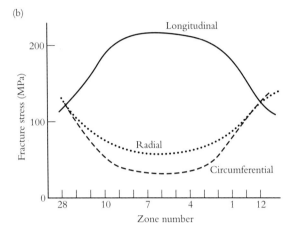

(c)

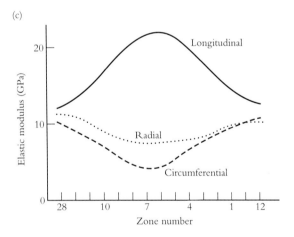

Figure 15.1 (a) Section of bovine tibia with specimen zones marked. (b) Regional variation of bone strength. (c) Regional variation of bone stiffness. From Pope and Outwater (1974), with permission.

small, with cruciate ligament tensions less than body-weight when walking (Morrison, 1968).

Buckling of a strut is resisted by a combination of the material stiffness and its geometrical distribution. The critical factor is the slenderness of the strut, the ratio of its

length to the cross-section. In this regard, the distribution of bone away from the central axis, to form a tube, is optimal. It can be imagined that a tendency to bend the axis of the bone is best resisted by having the tension in the bone material sited away from that axis, so as to give the tension a lever arm about the axis. Thus, a thin rod, compressed axially between its ends, will buckle far more readily than a tube of the same length with the same quantity of the same material.

Any eccentricity of the axial loading induces a bending moment which is superimposed on the stresses caused by the axial effect. The bending moment leads to a curvature along the bone, which is the first step towards a sudden collapse. In this context, most bones are subjected to both axial and bending forces, as the muscles pass alongside them. Further, the geometry of bones will often induce bending; for example, the femur is curved in the sagittal plane, and an axial impact such as a 'dashboard' injury will cause failure at the mid-shaft position, because the bending moment is greatest at that point, the end-load having impacted on to the femoral condyles posterior to the shaft axis.

Bending loads. The situation here is, in some ways, similar to that of resisting buckling. As a bone is subjected to a bending load, its central axis takes up a curvature. It follows that osteons on the outside of the bend are stretched, whereas those on the inside are compressed, and this axial deformation of the material leads to tensile and compressive stresses (and, hence, forces) respectively. It is this internal force distribution that resists the external bending moment applied to the bone (*Figure 15.2*). It is worth considering this in some detail.

If the bone has tensile stresses acting on the convex side of the bend and compressive stresses acting at the concave side, it follows that there must be a point at which there is a transition between the two extremes, where there will be no axial stress induced by bending; this is known as the neutral axis. It is always situated through the centroid (the 'centre of gravity' position) of the cross-section. A geometrical analysis shows that the deformation (i.e. the strain, or length change per unit length) depends linearly on the distance from the neutral axis, and so too does the stress, as long as the behaviour remains linearly elastic.

As with buckling, a given quantity of bone will resist bending most efficiently if it is distributed away from the neutral axis of bending, so that the force resulting from the stress in a given fibre in tension or compression has as

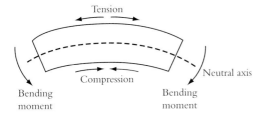

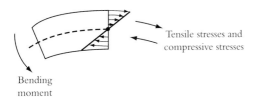

Figure 15.2 Stresses in bone due to bending. The bone fibres most distant from the neutral axis contribute most to resisting bending loads.

large a lever arm about the neutral axis as possible. This is why steel girders are often of a deep I section, with their material concentrated into the flanges at the top and bottom, away from the centre line. This section is optimal for withstanding bending loads acting in one direction; the circular sections of many bones reflect the imposition of loads from a range of directions, as well as the need to resist torsion. One location where bones do approximate to an I section is the ribs, near to the spine, where they are subjected to bending loads from the muscles attaching to them from the vertebrae. Their cross-section blends into a flatter profile anteriorly, reflecting a transition to shear loadings from the intercostal muscles. For a circular section bone subjected to a given bending moment, the peak stress will be inversely proportional to the diameter cubed, so it would seem at first thought to be optimal to have the largest diameter possible. There is, however, an optimum diameter for a given quantity of material (the weight of the structure is not a negligible consideration); eventually, as the material of a bone is spread to a larger diameter, the wall thickness will reduce to the point where it is becoming too fragile, and the wall may then fail by buckling, and so nature has reached an engineering compromise.

This mechanical theory has practical implications for the surgeon. For example, if the femur is subjected to an anteroposterior bending load *in vivo*, then there will be tensile stress in the anterior cortex and compressive stress in the posterior cortex. It will be relatively safe to drill a

hole for a bone screw on the lateral aspect, because this is on the neutral axis of bending, but much less advisable on the anterior aspect. This is only a hypothetical case, but the surgeon should be aware of this consideration when thinking about fixation of bones and the loads envisaged on them.

Torsion of bones. Torsion loading causes the bone to be twisted about its long axis: one end is rotated relative to the other, and a straight longitudinal fibre along one side of the bone will be deformed to take up a spiralling helical path. If two adjacent cross-sections of the bone are considered, and one is rotated relative to the other, corresponding points on the periphery of one will have moved circumferentially relative to the points on the adjacent section. This is a shear deformation, and it induces shear stresses in the bone (*Figure 15.3a*). The relative movement between points on the central axis is zero, so no shear stress is induced here, but the relative displacement increases with the radius from the axis, and so, too, do the shear deformations and shear stresses. Thus, the most highly stressed region is at the bone surface. This line of reasoning is exactly analogous to that already gone through for bending, and again it can be seen that a given fibre of bone will resist torsion best if it is positioned away from the central axis, so that it can have the best possible lever arm about the axis. It follows that the most efficient bone material distribution is as a tube, as we observe in nature.

The ability of a given cross-section to resist torsion depends on the geometry, and is expressed in terms of the 'polar moment of area', J, a mathematical term that derives from the distribution of the material away from the centroid axis. For a circular section, J depends on the diameter to the power of four, and the peak shear stress is inversely proportional to the diameter cubed; it is obvious that small changes to the diameter will have a large effect on the strength of a bone. This observation also explains why periosteal callus formation is able to stabilise a fracture of the shaft of a long bone after the deposition of a relatively small quantity of immature bone tissue.

If a bone is loaded until it fails in torsion, the resulting fracture morphology is usually known as a spiral fracture, and this is what occurs in the shaft of the tibia if a ski binding fails to release in a sideways direction. (In this context, the paragraph above explains why a good ski centre will measure the bone diameter when deciding how to set up the bindings for a customer.) Given that it

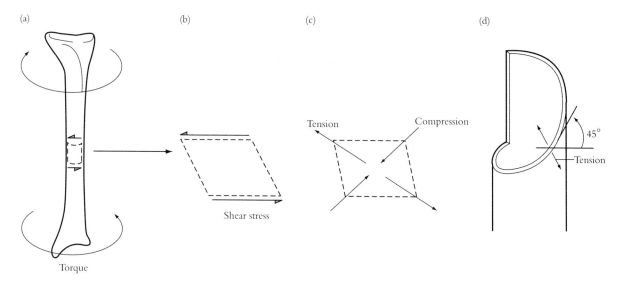

Figure 15.3 Shear of bone. (a) The torque twists the bone, imposing shear stresses on the top and bottom faces of the square element. (b) The shear stress deforms the previously square element. (c) Within the element, the shear deformation induces tensile and compressive stresses at 45° to the long axis. (d) The tension leads to a spiral fracture surface.

has just been shown that torsion induces shear stresses across a cross-section, the spiral fracture needs an explanation, which follows from consideration of the local bone deformation. If a small square element of bone is drawn on the surface, with its sides parallel and perpendicular to the long axis of the bone, and the bone is then twisted, the top surface moves sideways relative to the bottom surface, as explained above, due to the shear forces (*Figure 15.3b*). It is seen that the diagonals become longer and shorter, and this deformation induces tensile and compressive stresses in those directions in the element (*Figure 15.3c*). Thus, the bone sees the peak tensile stress acting in a spiral direction, at approximately 45° to the long axis, and the fracture is perpendicular to this (*Figure 15.3d*). Eventually, the fracture line propagates around the circumference, and the two ends are joined by a longitudinal split, as the circumferential strength is lowest (*Figure 15.3d*).

Investigations of bone torsion in the laboratory have shown that whole long bones can be twisted by approximately 25° before failure; Panjabi et al (1973) tested rabbit and Frankel and Burstein (1965) tested human tibiae. For a thin-walled structure, it can be shown that torsion resistance depends on the area enclosed by the cross-section, and so a tubular structure is very strong in relation to the mass of material. However, if the 'closed section' is converted into an 'open section', perhaps by

means of a saw cut through the cortex, there is a drastic reduction in torsion load capacity: Frankel and Burstein showed that the tibia then failed after only 6° of twist.

Strain rate sensitivity

It was noted above that bone exhibits viscoelastic behaviour, which implies that the properties are different at high and low speeds of testing. This is important, because most fractures *in vivo* will occur at high speed, owing to impacts.

Strain rate effects on the tensile strength of cortical bone were first shown clearly by Wright and Hayes (1976), who found that specimens exhibited plastic deformation at low speeds, but that this did not occur at strain rates above 0.174 per second, when brittle failure was seen at higher stresses. Both the ultimate tensile strength and the apparent modulus of elasticity increased with strain rate (*Figure 15.4*).

The amount of energy needed to cause a bone to fracture can be discerned from a measurement of the area under the stress–strain curve produced in a test to failure, as the energy is effectively a measure of work, which is a product of force and distance. Thus, as the strain rate increases, the height of the approximately triangular area under the graph will increase, as the ultimate tensile stress has been shown to increase. Also, the onset of fracture

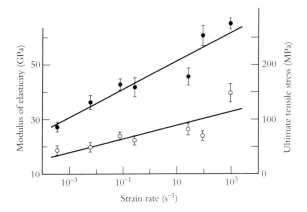

Figure 15.4   Effects of strain rate on the tensile strength (●) and apparent modulus of elasticity (○) of cortical bone. From Wright and Hayes (1976), with permission.

may be delayed slightly, in which case the deformation to fracture will also increase, and these effects combine to raise the amount of energy needed to cause fracture at high speed (*Figure 15.5*).

When investigating the effect of strain rate on torsion failure, Panjabi et al (1973) found that torsion stiffness did

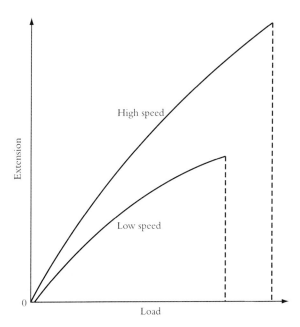

Figure 15.5   Failure energy of a specimen is inferred from the area under the tensile test curve. It is seen that the increases in failure stress and strain with increased strain rate lead to greater fracture energy needed in a high-speed impact. NB: Post-yield behaviour is not shown.

not change over the speed range of 0.003–13.2 radians per second. However, the torque and angle of twist to failure both rose by approximately 33%, and the energy absorbed before fracture rose by 67%.

Typical cortical bone properties

Reilly and Burstein (1974) suggested the use of the following values for calculations of cortical bone strength, which are based on the human femur:

- Yield stress: 100 MPa
- Ultimate tensile stength: 150 MPa
- Strain to failure 0.046 (there is no unit of strain)
- Modulus of elasticity: 14.1 GPa

Yamada's (1970) book contains details of the strength data then known for a number of individual bones, including the upper limb.

Material properties – cancellous bone

Trabecular architecture and function

It has long been realised that the trabeculae of cancellous bone are arranged systematically, and that the appearance is of arrays of bone struts oriented so that they can support the functional joint loads originating from the articular surfaces. The debate on the functionality of bone structure was really stimulated by the treatise on the 'Laws of bone architecture' written by Koch (1917), in which he performed an engineering analysis of the proximal femur and likened it to the design of a type of crane jib then in use, and this led on to analyses of trabeculae following 'stress trajectories', which attempted to prove Wolff's law linking bone structure to function (Murray, 1936).

Cancellous bone strength and energy absorption

Various workers have investigated the proportion of bones' strength that is contributed by the trabeculae. Weaver and Chalmers (1966) found that the cancellous bone inside vertebrae supported around 40% of the load, but suggested that it is probably not very meaningful to examine cancellous bone strength on its own, because it must surely act synergistically with the surrounding cortical shell. They pointed out that the strength of a solid piece of cortical bone beneath joint surfaces would be higher than needed to support the joint forces. Similarly, Hirsch and Brodetti (1956) hollowed out the trabeculae from the proximal femur, and found that the strength fell by only 30%. They, therefore, suggested that the main function was to absorb energy and, noting that some areas may be only 20% osseous tissue, termed the area 'quasi hydrostatic', well adapted for energy absorption.

The mechanism of energy absorption as trabecular bone collapses after yielding in compression was studied by Hayes and Carter (1976). They found that energy and yield strength increased linearly with apparent density, and that yielding occurred at 8% deformation. Post-yield behaviour was shown by scanning electron microscopy of specimens deformed by a range of strains to include buckling and fracture of the trabeculae, which would absorb energy and attenuate stress transmission.

It has been suggested that it is the response of cancellous bone to excessive loads that leads to the progression of osteoarthrotic changes in joints. The hypothesis is that cartilage damage, the initial lesion, allows the underlying subchondral plate to be subjected to stress concentrations, causing cancellous bone deformations that lead to local buckling fractures. As the micro-fractures heal, they do so by accretion of callus, and this thickening leads to increased cancellous bone stiffness. As a result of the increased stiffness, the sclerotic cancellous bone is less able to deform and spread the joint forces, leading to raised cartilage stresses. Thus, a vicious circle is initiated.

A comparison of tensile and compressive failure of cancellous bone by Carter et al (1980) showed that both modes of loading showed similar stiffness before yielding at approximately 6% strain. After this deformation, the bone kept on absorbing energy in compression, as described above, right up to the limit of the experiment at 50% deformation. It was shown that this allowed the bone to absorb more energy than would have been the case for a similar mass of cortical bone tested to fracture. (This principle of absorbing energy by prolonged buckling over large deflections is employed in the 'crumple zones' of motor vehicles to lessen the peak impact force.) However, when Carter and co-workers loaded cancellous bone in tension and the yield point was reached, the trabeculae tore apart, so they could not absorb further energy. Using these results, the authors estimated that a tensile fracture of the patella could be caused by 3 J of

energy, while a 10-mm crush fracture of a lumbar vertebral body would absorb 100 J. Although this difference would be accounted for partly by the difference in the cross-sections of the bones, this observation emphasised that relatively minor trauma can produce avulsion or other tension fractures through cancellous bone. This difference in fracture energy explains a number of clinical observations; at the radial head, for example, most fractures are tensile, with either a segment of the rim detached, or a bursting apart of several fragments, rather than a compressive crushing morphology (Amis and Miller, 1995).

Regional variation of material properties of cancellous bone

Even a cursory look at a radiograph shows marked regional variations in the cancellous bone density, so it is to be expected that there will be marked regional strength variations. This is important for many reasons: knowledge of the link between local bone architecture and loads applied in use will show the directions of forces acting on bone fragments that must be assembled and held together by fracture fixation devices, and knowledge of regional variations, for example across the tibial plateau, will be very useful when deciding on the positions of fixation stems of joint replacements.

At the proximal femur, for example, Brown and Ferguson (1980) examined the compressive strength of the cancellous bone of the head and neck. They found a large variation, with the strongest zone running from the superior aspect of the head across its diameter to the inferior aspect of the neck, corresponding to the radiographic density. The central area of the head required four times the force to crush it than the mean strength. Conversely, in Ward's triangle and in the intertrochanteric region, the strength was significantly lower.

Anisotropy of cancellous bone

The highly directional nature of cancellous bone strength was highlighted by Galante et al (1970), whose tests on fresh human lumbar vertebrae also demonstrated the dependence of strength on density (*Figure 15.6*). The results shown are not surprising, in view of the vertical loads acting between the vertebral endplates, and the associated vertical orientation of much of the trabecular architecture. Thus, although it is possible to relate bone

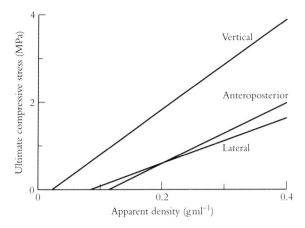

Figure 15.6 Effect of orientation and apparent density on the strength of lumbar vertebral bone. From Galante et al (1970), with permission.

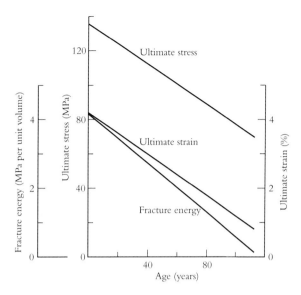

Figure 15.7 Changes in cortical bone properties with ageing. Regression lines from data of McCalden et al (1993), with permission.

strength to density (Rice et al, 1988), and this may be assessed *in vivo* by means of radiography or dual-energy X-ray absorption (DEXA) scanning, the highly anisotropic nature of cancellous bone means that the strength in a functional direction, aligned with the trabeculae, may be much greater than suggested from the global non-directional 'apparent density' assessment.

OSTEOPOROSIS: EFFECTS OF AGEING OR DISUSE

The chronic loss of bone material that accompanies ageing, particularly in females, is a major clinical problem. Not only is there the morbidity associated with the fractures that occur, but the weakened bone structure makes it even more challenging when attempting to obtain secure fracture fixation.

For cortical bone, the situation in ageing males is rather different to that in females, regarding both the tissue itself and the whole bone. For the tissue itself, McCalden et al (1993) found that the material of the human femoral cortex lost strength with increasing age, with ultimate stress, ultimate strain and energy absorption reducing by 5, 9 and 12% per decade, respectively. It was shown that increasing porosity of the bone accounted for 76% of these changes, and that microstructural changes, which might be expected to relate to changes in collagen or bone mineral particle morphology, correlated with por-

osity and thus had little independent effect. The magnitude of these changes with ageing are shown in *Figure 15.7*. When the increasing porosity with age was examined, it was found that female bones became porous at a significantly greater rate than male bones. Contrary to what might be expected, there was no significant change in mineralisation with age, and no correlation of mineralisation with changes in bone strength could be demonstrated across the population.

For the whole bone, Martin and Atkinson (1977) estimated the bending strength of the femur at four locations in 37 bones. They noted the increasing porosity with age in both sexes, but found that in men this was compensated for by an associated increase in the section modulus, which occurred by periosteal bone formation. In women, it was found that the section modulus decreased with age, and was caused by endosteal bone resorption; this effect exacerbated the degeneration of the material itself, leading to greatly reduced strength in old age. The changes in bone inner or outer diameter that produced these compensatory or exacerbating effects were small, but had a large effect, because the stress induced by a given bending moment acting on a circular section beam is inversely proportional to the diameter cubed.

For cancellous bone, Weaver and Chalmers (1966) showed that strength dropped with age in both the calcaneus and lumbar vertebrae. The loss of strength was more profound in women than in men, and was greater in the vertebrae (*Figure 15.8*). It was noted that the loss of strength was disproportionately large in relation to the proportion of bone mass lost, and this effect has been linked to the loss of trabeculae that are oriented perpendicularly to the predominant direction of loading. This occurs because these trabeculae are thinner when the bone is formed, and have a less direct function in supporting the load in use; as they are diminishing, so they lose the ability to stabilise the main trabeculae laterally, which allows the main trabeculae to fail by buckling. The tendency for a strut to buckle is increased by a diminution in cross-section, but is also proportional to the length squared. Thus, the loss of an intermediate stabilising trabecula would double the local distance between lateral supports, thus reducing the buckling load locally by 75%.

FATIGUE FAILURE

If a bone is subjected to a single episode of increasing stress, it will eventually yield and then fracture. It is possible, however, to cause bone fracture by imposing a number of cycles of a smaller load which would not have caused fracture if applied once. This process of damage accumulation is known as fatigue failure, and is well known in steel structures, for example. The situation *in vivo* is more complex than for a steel component, because the accumulation of micro-damage is counteracted by the normal processes of bone healing and remodelling, which may be stimulated particularly by local damage. It follows that the occurrence of fatigue fractures is associated with situations where the bone is subjected to a regime of relatively unremitting accumulation of loading cycles, so that the repair process is overwhelmed, as is the case when the army is 'toughening up' a recruit. In this situation, so-called 'marching fractures' can occur in the metatarsals or tibiae. It is generally the case that there is a relationship between the increasing severity of the loading cycle imposed on a material and the reducing number of load cycles that it can resist before failure, and this is shown in *Figure 15.9*.

Fatigue was studied extensively by Carter et al (1981), who demonstrated different fracture morphologies depending on whether the strain cycle acting on the

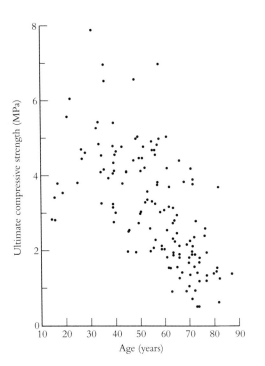

Figure 15.8 Change in vertebral compressive strength with age. From Weaver and Chalmers (1966), with permission.

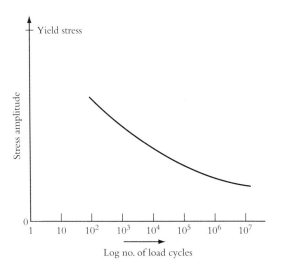

Figure 15.9 As the magnitude of the loading cycle reduces, so the specimen can withstand a greater number of load cycles before failure.

bone was predominantly tensile or compressive. Tensile deformations led to debonding of the cement line boundaries between osteons, whereas compressive fatigue damage was associated with numerous oblique microcracks that were influenced by the stress-concentrating effects of the central lacunae of the osteons. It was suggested that this fracturing morphology led to much greater cellular and vascular damage than occurred for a similar loss of structural integrity under tensile conditions. This observation could relate to the stimulation of bone repair by the cellular interactions in compression, and hence explain why tensile fatigue fractures are known to propagate to complete bone failure more readily than those in zones that are compressed *in vivo*.

EFFECTS OF SURGERY: HOLES AND CUTS IN BONES

Many surgical procedures involve saw cuts or the drilling of holes, which may have screws inserted into them. It is a well-known principle in engineering practice that any sudden change in the cross-section or shape of a uniform load-bearing component leads to localised high stresses, and it is possible to look up tables of stress concentration factors associated with common features. For example, a smooth round hole in a large sheet of material has a stress concentration factor of 3, which means that the stress at the edge of the hole will reach three times the nominal stress.

It is generally the case that the sharper the discontinuity, the greater the effect, and the ends of cracks, which have a geometry approaching an infinitely small radius, are theoretically the cause of nearly infinite stresses in blocks of material under load. This is not actually so, in view of elastic to plastic transitions, which limit the actual stresses at crack tips, but it is usually the case that, once a crack has started, failure can be expected at that site rather than elsewhere. This is complicated in a composite material such as bone, because the inhomogeneity encourages cracks to propagate longitudinally along osteonal boundaries, for example, reflecting the relative weakness in circumferential loading.

In bone, screw holes have their greatest effect in torsion; because tensile loads are carried along the osteonal structures, those near a hole at either side are little affected by direct tensile loads, or by tension induced by bending, as their fibres remain intact. In torsion, however, the shear stresses concentrated at points on the periphery of a drill hole tend to open up cracks between the osteons, and the circumferential strength of cortical bone is relatively low.

Burstein et al (1972) performed experiments on rabbit femora. Insertion of a screw led to a reduction of energy to failure in torsion of 74%. *In vivo*, this effect is usually overcome: if the screw is removed, the hole fills in, whereas if the screw is left *in situ*, the bone adapts to the stress raiser and lays down extra bone around the screw, restoring the intact strength. This effect was also seen by the author in experiments on artificial ligament anchors in sheep: when tested to failure immediately after placing the implants, the bones tended to fracture at the site of the anchor (6 mm diameter), whereas after 6 months or more *in vivo*, radiography showed endosteal bone deposition around the screw holes and there were no fractures at these sites.

If a hole must be made in the shaft of a bone, it is best kept to a rounded shape, and the area enlarged axially rather than circumferentially; sharp corners should *always* be avoided (Clark et al, 1977).

The large reduction of energy absorption before failure caused by screw holes can have dramatic consequences clinically, if the mechanical phenomena are disregarded. One such situation relates to the effect of transverse screws used to provide additional stability to bone fragments around intramedullary fixation devices. This situation is usually safe, but this was not the case for a proximal femoral device intended to stabilise subtrochanteric fractures. To provide rotational stability, a transverse screw was placed across the distal end of the intramedullary stem, at approximately one-third distance down the femoral shaft. Here, the bone was subjected to complex loads involving axial compression, bending and torsion, and the clinical use of this device led to spiral (i.e. torsional) fractures based on the screw hole. This situation was worsened by the screw being at the end of the intramedullary rod, where the stiffness discontinuity would have created additional stresses in bending.

BONE REMODELLING

This is an intriguing aspect of bone biomechanics, relating to the ability of the living bone to respond to the mechanical situation by adapting its structure accordingly. Such phenomena have long been recognised, and are studied routinely in the clinic, as fractures heal by callus formation, which then remodels and gradually diminishes in bulk as the cortical bone strength is re-established. The exact laws governing bone adaptation are not established, but it is generally accepted that bone reacts to disuse by losing material and strength, whereas it reacts to increased loads by hypertrophy. This follows from considerations of Wolff's law, and has been studied in relation to immobilisation after surgery and injury.

A dramatic demonstration of the power of bone remodelling was provided by Goodship et al (1979), who removed the ulnar diaphysis in young pigs. This led to the principal compressive strain in the radial shaft being increased by twice its normal value when walking, which precipitated a profound remodelling reaction. By 3 months after operation, the cross-section of the radius approached that of the radius and ulna combined in the normal limb, and the principal compressive strain was not significantly different to normal.

Although the above experiment was an extreme example, adaptive bone remodelling theory is currently being studied intensely, because it allows prediction of how the skeleton will adapt itself to the changing stresses imposed after an implant has been placed, for example. Thus, the prospect is that this analysis will be able to aid the prosthesis designer in avoiding the more obvious causes of disuse osteoporosis and resorption that can occur around implant fixation stems, due to stress shielding (Huiskes, 1993).

TENDONS AND LIGAMENTS

Structure and function

Ligaments and tendons both function by transmitting tensile forces, and their structures are adapted to that role. As with bone, the dominant tensile load-bearing material is collagen, which is arranged in longitudinal bundles of fibrils that are bound together into collagen fibre bundles by means of a complex mucopolysaccharide ground substance. As the scale of the material hierarchy increases, collagen fibre bundles are seen to be bound together into the orderly structures of the ligaments and tendons. Both structures can have discernible surface layers, which coat the load-bearing fibre bundles

and give coherence to the structure. For tendons, histological analysis of the epitenon layer shows it to contain some collagen, but not arranged into the disciplined lengthwise arrays of the main collagen bundles, and the collagen density is much lower than in the interior of the tendon.

Both tendons and ligaments have structures that vary along their length, both microscopically and on a macro scale, and both are well adapted to transmit forces from the soft tendon or ligament structure into the relatively rigid bone at the attachment site. This is accomplished by means of a multilayer stack of materials of progressively increasing stiffness: the tendon or ligament blends into a fibrocartilagenous layer, which passes through a transition into a mineralised or calcified form as it then approaches the bone itself. Histological examination shows that some collagenous fibres pass through these transitional layers and blend into the collagenous matrix of the bone trabeculae beneath the attachment site; these are usually known as Sharpey's fibres. In some situations, such as the medial collateral ligaments of the knee, the ligament approaches the bone surface tangentially, and so the fibres do not pass through all the transitions into the bone structure. Instead, they blend imperceptibly into the periosteum over a wide area.

These differences in insertion site morphology lead to distinct failure patterns if the structures are overloaded; for a structure that approaches the bone at a large angle, failure often includes a bone avulsion, and this occurs with the flexor digitorum profundus pulling from the distal phalanx in the 'rugby player's finger', which (for reasons unknown) usually affects the ring finger. This failure pattern is not seen in the 'tangential' fibre orientation, where, as might be expected, the failure takes a sliding path, and does not take bone with it.

Tendons, of course, transmit tensile forces from muscles to bones, and so their structures are different at each end. At the proximal origin within the fibres of a muscle, the tendon usually starts as a very thin collagenous sheet, and it is a matter for speculation as to exactly where the tendon starts. As the thin tendon sheet passes distally through the muscle, so it acts as a receptor for an increasing number of muscle fibres, and so, as one might expect, it gradually becomes thicker and/or wider to accommodate the muscle fibres and gain the necessary strength. With a unipennate muscle, the muscle fibres all approach the tendon from one aspect, and so the tendon sheet forms a part of the exterior surface of the muscle.

With bipennate and multipennate muscles, the tendon origins are buried within the muscle belly, and become visible distally only as thick tendons, as they emerge. The main part of the tendon is usually a well-organised and densely packed array of collagen fibres, and these are often seen to be taking a slow spiral path, rather than going in a straight line along the tendon. For the finger flexor tendons, this can be seen to be in the form of two bundles, side by side, which twist in opposite ways. Thus, when loaded, the collagen fibres are pulled closely together by this helical pathway, in the manner of fibres in a rope, thus gripping each other. This mechanism allows load to be transmitted from end to end, even if individual fibres are not long enough to pass from muscle to bone.

The collagen fibre arrangement of ligaments is not as well ordered as in the tendons, and this is discernible on visual examination, particularly for the cruciate ligaments once their synovial covering layer has been removed. This arises because bones that are linked by the two ends of a ligament often move greatly as the joint flexes and extends, and this causes one attachment to rotate relative to the other. Apart from other factors, this means that not all fibres can have the same tension as each other, except at one position, and that the attachments must be able to withstand loads from a range of directions.

These requirements are partly met by the fibre arrangements: they are usually grouped into fibre bundles, which can have distinct functions assigned to them at particular parts of the range of motion, arising from their length change patterns and relative orientations. Further, the cross-sections of ligaments are quite variable. The cruciate ligaments splay out as they approach the bone insertions, thus spreading the load over a large area of the bone; it can be seen that the fibre bundles separate and that there are spaces occupied by synovial tissue or ground substance. It could be hypothesised that the increased ground substance in ligaments, compared with tendons, is a functional response to the shearing actions between the different fibre bundles, as the attachments move relative to each other and different parts of the structure are tensed, acting as a lubricant layer. This splaying out means that there is less collagen per unit cross-section towards the attachments, and that the fibres are not aligned longitudinally. Hence, when loaded, the ligament shows non-uniform elongation, with the central region appearing to be stiffer and less extensible (Butler et al, 1985).

While the internal structures of ligaments are adapted to accommodate relative motions of the fibres across their broad cross-sections, tendons must often move greatly in a longitudinal direction relative to structures surrounding them, and this is allowed by means of a smooth epitenon layer on the tendon surface and other paratendinous layers separated by synovial fluid to form a sheath. Further, tendons must often change direction as joints move and the tendon passes over a pulley-like feature in the surface of a bone, at the dorsum of the wrist or medial malleolus, for example, or is suspended by a fibrous pulley or retinacular structure, as in the finger flexor tendons in their digital canals or at the wrist. Most anatomical texts describe all these areas as being coated by synovial tissue, to provide lubrication, but it is the author's observation that this is often not the case, with the delicate synovial cellular surfaces confined to the non-load-bearing zones. In contrast, the tendons are smooth surfaced and almost acellular for much of their length, and, where they bear against underlying structures, histological examination can reveal chondroid cells in their surfaces. This description accords better with the localised functional demands, as the tendons are relatively avascular in large zones that are distant from the vincula or sheath attachments, and the surfaces are subjected to compressive loading, allied to some shearing loads, during function. This is, of course, akin to articular cartilage, with nutrition by diffusion from synovial fluid.

Mechanical and material properties

As tendons and ligaments function to transmit tensile loads, this is the obvious manner in which to test their mechanical and material properties. This approach will be discussed in general terms first, and then in detail relative to each tissue type.

When a tendon or ligament is loaded in tension, the resulting force–extension graph is similar to that in *Figure 15.10*, in which the length of the curve has been split into a number of different zones of behaviour (Amis, 1985). In zone 1, the structure is seen to elongate easily at low extensions, with small load increments. However, as the elongation increases, so the gradient of the curve steepens, representing a steady increase in the load increment required to produce a given extension increment. In other words, the specimen is getting stiffer. This behaviour in tendons, which have a regular collagen structure, is explainable by reference to the micro-structure of the

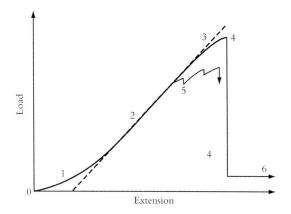

Figure 15.10   Load–extension curve for a ligament or
tendon.

tissue: when they are not under tension, the collagen
fibrils take up a crimped configuration, in which the
fibrils have a zig-zag path. As the tissue is tensed, so the
crimp is straightened out, and the increasing resistance to
elongation reflects this. Adjacent fibrils follow the same
crimp periodicity, and this gives rise to a characteristic
banded pattern when tendon fibres are viewed with
polarised light. When the fibres are loaded, the banded
pattern disappears as the fibres become straight. At this
point, further extension leads to elastic elongation of the
fibres alone, and this marks the transition into zone 2, the
linear elastic region of the graph in *Figure 15.10*. This may
occur at approximately 1% elongation in digital flexor
tendons (Pring et al, 1985).

The initial zone of increasing stiffness, often referred to
as the 'toe' region, is usually larger in ligaments than in
tendons, and may be 5% elongation. This is partly a
reflection of the less orderly arrangement of collagen
fibres in ligaments, but is due more to the fact that, in
most positions, not all of the ligament fibres will be
equally tensed or slack at the start of the test. Thus, as
the test starts to elongate the specimen, the load will be
borne only by the tightest fibres. As the bones move
apart, so those fibres are stretched and more fibres reach
the transition from being slack to resisting tension. This
progressive recruitment of fibres acts to extend the toe
region of the graph, and is believed to represent a means
for cushioning impact loads applied. This mechanism
might act at the knee, for example, when an impact to the
tibia will lead to recruitment of cruciate ligament fibres
(Zavatsky and O'Connor, 1992). This will be discussed in
more detail below.

The elastic behaviour zone (2) eventually blends into a
further zone (3) in which irrecoverable length changes are
imposed. This is seen in *Figure 15.10* as a dropping below
the straight elastic behaviour line. Eventually, damage
accumulates to the point (4) where sudden catastrophic
tensile failure occurs. In general, the failure stress depends
on the density of collagen in the cross-section, and values
of 80 MPa can be reached in digital flexor tendons. Thus,
with a cross-section of approximately 6 × 2 mm, they fail
at about 1 kN (Pring et al, 1985). (For comparison, mild
steel yields at 207 MPa.)

The nature of the microstructural events that take place
during the elongation to failure are rather complicated
and not properly understood, partly because of the nature
of the composite material. Collagenous fibrils embedded
in ground substance are loosely analogous to threads in
treacle, and so it is easy to imagine that the rate at which
deformation occurs will influence their behaviour: there
will be some combination of elasticity displayed by fibre
stretching, but also an effect due to the viscosity of their
surroundings. This is 'viscoelasticity', and it has implications for whether a given deformation may be recovered
fully if applied and released rapidly, before irreversible
slippage has occurred, or whether, at the other extreme,
maintenance of the same peak load for a long time might
lead to gradual creep elongation and rupture. It follows
that a given structure might display a whole range of
deformation graphs, depending on both the speed of
application and the immediate prehistory of loading
events.

This effect is often allowed for when testing ligaments
in the laboratory, when they are usually subjected to a set
of preconditioning load cycles, which do not reach a
damaging level, but take out much of the toe region. As
the cycles run, it is apparent that the hysteresis in the
ligament decreases rapidly, and that the resting length and
stiffness are increased (*Figure 15.11*). This is probably
what athletes do to their ligaments when 'loosening up';
the ligaments will literally be working in a slightly slack
state. This observation implies that athletic activities rely
on coordinated muscle actions to stabilise the joints, and
not the passive ligament tensions, except as 'check reins' if
motion tends to leave a normal envelope. The area
bounded by the hysteresis curve represents energy dissipated as the structure deforms (reflecting viscous
effects), so the structure becomes more efficient, energy-
wise, after 'conditioning': it acts more like a spring, which
stores and releases energy elastically.

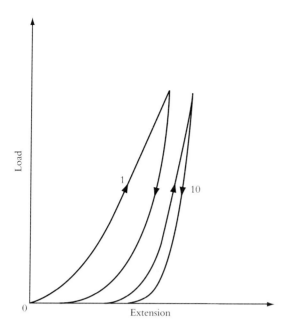

Figure 15.11 Conditioning of ligaments by load cycles, showing the first and tenth load cycles.

Some ligament investigators have described a 'yield point' in the load–extension graph, which is seen to be a sudden drop, or series or small drops, in the graph as ultimate failure occurs see (zone 5 in *Figure 15.10*). This is not a property of the tissue, but a reflection of the test set-up, and relates to a lack of uniformity of fibre tension across the cross-section of the ligament when tested. The drops are caused by sequential localised failures of particular bundles of fibres which have reached their ultimate strain before the rest of the structure. This is not surprising if the geometry of a structure such as a cruciate ligament is considered, which may have a bone attachment 25 mm across, and fibres spreading out to it in a range of directions; some are probably going to be loaded more than others, leading to a progressive tearing failure across the attachment. It has been shown that, by testing functional areas of the posterior cruciate ligament separately, it is possible to avoid these premature failures, and thus approach closer to the true ultimate strength of the structure (Race and Amis, 1994). A linked effect is that the elongation recorded up to the failure point will be lower if the fibres are well aligned when loaded, as a broadly fanned-out ligament will allow some attachment separation by swinging of the fibres, rather than elongation.

Finally, the graph shows another zone (zone 6 in *Figure 15.10*) of low resistance to elongation after the ultimate rupture has occurred. If a ligament is examined in this state, it appears to be intact, and this has caught out many an arthroscopic investigator who did not also pull on the ligament with a hook. The failure mechanism is one of interstitial fibre failures but not of complete lengthwise separation, and zone 6 reflects the viscous load required to cause the fibres to slide past each other before parting company.

Non-uniformity of fibre tension across the ligament is especially marked in the broad cruciate ligaments: when the knee is at full extension, the anterior cruciate ligament (ACL) has all its fibres tight. However, although there is much talk of 'isometricity', which means that the ligament fibres remain at a constant length as the knee flexes, this can be true only at a point; elsewhere, the fibre attachments will effectively circle around the 'isometric' spot as the knee flexes and extends. In the ACL, the isometric area has most frequently been identified at the anteroproximal corner of the femoral attachment (Amis and Zavras, 1995), and this means that the posterior bulk of the ACL swings towards the tibial attachment with knee flexion, thus slackening (*Figure 15.12*). Meanwhile, this leaves the relatively isometric anterior fibres in a state of constant tension. The implication of this observation is that it is the anterior fibres of the ACL that are most important, and which the surgeon should aim to reproduce. This suggestion is supported by the finding that the anterior fibres have superior material properties in both of the cruciates, which might reflect greater duty *in vivo*.

A practical consequence of the lack of uniformity in ligament fibre elongation at certain joint positions is that

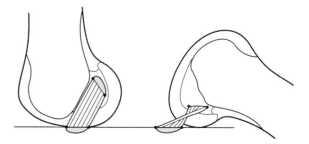

Figure 15.12 The fibres of the anterior cruciate ligament are all tensed at full knee extension, but the posterior fibres slacken as the knee flexes. From Amis and Zavras (1995), with permission.

this can lead to partial ligament ruptures. For the ACL and medial collateral ligament of the knee, for example, an injuring event when the knee is flexed may well rupture the anterior fibres but leave the posterior fibres intact. A corollory of this is that the Lachman sign may be negative (because knee extension will have tightened up the intact posterior fibres) when the anterior drawer test at 90° flexion may be positive, allowing tibial subluxation until the posterior fibres have been tensed.

As some joint positions lead to non-uniform ligament fibre tensions across the width of the structure, it follows also that failure may well occur as a sequential tearing, as noted above, and this is reflected by lower failure loads. For the ACL, the failure strength at 90° flexion may be only 40% of that recorded at full knee extension. Furthermore, the failure mode will vary, with progressive tearing of the femoral attachment at 90° flexion and interstitial fibre failures at a higher load in full extension.

Partial ruptures can also be caused by the spectrum of fibre lengths within a given ligament, and this is clear for the medial collateral ligament of the knee, which has a relatively short group of fibres on the deep aspect, and long superficial fibres, which pass down to the tibial shaft. It is generally the case that ligament fibres will elongate to a strain limit before failure, typically 20–25% elongation. If a valgus injury causes the knee to open medially as in *Figure 15.13*, it can be seen that the deep fibres will be past the point of failure at 30% elongation, whereas the superficial fibres remain intact at 15% (Amis, 1985).

Strain rate effects

It has been noted above that ligaments respond viscoelastically, and this was investigated by Noyes et al (1974). It was found that for a 100-fold increase in test speed, with the higher being representative of trauma, the failure load increased by 21%, extension to failure by 31% and energy to failure by 31%, while a 20% increase in stiffness has also been found for a similar speed range. One side-effect of different injury speeds is that the failure mode may change, although the injury mechanism remains the same. It was shown earlier that bone is more sensitive to strain rate than has just been reported for ligaments. The consequence is that the bone becomes stronger, in relation to the ligament, as the injury speeds up. Thus, a slowly applied force might cause a bone avulsion, whereas a rapid event may lead to ligament fibre failure, and this change was demonstrated clearly by Noyes et al (1974).

Age and disuse effects in ligaments

It is well known that the morphology of ligament tissue changes with ageing: the collagen fibres enlarge, and hence the water content and ground substance diminish. The result of this change is that the material becomes stiffer and fails at a lower strain. This may be magnified by changes in the underlying bone structures, allowing avulsion failure at lower forces. After reaching maturity, further ageing leads to ligament degeneration, which is

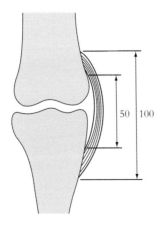 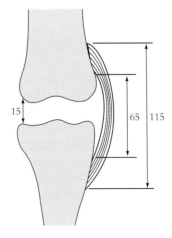

Figure 15.13   The deep fibres are ruptured as the bones move apart, whereas the superficial fibres remain intact, if failure occurs at 20–25% elongation.

reflected by greatly reduced failure strength. Noyes and Grood (1976) investigated the human ACL, and found that specimens from subjects aged 16–26 years were 2.4 times as strong as those from people aged 48–83 years, with the failure mode changing from ligament fibre rupture to bone avulsion. Further work with young specimens (Hollis et al, 1988) showed that the ACL has a mean strength of 2.5 kN in the third decade, with strength falling most rapidly immediately thereafter.

Disuse effects can be as profound as those associated with ageing. Although ligament tissue, being relatively avascular, has a low rate of metabolism, the strength of the construct is also limited by the underlying bone, and this is where the main changes occur. Laros et al (1971) showed that 9 weeks in a plaster cast caused the medial collateral ligament of the canine stifle ('knee') joint to lose 39% of its strength, principally due to subperiosteal bone resorption. Although muscle weight returned to normal by 12–18 weeks after activity recommenced, bone remineralisation was not complete at 24 weeks and ligament strength was still not normal at 30 weeks. This has obvious implications for postoperative rehabilitation.

Joint stabilisation mechanics

Having examined the ligaments as isolated entities, it is appropriate to consider their function as an integral part of the whole joint. In general, the form of the ends of bones is adapted both to carry the compressive joint forces and also to allow such stability as is needed, bearing in mind the ranges of motion at each joint. Because the ligaments are passive structures, they can act only when the bone attachments have moved apart in order to tense them. In part, this can happen as part of normal joint motion, when the joint reaches its limit of any arc of movement, and in other situations the ligament may attach close to a relatively constant axis of rotation, and thus be able to remain at or close to a tensed state throughout. It is not possible for a ligament to undergo any great length change as part of normal joint motion, while remaining tensed, because strains greater than about 5% lead to length changes that require some time in order for the tissue to relax to its original length, or may even be irreversible if too great. Thus, ligament fibres that attach away from the axis of rotation will inevitably become slack for part of the arc of motion. This has already been described with reference to the posterior fibres of the ACL.

Observation of the form of bone ends shows that the ligaments are attached in such a way as to give them the best mechanical advantage: hinge-like joints, such as interphalangeal joints, are widened along the rotation axis, and often have a bicondylar form. Thus, any moment tending to cause a valgus or varus angulation will allow the restraining collateral ligament to function with a large moment arm, normally the distance between the ligament on one side of the joint and the centre of rotation of the opposite condyle. Similarly, joint motion is often limited by a thin capsular sheet of ligamentous tissue and, to obtain the best mechanical advantage, the capsule is forced to bulge over the joint surfaces, again giving a large moment arm. This is the case at the anterior capsule of the elbow, for example.

The width of the joint surfaces, when compared to the diameter of the adjacent bone shaft, also helps the joint to withstand torsion loads. It was shown earlier how bone resists torsion best if it is disposed centrifugally, away from the central rotation axis, and the same is true for the soft tissues that link the bones. Thus, at the knee, it is the collateral and adjacent capsular tissues that resist torsion, and not the cruciates, despite there having been much talk of their role when twisted together – they are simply too close to the axis to act effectively (Amis, 1985), although their tension may restrain the bones from 'climbing uphill' over the tibial spines as they try to rotate.

Primary and secondary ligamentous restraints

The discussion above has concentrated on the primary actions of ligaments about the joints, but they do not act in isolation as the bones are moved relative to each other, so, although there may be a 'primary restraint' against a particular subluxation or deformity, there will often also be 'secondary restraints' acting to resist the same load. This nomenclature has gained most widespread usage at the knee, where there are sufficient ligaments for their actions to duplicate each other to some extent. For example, the ACL is commonly cited as the primary restraint against anterior subluxation of the tibia relative to the femur, whereas the medial collateral ligament (MCL) is described as a secondary restraint against the same tendency. *Figure 15.14* shows why this is the case: the relatively more efficient orientation of the ACL means that it is elongated to a greater strain, for a given displacement, than is the MCL.

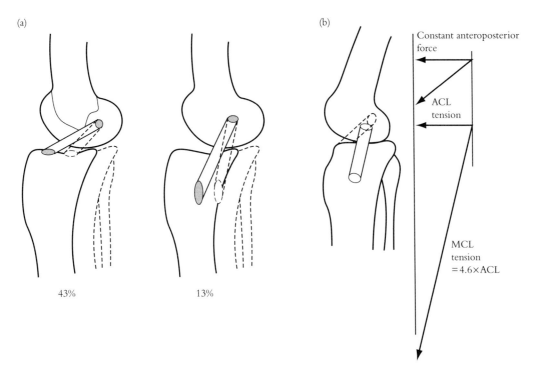

Figure 15.14 Primary and secondary restraints. (a) The anterior cruciate ligament (ACL) is oriented more efficiently to resist the load, and is also stretched by a greater percentage, so the ACL tension builds rapidly; it is thus the primary restraint. (b) In the absence of the primary restraint, the secondary ligament must exert a much larger tension in order to restrain the same anteroposterior force, and this may lead to stretching. MCL, medial collateral ligament.

Given that the ACL is a stronger and stiffer structure, it is clear that the restraining force will build up much more rapidly in the ACL than in the MCL. Further, this is compounded by the ACL having an orientation that allows a large proportion of its tension to resist the subluxation, whereas the MCL acts nearly perpendicularly to the displacement, and is thus relatively inefficient. Consideration of the force vector diagrams shows that the tension in the MCL must be much greater than that in the ACL to resist the same subluxing force, and this explains why secondary restraints may act adequately in the short term, but tend to be stretched with use.

CONCLUSIONS

The overwhelming impression gained from close study of the load-bearing tissues, from the viewpoint of an engineer, is that the body is beautifully adapted to its role. This is apparent from the large-scale shapes of the

bones down to the micro-structure of the tissues, and an understanding of the histology often leads to understanding of the mechanics and failure mechanisms. It has sometimes been the case that surgeons have seen fit to dispose of parts of our load-bearing anatomy, thinking that their role was not important, but study of the biomechanics has led to a greater understanding of their significance. This is exemplified by the menisci, of course, but the lesson is a general one: Wolff's law will be obeyed, it seems, so musculoskeletal tissues are not there unless they have a role to play. It is hoped that some of the thoughts outlined in this chapter will guide future surgeons to a greater appreciation of some of the factors involved.

REFERENCES

Amis AA. The biomechanics of ligaments. In: Jenkins DHR (ed.) *Ligament Injuries and their Treatment.* London: Chapman and Hall, 1985: 3–28.

Amis AA, Miller JH. The mechanisms of elbow fractures: an investigation using impact tests in-vitro. *Injury* 1995; **26**: 163–168.

Amis AA, Zavras TD. Isometricity and graft placement during ACL reconstruction. *The Knee* 1995; **2**: 5–17.

Brown TD, Ferguson AB. Mechanical property distributions in the cancellous bone of the human proximal femur. *Acta Orthop Scand* 1980; **51**: 429–437.

Burstein AH, Currey J, Frankel VH, Heiple KG, Lunseth P, Vessely JC. Bone strength: the effect of screw holes. *J Bone Joint Surg [Am]* 1972; **54A**: 1143–1156.

Butler DL, Grood ES, Noyes FR, Sodd AN. On the interpretation of our anterior cruciate ligament data. *Clin Orthop* 1985; **196**, 26–34.

Carter DR, Schwab GH, Spengler DM. Tensile fracture of cancellous bone. *Acta Orthop Scand* 1980; **51**: 733–741.

Carter DR, Caler WE, Spengler DM, Frankel VH. Fatigue behaviour of adult cortical bone: the influence of mean strain and strain range. *Acta Orthop Scand* 1981; **52**: 481–490.

Clark CR, Morgan C, Sonstegard DA, Matthews LS. The effect of biopsy hole shape and size on bone strength. *J Bone Joint Surg [Am]* 1977; **59A**: 213–217.

Frankel VH, Burstein AH. Load capacity of tubular bone. In: Kenedi RM (ed.) *Biomechanics and Related Bioengineering Topics*. Oxford: Pergamon, 1965: 381–396.

Galante J, Rostoker W, Ray RD. Physical properties of trabecular bone. *Calcified Tissue Research* 1970; **5**: 236–246.

Goodship AE, Lanyon LE, McFie H. Functional adaptation of bone to increased stress. *J Bone Joint Surg [Am]* 1979; **61A**: 539–46.

Hayes WC, Carter DR. Postyield behaviour of subchondral trabecular bone. *J Biomed Mater Res* 1976; **7**: 537–544.

Hirsch C, Brodetti A. The weight bearing capacity of structural elements in femoral necks. *Acta Orthop Scand* 1956; **26**: 15–24.

Hollis JM, Lyon RM, Marcin JP, Horibe S, Lee EB, Woo SL-Y. Effect of age and loading axis on the failure properties of the human ACL. *Translations of the 34th Annual Orthopaedic Research Society Conference* 1988; **13**: 81.

Huiskes R. Stress shielding and bone resorption in THA: clinical versus computer simulation studies. *Acta Orthop Belg* 1993; **59**: 118–129.

Koch JC. Laws of bone architecture. *American Journal of Anatomy* 1917; **21**: 177–298.

Laros GS, Tipton CM, Cooper RR. Influence of physical activity on ligament insertions in the knees of dogs. *J Bone Joint Surg [Am]* 1971; **53A**: 275–286.

Martin RB, Atkinson PJ. Age and sex-related changes in the structure and strength of the human femoral shaft. *J Biomech* 1977; **10**: 223–232.

McCalden RW, McGeough JA, Barker MB, Court-Brown CM. Age-related changes in the tensile properties of cortical bone. The relative importance of changes in porosity, mineralisation and microstructure. *J Bone Joint Surg [Am]* 1993; **75A**: 1193–1205.

Morrison JB. Bioengineering analysis of force actions transmitted by the knee joint. *Biomed Eng* 1968; **3**: 164–170.

Murray PDF. *Bones*. Cambridge: Cambridge University Press, 1936.

Noyes FR, DeLucas JL, Torvik PJ. Biomechanics of anterior cruciate ligament failure; an analysis of strain rate sensitivity and mechanisms of failure in primates. *J Bone Joint Surg [Am]* 1974; **56A**: 236–253.

Noyes FR, Grood ES. The strength of the anterior cruciate ligament in humans and rhesus monkeys: age-related and species-related changes. *J Bone Joint Surg [Am]* 1976; **58A**: 1074–1082.

Panjabi MM, White AA, Southwick WO. Mechanical properties of bone as a function of rate of deformation. *J Bone Joint Surg [Am]* 1973; **55A**: 322–330.

Pope MH, Outwater JO. Mechanical properties of bone as a function of position and orientation. *J Biomech* 1974; **7**: 61–66.

Pring DJ, Amis AA, Coombes RRC. The mechanical properties of human flexor tendons in relation to artificial tendons. *J Hand Surg [Br]* 1985; **10B**: 331–336.

Race A, Amis AA. The mechanical properties of the two bundles of the human posterior cruciate ligament. *J Biomech* 1994; **27**: 13–24.

Reilly DT, Burstein AH. The mechanical properties of cortical bone. *J Bone Joint Surg [Am]* 1974; **56A**: 1001–1022.

Rice JC, Cowin SC, Bowman JA. On the dependence of the elasticity and strength of cancellous bone on apparent density. *J. Biomech* 1988; **21**: 155–168.

Swanson SAV. Biomechanical characteristics of bone. In Kenedi RM (ed.) *Advances in Biomedical Engineering*. New York: Academic Press. 1971: 137–187.

Weaver JK, Chalmers J. Cancellous bone: its strength and changes with ageing and an evaluation of some methods for measuring its mineral content. Part 1: Age changes in cancellous bone. Part 2: Osteoporosis. *J Bone Joint Surg [Am]* 1966; **48A**: 289–308.

Wright TM, Hayes WC. Tensile testing of bone over a wide range of strain rates: effects of strain rate, microstructure and density. *Medical and Biological Engineering* 1976; **14**: 671–679.

Yamada H. *Strength of Biological Materials*. Gaynor Evans (ed.) Baltimore: Williams and Wilkins. 1970.

Zavatsky AB, O'Connor JJ. A model of human knee ligaments in the sagittal plane. Part 2: Fibre recruitment under load. *Proc Inst Mech Eng [H]* 1992; **206**: 135–145.

16

Tribology of Natural and Artificial Joints

John Fisher

INTRODUCTION

Tribology is the study of friction, wear and lubrication which occur when one solid rolls or slides against another. This relative movement of two solids in contact occurs in many areas of engineering, and is an important aspect of biomechanical research into articulating joints. An analysis of the lubrication of normal and abnormal joints, and wear in artificial joints, has provided significant understanding of the mechanical function of joint surfaces and the constraints required in the design of artificial joints. In this chapter the application of the concepts of friction, wear and lubrication to normal and artificial joints will be discussed.

Friction

Friction can be defined as the tangential resistance acting on one solid body sliding over another. Consider the situation illustrated in *Figure 16.1*, in which a body of weight W is resting on a flat horizontal surface. The force required to move the body along the surface is proportional to the weight, and is described by the equation:

$$F = \mu W$$

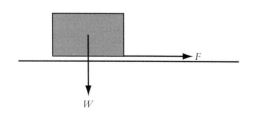

Figure 16.1   Frictional force required to move a body of weight W across a flat horizontal surface.

where the constant of proportionality, μ, is the coefficient of friction.

Frictional forces are caused by many factors at a macroscopic, microscopic and molecular level. Even though surfaces may look smooth, at a microscopic level they will exhibit surface roughness, which will contribute to friction, as will intermolecular attraction and electrostatic effects. Friction is highly dependent on the lubrication regime, with both solid and fluid layers and films between articulating surfaces having a dramatic effect on both friction and wear.

Wear

Wear is defined as the progressive loss of material from the surface of a body due to relative motion at that surface. As with friction, there are many physicochemical processes that lead to surface damage and wear. Abrasion, adhesion, fatigue and corrosion can all contribute to wear. Once the wear process starts to occur, the particles generated by the wear can themselves create surface damage, accelerating the wear rate.

Lubrication

The primary function of a lubricant is to reduce friction, or wear, or both by its application to the surfaces in relative motion. Lubricants may be solid (talcum powder), liquid (engine oil, synovial fluid) or gaseous. In the simplest engineering system, a fluid film of constant viscosity separates two rigid solid surfaces (*Figure 16.2a*). The thickness of the lubricant is sufficient to separate the surfaces, and friction is due to shear of the viscous lubricant. This is called fluid film lubrication.

As the thickness of the lubricating film approaches the dimensions of the surface roughness, then the process of

(a)

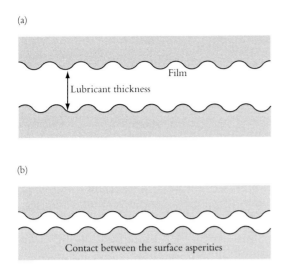

(b)

Figure 16.2   Diagrams showing the separation of two surfaces for (a) fluid film or hydrodynamic lubrication and (b) boundary lubrication.

boundary lubrication starts to occur (*Figure 16.2b*). In this situation, friction depends on the chemical properties of the surfaces and the mechanical nature of the interface. Articular cartilage surfaces are much more complex than most engineering systems, as the viscosity of synovial fluid is a function of shear rate, articular surfaces are not rigid, and cartilage is itself permeable to small molecules in the synovial fluid.

NATURAL SYNOVIAL JOINTS

Tribology of natural synovial joints has been studied extensively over the past 30 years. The tribological requirements for the natural joints are extremely demanding. In the lower limb, loads of up to four times body-weight are transmitted through the joints during normal walking, and even higher loads are experienced during running, jumping or climbing stairs. The loading regimes are complex, motions are highly variable, duty cycles are demanding and the life expectancy is greater than 70 years or 100 million cycles. It is therefore not surprising that the tribological design of the natural synovial joint is very sophisticated and it has taken extensive fundamental research to understand the func-

tion of the normal synovial joint, let alone its disease processes and states.

The main elements that influence the tribological function of the natural joints are the articular cartilage (and in the knee the menisci) and the synovial fluid. Other components, such as the subchondral bone, the synovial capsule, and the soft tissues and ligaments, may also directly influence the tribological conditions, particularly with respect to load-bearing and kinematics or motion. The loading patterns in the hip and knee were described extensively in research by Paul and co-workers during the 1960s and 1970s (Paul, 1967).

In the hip, the loading pattern during the stance phase of the walking cycle has two peaks, one at heel strike and one at toe-off, where the load typically reaches four times body-weight, and in between the peaks the loading drops to approximately twice body-weight. The peaks are associated with inertial forces, that is acceleration and deceleration of the body segments, as well as static forces. The static forces alone, which can be determined during a one-leg stance, are twice body-weight, owing to the moments involved in the lever actions of the muscle forces about the joint which are necessary to counteract and the forces associated with the body masses. During the swing phase of walking, the forces across the joints are much smaller, and are often quoted in the range 60–100 N, that is about 10% of body-weight.

The force fields during a simple activity like walking are extremely complex, three dimensional and time dependent in nature, and clearly vary considerably as the speed of walking, stride length and gait alter. Paul (1967) also defined the complex three-dimensional motions in the hip and knee during walking in terms of flexion–extension, abduction–abduction and rotation. The main articulation during walking comes from flexion–extension, with an angular motion of between 45° and 60° per stride, which can result in average sliding velocities at the hip of up to $50 \, \mathrm{mm \, s^{-1}}$ with peak values of two to three times that value.

In the knee, the motions are more complex, with the femoral component initially rolling over the tibial component at the start of flexion, which results in translation of the centre of rotation and then subsequently the femoral component rotates about a fixed point and slides over the tibial component. The exact combinations of these motions are controlled by the ligaments. In both the hip and the knee, the combination of complex motions and a three-dimensional force field, which varies both spatially and temporally, means that the actual contact zone between the two articulating surfaces (femoral head–acetabular cup or femoral condyles–tibia) varies during the activity. This clearly has a significant influence on the tribological conditions at the articulating surfaces.

The durability of the natural joint depends primarily on its ability to transmit these loads and also to articulate with low levels of friction and wear. The mechanical properties of the articular cartilage – the synovial fluid, the lubrication regimes and the friction, which are key determinants of the tribological function – are described in detail in the following sections.

ARTICULAR CARTILAGE

The elasticity or compliance of articular cartilage and its ability to deform and transmit loads with relatively low levels of stress is one of its most important and often frequently overlooked properties. The geometry of articulating surfaces in natural joints in the body cannot be perfectly conforming (or matching) owing to the complexity and range of movements that are required. When two non-conforming surfaces come into contact they touch at a point or over a very small area. If the articular cartilage were stiff like cortical bone, it would not deform much and the loads would be transmitted over small areas resulting in very high levels of stress.

The elasticity of cartilage (modulus of elasticity in the range 2–20 MPa) allows the material to deform as the load applied across the joint increases, and hence the stress level remains relatively low. For example, in the hip at peak load during walking (2500 N) the contact area may increase to greater than 500 mm^2, resulting in average stresses of less than 5 MPa.

It is important to recognise that a thin layer of articular cartilage which is 2–4 mm thick could not support this level of stress level on its own, as it would deform to extremely high levels of strain which would cause it to fatigue and fail. In the body, the thin cartilage layer is integrated to the subchondral bone, and it is this composite structure of compliant layer integrated to a stiff rigid substrate that enables the loads and stresses to be transmitted.

One simple engineering model that has been used to represent articular cartilage is a thin layer of hard rubber bonded to a stiff substrate. As an increasing load is applied to the rubber, the width of the contact area grows to many times the thickness of the compliant layer, and under these conditions much of the load is transmitted through the compliant layer in a hydrostatic compressive stress field, which is less damaging to the compliant layer. However, there are high levels of shear stress at the interface between the compliant layer and subchondral bone, where the compliant layer is constrained. Furthermore there are high levels of tensile stress at the edge of the contact area close to the surface. Both these shear and tensile stresses are considered potentially damaging to the compliant cartilage. This elastic model is only a simple representation of the much more complex structure and properties of articular cartilage.

Articular cartilage comprises of 80% water with the remaining 20% being made up of a collagen fibre network and proteoglycan matrix. The proteoglycan matrix is highly hydrophilic and is able to retain water in the cartilage and resist the flow of water through the cartilage even under heavy compressive loading. The biphasic nature and properties of articular cartilage have been extensively researched and described by Mow (1986), and these properties have proved to be extremely important, not only in carriage and transmission of load, but also in reducing friction during articulation.

The collagen fibre network forms the core of the solid phase of the cartilage. The fibres run perpendicular to the interface of the subchondral bone, where they become calcified and integrated with the bone. The orientation of the fibres changes as the articulating surface of the cartilage is approached, and close to the surface they run parallel to the surface. The collagen network is thought to have a waviness on the surface with an amplitude of the order of 1–5 μm, with a wavelength of 100 μm. These fibres can sometimes make the surface appear microscopically rough, but this is often as a result of removal of the ground substance and surface layer, which effectively smooths the surface.

The protein or proteoglycan network is integrated with the collagen network and retains the high water content in the cartilage through its biochemical attraction. A simple model has been used to describe how the proteoglycan can attract water into the articular cartilage, swelling it, until the collagen network is in tension and an equilibrium position is reached. Clearly the biomechanical and biochemical interactions of the biphasic cartilage are extremely complex and have been explained in detail by Mow (1986).

When load is applied to biphasic cartilage, for a very short period of time after application of the load, it behaves like a layer of incompressible elastic rubber, that is it deforms by changing its shape. Theoretically this type of deformation occurs instantaneously, but it is often used to describe deformations that occur up to 100 ms after the application of load, as this length of time can be required to measure the deformation practically. This can be described as phase I of the deformation, that of a linear elastic solid.

Some workers have indicated that it is reasonable to use this model for the deformation of cartilage for the periods of loading that occur during normal walking (typically 500 ms), but this is clearly not the case as almost immediately after the load application, fluid starts to flow through the cartilage matrix and the subsequent deformation is controlled by the flow of fluid out of the cartilage. The resistance to flow is controlled by the permeability of the cartilage and the hydrophilicity of the proteoglycan matrix. Hence, the biphasic properties of the cartilage are most important in determining both the deformation of the cartilage and also how the load is carried in cartilage. In the biphasic model of the cartilage, the initial application of load results in a change in shape of the material and also in pressure gradients being set up in the fluid phase of the material; it is these pressure gradients that cause the flow of fluid out of the cartilage resulting in the second phase of deformation.

After the initial application of load, at the start of the second phase of deformation, pressure gradients in the fluid phase are a maximum and the rate of flow of fluid is greatest. At this point it has been shown that a large percentage of the load is carried by the fluid phase of the biphasic cartilage (Wayne, 1995). Hence it has been predicted that the stresses in the solid phase, the collagen fibres, are very different from those predicted by a single solid phase elastic model. As the load continues to be applied, the cartilage continues to deform at an ever-decreasing rate until finally the equilibrium position is reached after 45–60 minutes when no further fluid flow occurs and all the load is carried by the solid matrix (phase III). The importance of the biphasic properties of articulating cartilage in both load carriage and lubrication cannot be over-emphasised.

FRICTION AND LUBRICATION

Lubrication of the articulating cartilage surfaces and the resulting coefficient of friction are very important for the long-term wear and durability of natural synovial joints. Increased levels of the coefficient of friction not only cause surface shearing, damage and fibrillation at the surface, but also markedly alter the overall stress distribution in the cartilage layer, increasing shear stresses at the interface between the cartilage and subchondral bone and also raising the level of tensile stresses in the collagen close to the surface at the edge of the contact. These can all lead to fatigue damage.

It is difficult to know precisely what is an acceptably low value for the coefficient of friction for articular cartilage, as this may depend on many factors. Generally speaking, if the coefficient of friction is below 0.01, the frictional forces are unlikely to cause direct damage, but if the coefficient rises above 0.1 it is likely to play a significant role in deterioration of the cartilage. Many people may suggest that values of friction above 0.02, or 0.05, are potentially damaging to long-term integrity.

There has been a long debate over the past three decades as to the mechanisms of lubrication in natural synovial joints that can produce coefficients of friction less than 0.01. It is now clear that there must be a number of different lubrication mechanisms involved, each providing a different contribution under the various loading conditions (Murakami, 1990). Traditionally engineers have considered both the nature of the lubricant and also the surface topography in order to determine the lubrication mechanics and friction. If the articulating surfaces are separated by a continuous film of lubricant, this is termed fluid film lubrication, and the coefficient of friction, which is generally very low, is determined by the shearing of the fluid film (see *Figure 16.2*). If the fluid film becomes thin, the asperities or peaks on the surface layers break through the film and direct contact between the surface layers occurs and the contact enters the mixed and boundary lubrication regimes. Under these conditions, where the surface comes into direct contact, adhesive friction or deformation friction starts to raise the coefficients of friction, and the material properties and surface chemistries of the materials themselves become important.

In cartilage, where the material has such a high water content, the biphasic properties of the material are also a key element of the lubrication mechanics in the mixed lubrication regime. Furthermore, the biochemical inter-actions and molecular layers that form between the articular cartilage and the synovial fluid are also very important in the boundary lubrication action.

The next four sections explain the various lubrication mechanisms and the contributions they make to reducing friction under different conditions in natural synovial joints.

Elastohydrodynamic fluid film lubrication

In many engineering bearings, friction and wear are kept to very low levels by a continuous film of thick (viscous) lubricant or oil which separates the moving surfaces of the bearings. This is termed fluid film lubrication. To prevent contact between the surfaces, the thickness of the fluid film (h) has to be at least three times the average combined surface roughness (R_a) of the bearing surfaces. It has been proposed that this mechanism can lubricate the natural synovial joint (Unsworth, 1993) and that the film of fluid that separates bearing surfaces is between 0.5 and 2 μm thick and is generated by either squeeze film action or entraining action. Both mechanisms are depen-dent on the viscosity of the synovial fluid, which can vary between 1 and 100 times that of water depending on the hyaluronic acid content and the shear rates. The squeeze film action is important when load is applied during dynamic loading; the viscosity of the lubricant helps to preserve the lubricating film between the surfaces as the two surfaces approach.

Jin et al (1992) have recently predicted that, in the hip, after 0.5 seconds of load, the thickness of the lubricating film is between 0.6 and 2 μm. When relative sliding of the surfaces occurs, then the entraining action can also produce a film of lubricant between the surfaces, and Jin and co-workers (1993) have predicted a film thickness of 0.5–1.8 μm for normal walking in the hip depending on the viscosity of the synovial fluid. Similar values have been predicted in the ankle (Medley et al, 1984).

Both cyclic loading and motion occur during active walking, and these mechanisms may well contribute to reducing friction during this activity by promoting fluid film lubrication. However, the film thicknesses predicted (0.5–2 μm) are similar to the surface roughness of the collagen network on the cartilage surface (1–5 μm) and hence, theoretically, full fluid film lubrication is not expected. However, Dowson and Jin (1986) have pro-posed that the cartilage surface is effectively flattened by microelastohydrodynamic action to preserve the fluid film.

An alternative explanation for preservation of the fluid film comes from more recent analysis of the surfaces of cartilage where the surface layers of proteoglycan and lipids have been preserved and much smaller surface roughness values were indicated. It always has to be recognised that a biological surface-like cartilage will have a degree of waviness even though its actual rough-ness is (R_a) is very small. If elastohydrodynamic fluid film lubrication is effective in the natural synovial joint (and conclusive evidence has still to be obtained for this), it will be effective only during active walking or running under conditions of cyclic loading and high relative sliding velocities. For the remainder of the time (more than 95% of the lifetime) other lubrication mechanisms must protect the articular cartilage surface.

Boosted lubrication

The boosted lubrication of ultrafiltration mechanism was proposed by Walker et al (1968). Essentially this mechan-ism protects the articular cartilage surface by formation of a viscous gel of high molecular weight protein from the synovial fluid. As the lubricating films start to become very thin, the water in the synovial fluid enters the permeable cartilage, leaving behind the hyaluronic acid, and the high molecular weight proteins form a highly viscous lubrication layer. This mechanism may extend the conditions during which the cartilage surfaces remain completely separated by a film of lubricant.

Biphasic lubrication

McCutcheon (1959) proposed that because cartilage had such a high water content it was inherently self-lubricat-ing, and that water could flow from the material to lubricate the surfaces. This was termed 'weeping' lubrica-tion. More recently, this 'weeping' explanation has been questioned as two separate studies have shown a net flow of fluid into the cartilage from the surface film (Mow, 1986; Jin et al, 1992). However, the self-lubricating concept has been developed through the biphasic model (Mow, 1986; Wayne, 1995) and current understanding that the majority of the load is carried in the fluid phase for long periods of time after the application of load has

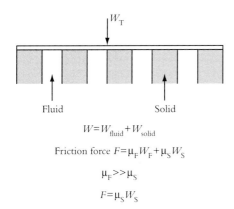

$$W = W_{\text{fluid}} + W_{\text{solid}}$$

Friction force $F = \mu_F W_F + \mu_S W_S$

$$\mu_F \gg \mu_S$$

$$F = \mu_S W_S$$

Figure 16.3   Simple representation of biphasic lubrication in articular cartilage.

recently been reinforced by an extensive study of friction under extended loading periods (Forster et al, 1995).

In this study friction was less than 0.01 after 5 seconds of loading and remained below 0.05 for periods of loading up to 2 minutes, for cases where there was either no surface lubricant, Ringer's solution or synovial fluid on the surface. Furthermore, it showed that if the force vector moved, so moving the area of contact on to a fully hydrated cartilage, friction was again reduced to below 0.01. This experimental study showed that the intrinsic mechanism of the biphasic cartilage can maintain low friction under extreme loading conditions, with limited or no motion. Most importantly, it demonstrated that the biphasic mechanics and properties of the cartilage are likely to play a critical role in the long-term tribology and durability of articular cartilage.

Boundary lubrication

In a number of different parts of the body, phospholipids (Hills and Butler, 1984) or glycoprotein complexes (Linn and Radin, 1968) have been cited as an effective boundary. More recently, both these have also been shown to reduce friction in articular cartilage contacts. However, the relative importance of these boundary layers has still to be quantified, although it is likely that they will become more important after prolonged periods of loading when the reduction in friction by the intrinsic biphasic mechanism is less effective.

LONG-TERM DURABILITY, WEAR, DAMAGE AND DEGENERATION

A good number of clinical studies have reported surface damage and fibrillation as well as defects of the cartilage at the interface with the subchondral bone. Both these could be caused by high levels of friction. Alternative damage or degenerate processes could also produce these effects, which would result in higher friction. A reduction in the viscosity of synovial fluid has been found in patients with both osteoarthritis and rheumatoid arthritis, and is likely to produce less effective elastohydrodynamic film lubrication; but whether this produces a significant increase in degenerative processes is still unclear. Some centres claim that injection of hyaluronic acid to increase the viscosity of the synovial fluid, and perhaps produce beneficial boundary lubrication, produces improved lubrication and lower friction, but the long-term benefits of this type of treatment have still to be proved.

Clearly, what is important in articular cartilage is the intrinsic biphasic lubricating properties; disease or degenerative processes that influence the elasticity, permeability, water content and hydrophilicity are likely to result in increased mechanical damage.

The articular cartilage and synovial joint remains a remarkable articulating bearing surface with low friction and wear, and in many patients extensive and acceptable lifetimes.

TOTAL ARTIFICIAL JOINTS

Total replacement joints have been used successfully in the hip and knee for over 30 years. It is estimated that over 1% of the population of the UK have had a joint replacement. The majority (over 95%) of these joint replacements comprise a highly polished metallic femoral component articulating against an ultra-high molecular weight polyethylene (UHMWPE) acetabular cup or tibial plateau. During the 1980s little attention was paid to the tribological performance of these devices as it was considered that the majority would survive over 20 years without wearing out.

During this period, more concern was expressed about the then perceived causes of loosening such as stress shielding causing bone resorption, cement on bone inter-face failure and the introduction of new bioactive sur-faces. However, it has been widely recognised in the past 5 years that wear debris, and in particular UHMWPE wear particles, are a major cause of osteolysis and loosen-ing of prosthetic devices (Amstutz, 1991). This has led to a renewed interest in the tribology of total artificial joints (Fisher and Dowson, 1991; Fisher, 1994). In particular, factors that can cause increased wear rates in UHMWPE and an increased number of wear particles have been investigated and identified. Alternative bearing surfaces, such as metal on metal, ceramic on ceramic and cushion form bearings, are also being considered. The following three sections deal with tribological considerations of each of these types of bearing.

WEAR OF ULTRA-HIGH MOLECULAR WEIGHT POLYETHYLENE

Total replacement joints manufactured from UHMWPE do not benefit from fluid film lubrication as has been proposed for the natural synovial joint. Under active walking conditions in the artificial hip, the lubricating film thickness is likely to be less than 300 nm, whereas the roughness or waviness of the polyethylene surface is of the order of 1 μm; hence direct contact between the surfaces occurs as the bearing operates in the mixed lubrication regime. This results in the wear of the UHMWPE, and in artificial hips this penetration is typically less than 200 μm per year. Hence the wear life of the polyethylene, which is always thicker than 4 mm, is expected to be greater than 20 years of linear penetration. However, there is currently widespread concern about the effect of polyethylene wear debris producing adverse tissue reactions, bone resorption, and long-term failure and loosening.

Clinical studies show that in cases of severe wear rates, this can occur in under 10 years, while with moderately high wear rates the problem manifests itself in the second decade. Other studies show high clinical success rates, greater than 70%, for hips for implant durations in the range of 15–20 years. Typical average UHMWPE clinical wear rates for hips have been reported as 80 mm^3 per million cycles for 32-mm diameter metallic heads, to 30–40 mm^3 per million cycles for 22-mm diameter metallic

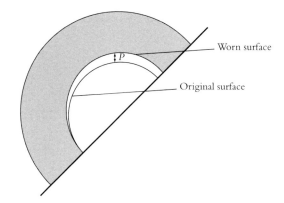

Figure 16.4 Penetration of a femoral stem into an acet-abular cup due to wear at the surface of the cup. P = linear penetration.

heads. In any one clinical group there is a vast range of wear rates, extending from a few millimetres cubed per million cycles to over 200 mm^3 per million cycles. Clinical studies also indicate a 50% reduction in wear rates with the use of alumina ceramic femoral heads compared with metallic femoral heads, although they have been widely used only in the sizes 28 and 32 mm diameter.

In the knee, the clinical prediction of wear rates is less well understood. There have been extensive case study reports of structural fatigue failure and delamination in the first 10 years in knees, and this has resulted in a move towards more conforming designs, less translation of the contact area on the polymer tray, designs that prevent extreme posterior or anterior loading, designs that are more tolerant of surgical misalignment, and an improve-ment of techniques for correct placement. In the absence of this early structural fatigue, many of the more con-forming knee designs are showing high success rates beyond 10 years. In these situations, surface wear and wear debris-induced osteolysis might be expected to play an important role in the second decade of the lifetime of the device, as has been found in hip prostheses.

Much attention has been focused on retrieval analysis of wear particles and retrospective investigation of cellular reactions in retrieved tissues that may have produced osteolysis. In most cases, these are retrospective analysis of failure of designs that predominated during the 1970s and 1980s. The vast majority of these research studies have been carried out in North America. Analysis of poly-ethylene particle distribution using isolation techniques has shown that distributions peak in the size range of

0.5–1 μm, although small differences have been found in studies between different centres.

From these studies, groups have used the mode or the median of the two-dimensional size distribution to predict that the total numbers of particles generated per year are in the range 10^{10} to 10^{12}. Unfortunately, these calculations may be erroneous as they disregard the larger particles that occur extensively and may account for a significant mass of the debris. Most importantly, in presenting only a frequency distribution for the particles, researchers have failed to recognise that this does not give a correct indication of the total number of particles, and therefore cannot be used to predict differences between different designs, materials and clinical outcomes. In general, current studies do not consider that there may well be significant differences in the total numbers of wear particles produced, even though total wear volumes and the modes of the particle size distribution are similar.

Studies of biological reactivity have led to a focus on the smaller particles (around or below 1 μm in size), as they have been found to activate macrophages, which in turn may mediate osteoclast activity to cause bone resorption. Attention has also been focused on the influence of particles on osteoblasts and new bone formation. Furthermore, it is important not to overlook the role of the giant cells and their reaction to larger particles.

The exact biological pathways that can lead to resorption are currently receiving a lot of attention, but the complexity of the *in vivo* situation makes fundamental understanding difficult, and more researchers are turning to the use of *in vitro* cell culture models to investigate these reactions in a more controlled manner. To date, however, little *in vitro* work has been reported using realistic UHMWPE particles. Retrospective analysis of clinical retrievals is extremely useful in defining the problems, but with so many different variables influencing outcome, it is often difficult to establish fundamental knowledge of how different tribological design variables, material combinations and operating conditions influence the important clinical outcome parameters such as wear volume, number of particles, particle size distribution and biological reactions. It is in this area that carefully controlled *in vitro* studies are particularly valuable.

The wear of UHMWPE has been studied extensively in laboratory wear testers and simulations in the past 5 years. Volumetric wear rates have been studied primar-

ily, although researches are now moving towards other outcome parameters such as number of particles.

Two factors have been shown to be particularly important in influencing volumetric wear rates of polyethylene in the hip. They are the counterface topography of the femoral surface and degradation of the polyethylene following irradiation. A fivefold increase in surface roughness of the femoral head or a single 2-μm deep scratch can produce a 30-fold increase in volumetric wear rates. Clinically, metallic heads may be implanted smooth ($R_a < 0.5 \mu$m) but are damaged by third body particles (contaminants) such as bone, bone cement, metallic or hydroxyapatite (HA) particles, resulting in increased long-term wear rates. Alumina ceramic femoral heads are thought to be more resistant to this damage, and this may explain lower clinical long-term wear rates of polyethylene. Zirconia ceramic heads are now being introduced widely as they are tougher than alumina and less likely to fracture; however, their damage resistance has still to be established.

The influence of ageing and degradation following γ irradiation has received a lot of attention in the past 2 years. Degradation of mechanical properties such as ductility and toughness, as a result of oxidative chain scission, increased crystallinity and reduced molecular weight, has been reported widely. In addition, in simple wear tests, immediately irradiated material demonstrates a 50% increase in wear compared with that in non-irradiated material, whereas material that has aged for 5 years after irradiation shows a 300% increase in wear rate compared with non-irradiated material. Degradation and reduction in the fatigue strength of UHMWPE may also be responsible for delamination failures in knees with high contact stresses. Many manufacturers are moving towards inert packaging, sterilisation in inert atmospheres and, in some cases, ceasing to use γ irradiation for sterilisation.

It is interesting to note that, in recently published hip joint simulator studies from Leeds, volumetric wear rates of 25 mm^3 per million cycles were found for 32-mm diameter cups sliding on metallic and zirconia ceramic heads, whereas volumetric wear rates of less than 10 mm^3 per million cycles were found for 22-mm diameter heads. In each case the studies were run in a physiological hip joint simulator in the anatomical position, the head remained undamaged at the end of the test and the polyethylene was not aged or degraded. These findings can be compared with average clinical wear rates of 80 and $40\,mm^3$ per year, respectively for 32- and 22-mm diameter metallic femoral heads where the counterface may have been damaged and polyethylene may have been degraded with age.

It is not known at present what the clinical lifetime of prostheses would be if the polyethylene wear rates clinically were less than $10\,mm^3$ per year. However, these recent laboratory studies indicate that low volumetric wear rates of less than $10\,mm^3$ per year, which corresponds to penetration rates of about $50\,\mu m$ per year for a 22-mm diameter head, could be realised with appropriate designs and material preparation and sterilisation. This may extend the osteolysis free life in hip prostheses to well beyond the second decade.

METAL ON METAL AND CERAMIC ON CERAMIC BEARINGS

There is renewed interest in these alternative bearing materials for the hip. Ceramic–ceramic bearings have been used in a number of centres in Europe (Sedel, 1992), and one centre has reported good 10-year results with wear rates as low as $1\,mm^3$ per year, penetration rates of the order of a few micrometres. However, the success of such bearings is highly dependent on the tribological design, precise manufacturing and extremely good control of the material quality. Furthermore, the designs seem particularly sensitive to accurate surgical placement, with misalignment of the cup causing catastrophic failure. It remains to be seen whether good results from one centre can be repeated elsewhere, or whether the widely experienced early catastrophic failures are the norm.

Metal on metal hip prostheses have also received a lot of attention recently (Muller, 1995). The Sulzer product now has 4–5 years of follow-up in a selected group of patients, and the wear rates are low – 1–$2\,mm^3$ per year. Depending on the reference value taken for polyethylene, this may be between 5 and 50 times less than current prostheses using polyethylene. However, the clinical problem is osteolysis, not volumetric wear rates, and the amount of osteolysis depends on the number of particles, the particle size and reactivity. It is generally accepted that the metal particles are smaller in size than UHMWPE particles, and this may well result in more wear particles per unit wear volume.

As with ceramic–ceramic bearings, the wear rates of metallic–metallic bearings are highly dependent on tribological design and manufacture. Furthermore, the biological reactivity of metallic debris has still to be determined. A number of the particles are in a size range where they will activate macrophages, but the smaller particles of less than 250 nm may well react directly with other cell types and be transported extensively throughout the body. Evidence of metallic particles in lymph nodes has already been reported. If metal on metal bearings are to become more widely used in hip prostheses, the response to metallic debris will become a focus of much research.

FUTURE CONSIDERATIONS, CHALLENGES AND EVALUATION

Tribology of artificial joints is at an interesting and challenging crossroads. One safe and conservative approach is gradually to reduce the wear rate of polyethylene and wear debris-induced osteolysis by using improved designs and materials, building on the broad knowledge that has arisen from recent research and clinical experience. A much more radical and high-risk approach is to utilise alternative materials such as ceramic–ceramic, metal on metal, or compliant cushion form bearings where potential clinical problems may still have to be defined. It may take a further 20 years of clinical practice to determine which of these is the best approach.

The challenge therefore lies not only in producing the technologically advanced solutions and demonstrating their potential benefits through independent laboratory simulations, but in conducting carefully controlled clinical trials with good clinical follow-up, where the complex tribological and biological interactions that lead to osteolysis and failure can be investigated thoroughly.

REFERENCES

Amstutz HC. Mechanical and clinical significance of wear debris induced osteolysis. *Clin Orthop* 1991; **276**: 7–17.

Dowson D, Jin ZM. Micro elastohydrodynamic lubrication in synovial joints. *Engineering in Medicine* 1986; **15**: 63–65.

Fisher J. Wear of ultra high molecular weight polyethylene in total artificial joints. *Current Orthopaedics* 1994; **8**: 164–169.

Fisher J, Dowson D. Tribology of artificial joints. *Proc Inst Mech Eng [H]* 1991; **205H**: 73–79.

Forster H, Fisher J, Dowson D, Wright V. The effect of stationary loading on the friction and boundary lubrication of articular cartilage in the mixed lubrication regime. In: Dowson D, Taylor CM et al (eds) *Lubricants and Lubrication.* Amsterdam: Elsevier, 1995: 71–84.

Hills BA, Butler D. Surfactants identified in synovial fluid and their ability to act as boundary lubricants. *Ann Rheum Dis* 1984; **43**: 641–648.

Jin ZM, Dowson D, Fisher J. The effect of porosity of articular cartilage on the lubrication of a normal hip joint. *Proc Inst Mech Eng [H]* 1992; **206H**: 117–124.

Jin ZM, Dowson D, Fisher J. Fluid film lubrication in natural hip joints. In: *Tribology Series 25. Thin Films in Tribology.* Amsterdam: Elsevier, 1993: 545–555.

Linn FC, Radin EL. Lubrication of animal joints III. *Arthritis Rheum* 1968; **11**: 193–205.

McCutcheon CW. Sponge hydrostatic and weeping bearings. Nature 1959; **184**: 1284–1285.

Medley JB, Dowson D, Wright V. Lubrication models for the human ankle joint. *Engineering in Medicine* 1984; **13**: 137–151.

Mow VC. Biomechanics of articular cartilage. In: Nordin, Frankel (eds) *Basic Biomechanics of the Musculoskeletal System.* London: Leafebeyer, 1986: 31–58.

Muller EM. The benefits of metal on hip replacements. *Clin Orthop* 1995; **311**: 54–59.

Murakami T. The lubrication of natural synovial joints. *Jpn Soc Mech Eng* 1990; **33**: 465–474.

Paul JP. Forces transmitted by joints in human body. *Proc Inst Mech Eng* 1967; **181(3J)**: 8–21.

Sedel L. Ceramic hips. *J Bone Joint Surg* 1992; **74**: 331–332.

Unsworth A. Tribology of human and artificial joints. *Proc Inst Mech Eng [H]* 1993; **205H**: 163–172.

Walker PS, Dowson D, Longfield MD, Wright V. Boosted lubrication in synovial joints. *Ann Rheum Dis* 1968; **27**: 512–520.

Wayne JS. Load partitioning influences the mechanical response of articular cartilage. *Ann Biomed Eng* 1995; **23**: 40–47.

17

Applied Biomechanics of Prosthetic Joint Replacement

Andrew J Forester and Edward RC Draper

INTRODUCTION

Attempts to improve the function of joints following trauma or degenerative changes have received attention from surgeons for many centuries. Treatment with rest and the use of a walking aid remains a mainstay of early management, as does the use of heat or cold, physiotherapy and acupuncture. Surgical treatment by joint debridement treats radiological findings by removal of osteophytes and loose debris in the joint. This often produces some temporary relief of symptoms but fails to address the pathology. Osteotomy has also been used successfully to realign joints in order to transfer load to a relatively undamaged area of the articular surface.

It is from the nineteenth century that the evolution of modern joint replacement may be traced. Resurfacing arthroplasty with fascia lata, split skin and chromicised pig bladder has proved of value. However, the modern era of joint replacement commenced with Sir John Charnley and other pioneering surgeons who developed metal and plastic implants to reconstruct arthritic joints.

Replacement of joints with implants is now very successful, with over 90% of patients receiving hip or knee replacements achieving a good or excellent result. In the more elderly patients, or those with limited functional demands, arthroplasty may be successful for 15–20 years. In patients who are more active, the initial good result may deteriorate with time such that the joint may require revision, which is frequently highly technically demanding.

More recently interest has been concentrated on the resurfacing of the articular surface of joints with 'normal' cartilage, seeking to address the root problem of repairing damaged cartilage.

There is still no consensus on the design of the 'ideal'

prosthesis, and until the recent changes to the regulations controlling the manufacture of medical devices in Europe (Council Directive, 1993) and USA, it was possible to design, manufacture and implant a prosthesis without formal controls.

This chapter aims to describe some of the changes in stresses that joint replacement generates and to discuss the accumulated literature concerning many of the controversies in prosthetic joint replacement. It deals largely with hip and knee replacement, and to a lesser extent shoulder and elbow replacement. For information concerning the replacement of the joints of the hand or wrist, which are beyond the scope of this text, the reader should consult one of the standard textbooks on the subject. Replacement of the ankle joint should be considered as being experimental until results of good long-term prospective trials of the available prostheses have been published.

General considerations

Prosthetic joint replacement alters the magnitude and direction of stresses applied to the joint. Knowledge of these is essential if catastrophic failure is to be avoided. Normal joint function demonstrates that trabeculae are aligned to resist the maximum stresses and that lubrication maintains a low frictional resistance. However, prosthetic joints are only minimally compliant compared with normal joints and therefore stresses are transmitted directly to the tissue interfaces.

Fixation

Anchorage to the skeleton should be as rigid as possible to ensure that the result will be pain free. Although there has been a vogue for the use of uncemented components, the 'gold standard' remains fixation with polymethylmetha-crylate bone cement, which acts as a grout. Numerous techniques have been described to improve the mechanical characteristics of bone cement and to ensure an even cement mantle. Cement stresses will be higher with a thin mantle and, if incomplete, may lead to failure.

Variables

It is important to remember that in any joint replacement surgery the key variables are dependent on:

- Prosthesis geometry
- Choice of material
- Operative procedure

HIP REPLACEMENT

Historical perspective

The first total hip replacement was performed by Gluck in 1890 using ivory, holding the prosthesis in place with glue. Delbet, in 1919, used a rubber component but these early attempts were unsuccessful. However, in 1939 Smith-Petersen described an interpositional (mould) arthroplasty. Initially this was made of glass, but he modified this over a period of time to celluloid, Pyrex, Bakelite and finally Vitallium. Progress through the late 1930s and 1940s was rapid, with McKee and Watson-Farrar (1966) describing a metal-on-metal hip and Charnley (1967) a metallic femoral component and a low-friction high molecular weight polyethylene acetabular cup. Charnley used polymethylmethacrylate for fixation of his components, and it is his prosthesis that remains the gold standard in hip replacement. There are now approximately 40 000 total hip replacement operations performed each year in the UK, with the rate of revisions being quoted as between 10 and 15%. Murray et al, in 1995, compared available hip replacements and their clinical performance, and concluded that there is little evidence that newer (and more expensive) implants give better results than the established designs.

Controversies

A number of controversies exist in the design of the femoral implant for hip arthroplasty, such as:

- Stem size and length
- Surface finish
    (a) In cemented components, should this be matt or polished?
    (b) In uncemented components should this be porous coated or hydroxapatite coated?
- Collared or collarless prosthesis?
- Cross-section of femoral prosthesis
- Femoral head size
- Modularity
- Femoral neck anteversion
- Choice of material

With the acetabular component controversies include:

- Should a polyethylene component be all polyethylene or metal backed?
- Thickness of polyethylene liner/cup
- Methods of fixation

The most important of these factors are addressed in the following section.

Femoral component

Design aspects of femoral components may be conveniently divided into considerations of the head, neck, collar and stem.

Femoral head

Although the surface finish and sphericity of the prosthetic femoral head is important, there are many biomechanical factors that must be considered when choosing a femoral head size in order to obtain a low-friction hip replacement. These include friction, wear, torque, force transmission, range of motion and stability. A variety of femoral head sizes are currently available, with head diameters of 22, 26, 28 and 32 mm. When Charnley designed his hip replacement, he chose a head size of 22 mm as a trade-off between friction (which varies directly with head size) and wear (which varies inversely with head size). It has subsequently been shown that the wear rate of a 22 mm femoral head on high-density polyethylene is greater than that of a 32-mm head. However, because of the increased surface area of the 32-mm cup, the wear debris is in fact greater with the larger head.

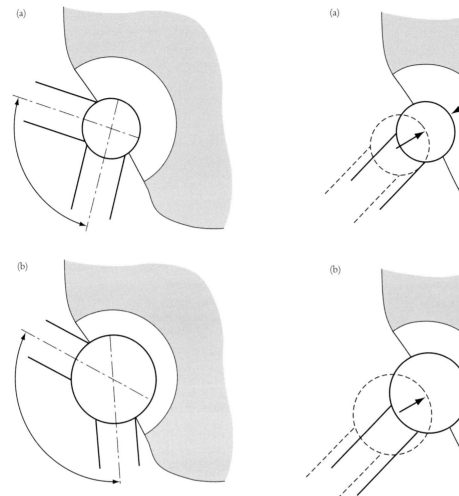

(a)

(b)

Figure 17.1   Greater range of motion is allowed by the use
of a large femoral head.

(a)

(b)

Figure 17.2   Effect of femoral head diameter on the
displacement necessary for dislocation.

Range of motion. Provided the femoral head neck length
remains constant, larger femoral heads provide a potential
greater arc of motion (*Figure 17.1*). However, clinical
data documenting the arc of motion for 22, 28 and 32-
mm femoral components would suggest that the motion
obtained following surgery is essentially the same for all
three, and that it is the preoperative range of motion that
more accurately determines motion following joint
arthroplasty.

Dislocation. For the prosthetic femoral head to dislocate
from a hemispherical acetabular socket, a displacement
must occur that is equal to half the diameter of the head.
Therefore, in theory, the 32-mm implant should provide

greater stability to the replaced joint because 16 mm of
translation is required for dislocation compared with
11 mm for the 22-mm implant, as shown in *Figure 17.2*.
There is no strong evidence to support any advantage of
one head size over the other in clinical trials. The main
variables affecting dislocation are previous surgery, the
choice of surgical approach and, if a trochanteric osteotomy has taken place, non-union of the trochanter.
Clinical work in this field is complicated by the fact that
different prostheses have been studied with various
surgical approaches and, when those variables are taken
into account, there is little to support using a larger
femoral head size.

Transmission of force. Frictional torque is the **indirect** force that is suggested as the main reason for the fatigue loosening of the acetabular component and, although hip arthroplasty with a metal and UHMWPE bearing has been designed as a low-friction implant, the coefficient of friction is still 40 times greater than that in the normal joint.

The frictional torque, F, between the acetabular component and the pelvis in which it is sitting is dependent on the size of the femoral head (r) and the outside diameter of the acetabulum (R), represented in the formula:

$$F = (\mu \times W)\, r/R$$

where W is the overall force experienced at the joint surface of the hip.

To reduce the chance of loosening, it is best that this frictional torque is as low as possible, which can be done by reducing the diameter of the femoral head and increasing the diameter of the acetabular component, as shown in *Figure 17.3*. This has implications for the thickness of the acetabular cup, with a thicker cup being associated with a lower frictional torque. This may also be mimicked by using a thinner acetabular component with a metal backing.

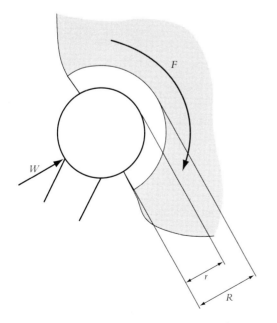

Figure 17.3   Loosening torque on the acetabular component of total hip replacement.

These findings have to be considered against **direct** force transmission, and it has been shown that surface stresses are reduced by increasing the thickness of the polyethylene component to at least 8 mm. These investigations have also demonstrated that there are greater surface stresses with the 22-mm head than for the 28-mm head diameter. Although the surface stresses are important, stress transmission across the joint replacement is an important consideration but is difficult to assess because it is multifactorial. Factors that influence it include the thickness of the cement mantle, thickness of the acetabular component, whether the acetabular component is metal-backed and the quality of the acetabular bone.

At the acetabulum, compressive stresses occur in the mid-portion of the weight-bearing surface of the implant and tensile stresses at the periphery. Thickness of the cement mantle influences bone cement stresses and these decrease as the cement thickness increases from 1 to 5 mm (Carter et al, 1982). A smaller femoral head will allow for a larger thickness of polyethylene, but the effects of a larger femoral head size may be reduced by using a metal-backed component. As the larger 32-mm head size produced a greater stress transmission, and the smaller 22-mm head size causes increased surface stress and wear, experimental evidence would suggest that intermediate femoral head size (26 or 28 mm) may be more favourable.

Friction and wear. Surface finish is important for wear, and current joint replacement implants (metal on polyethylene) are finished to tolerance of approximately $0.02\,\mu$m. These implants have a coefficient of friction (μ_s), in the order of 0.1–0.2, compared with metal-on-metal implants for which the coefficient of friction is approximately three times greater.

Wear volume is proportional to load and sliding distance and represented in the relationship:

$$V = kWL$$

where V is wear volume, k is the coefficient of wear, W is applied load and L is distance. This would suggest that, because the larger femoral head has a greater range of motion, it will generate a greater amount of wear particles as it will travel a proportionally greater distance. The important factors in friction with the metal–polyethylene bearing are diameter of the femoral head, surface finish, sphericity and clearance between the two components. In the laboratory it has been shown that the 28-mm implant shows less wear than either the 22- or 32-mm implant.

Wear debris has become an increasingly important topic in recent years and the biological response to wear debris has been related to an increased incidence of loosening, proximal femoral resorption and lysis. It would seem, both from clinical and theoretical applications, that the 28-mm head size generates less linear wear than the 22-mm head, and less wear volume than the 32-mm size. A 28- or 26-mm femoral head has a similar stability to the 32-mm implant, has less frictional torque than the 32-mm implant, and has a better stress transmission than either the 32- or 22-mm implant. It has more favourable wear characteristics than either the 32- or 22-mm implant.

Femoral neck

The most important features of design of the femoral neck are its geometry, the neck-stem angle, length and the neck-stem offset. Clearly the cross-sectional area of any prosthesis intended as a hip implant must be sufficient to withstand the bending moments that will be applied during walking. It should have a design that will not impinge on the acetabular component, so restricting motion and leading to loosening. Most hip implants currently available have a neck-stem angle of 135° and an average neck length of 35 mm. Most designs incorporate a difference in the neck length, either by providing a range of fixed head prostheses or by being modular in design, allowing appropriate tensioning of the prosthesis. It has become increasingly recognised that it is the balance of the soft tissues and joint arthroplasty that contributes significantly to success, and that appropriate tensioning of the soft tissue envelope at surgery is of paramount importance. It is also important to recognise that, if the neck length is too short, the prosthesis may impinge on the acetabulum or pelvis and dislocation may result as the prosthesis is levered out. This is illustrated in *Figure 17.4*.

The neck offset is important in the design of the prosthesis and is related to the neck-stem angle and neck length, and will affect the mechanical function of the hip (see *Figures 17.5* and *17.6*). If the offset is too small, there will be a reduced moment arm of the hip abductors, and a permanent limp will result. If the offset is too large, there may be an increased bending moment during weight-bearing, which may lead to fatigue fracture.

(a)

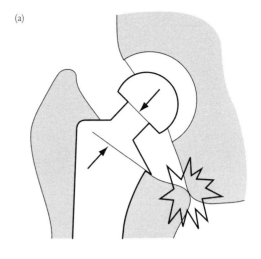

(b)

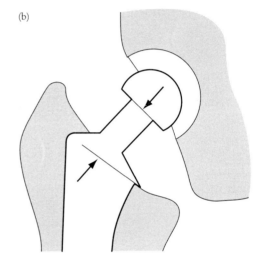

Figure 17.4   Problems of impingement with short femoral necks.

In modular prostheses it is important that the Morse taper is machined to a high specification such that accurate mating is obtained. Some implants include machined ridges on the tapers, which improve the fit with its mating surface. It has been shown that, when the head of the modular prosthesis is fitted to the neck, the two bearing surfaces must be dry or disassociation may occur. Severe wear may occur at the taper, particularly if the manufacturing tolerances are not stringent. It is clearly important to ensure that the materials meet the same specifications for composition and moduli.

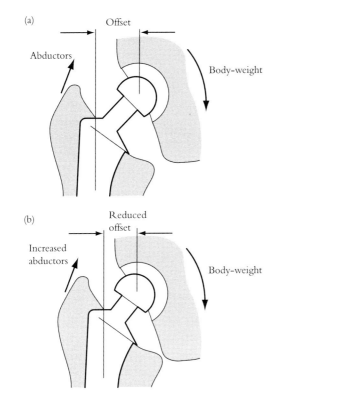

Figure 17.5   Effect of reduced moment arm increases hip abductor forces.

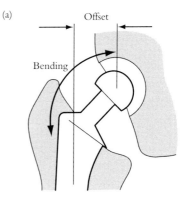

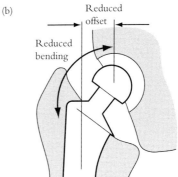

Figure 17.6   Increased bending moment with longer femoral necks.

Femoral collar

The collar has remained a continuing area of controversy (Crowninshield et al, 1981). It has been claimed that in collared prostheses (which are fixed with bone cement) the collar functions to provide some cement pressurisation (although there is little evidence to support this) and to serve as a 'stop' to insertion at the calcar femorale. In addition, it is suggested that the femoral collar allows load transfer through the calcar to the femoral shaft. However, this does not occur if the cement immediately below the collar fails. Instead, the collar may act as a fulcrum for motion of the femoral component producing a 'wind-screen-wiper effect' at the distal part of the prosthesis, leading to failure.

Collarless designs allow a gradual subsidence of the stem, thereby producing a tighter fit within the femur, but are subject to higher hoop stresses (circumferential tensile stresses) in the proximal bone and cement. There is, as yet, no consensus on whether the prosthesis should be collared or collarless.

Femoral stem

The main features of interest in the femoral stem are its material properties, surface finish and geometric parameters, such as its size, length and cross-sectional shape. Early designs utilised a curved femoral stem but these were largely abandoned in favour of a straight stem because an even cement mantle could not be obtained with curved stems, leading to implant loosening. It appears that a straight, slightly tapered, stem is optimal, allowing pressurisation of cement and the maintenance of a uniform cement mantle. In theory, the longer the stem the greater the distribution of load, thereby reducing the stresses within the cement mantle.

For primary total hip replacement a stem length of between 100 and 130 mm seems optimal, as a longer stem leads to higher stresses in the stem with distal stress transfer and stress shielding in the proximal bone, whereas a shorter stem produces high proximal stresses (*Figure 17.7*), which may approach or exceed the tensile strength of the cement and/or bone. Clearly the stem length is not

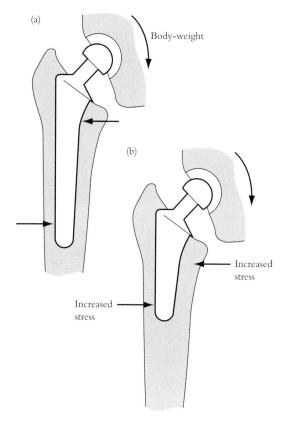

Figure 17.7 Increased proximal stresses due to short femoral stem.

dictated by these factors alone, but by the individual aspects of each case.

The cross-sectional shape of the femoral stem defines its structural qualities, such as strength and stiffness, as well as the material properties of the implant used. The principle of importance with regard to stem cross-section is that sharp corners should be avoided because they produce stress concentrations. Stems with a thick medial aspect produce less compressive stresses in cement, whereas those with more material laterally are more resistant to bending and produce less tensile stress in the cement mantle. For cemented stems, the cement is approximately three times stronger in compression than in tension, and therefore the final cross-section or shape must take this into account.

Material properties of femoral implants

The stiffness of a material is defined by its Young's modulus. For titanium alloys this modulus is approxi-mately half that of steel, but still four times that of cortical bone and 12 times greater than that of bone cement. These more flexible components, such as titanium alloy, tend to transfer load proximally and are probably advan-tageous for femoral components used without cement. For cemented devices, material properties of the bone cement are more important than those of the prosthesis and a more rigid material, such as a cobalt chrome alloy, is used.

Fatigue failure of a component, due to a cyclical loading, is dependent both on implant design and on its material properties. It is important to note that the fatigue strength of implant material may be altered by heating. In particular, preparation of the stem for porous coating may alter its expected performance dramatically.

Fixation of the femoral component

Femoral fixation falls into two general groups: fixation using polymethylmethacrylate bone cement or non-cemented techniques. Traditionally it has been taught that uncemented prostheses are more suitable for younger patients in whom revision may be expected, but clinical experience has not supported this view.

Cemented components. The use of polymethylmethacry-late bone cement as advocated by Charnley has been recognised to be the weak link in the bone–cement–prosthesis composite, because it has unfavourable physical properties (low tensile strength and fatigue strengths), Young's modulus one-third lower than that of cortical bone, and low fracture toughness. Although other poly-mers have been investigated for their potential use in implant fixation, they have been found to have unfavour-able physical or biological properties. Other methods of improving bone cement have been implemented. Low-viscosity cement was introduced to improve cement penetration into trabecular bone, but it has a lower fatigue strength. The addition of carbon fibres to the cement has been tried. While this increases the fatigue strength of the cement and fracture toughness, it increases the viscosity and reduces the penetration into bone. The preparation of bone cement has also been investigated. Vacuum mixing and centrifugation of the cement reduce the porosity and increase the tensile and fatigue strength.

Uncemented components. Uncemented components rely on fixation by filling the femoral canal either by a macrolock or by coating of the femoral stem with beads of metal or ceramic in order to encourage tissue ingrowth. Studies have shown that pore size of between 2 and 400 μm is optimal for ingrowth. However, for this ingrowth to occur, there must be rigid fixation largely to eliminate micro-motion. There have been many reports in the literature detailing the extent of bone ingrowth into porous-coated prostheses. They show that most ingrowth is fibrous. More recent designs have included porous coating only on the proximal portion of the implant, as ingrowth of the distal stem is considered to be undesirable, transferring stress distally under load. There are many areas of controversy in uncemented femoral fixation which will be resolved when the results of further studies are available.

Acetabular component

The design of the acetabular component for hip joint replacement has been a topic of controversy, with most design developments seeking to improve acetabular fixation. Radiographic studies have shown a high incidence of bone cement lucency, ranging from 25 to 100% in long-term studies. For cemented components, the thickness of the polymethylmethacrylate layer and the preparation of the acetabular bed have attracted interest. It has been shown that cement fixation is improved if the subchondral bone plate is preserved. There is evidence that at least 3 mm of cement thickness is needed for cemented metal-backed polyethylene implants. Some manufacturers of prostheses have addressed this by the addition of studs to ensure a reliable cement mantle thickness.

Acetabular design in the normal hip joint

The resulting force from loading is in the mediosuperior direction. The stresses in the normal acetabulum are less on the pelvic aspect than on the acetabular aspect of the bone. It has been shown that cancellous bone does not ideally withstand stresses transmitted from a prosthetic implant and that maintenance of the subchondral bone plate is important. Fixation is improved by using small drill holes to provide fixation for the implant while maintaining the subchondral bone.

Following hip replacement, compressive stresses occur at the apex of the prosthetic implant with tensile forces at the periphery, which may result in buckling of the prosthesis, as shown in *Figure 17.8*. An increased

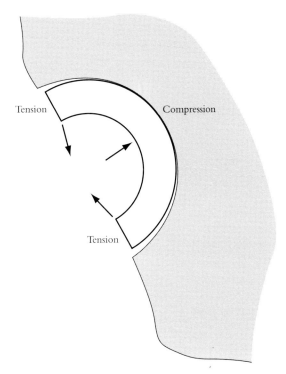

Figure 17.8 Buckling of acetabular component due to compression and tension.

cement mantle reduces these stresses, resulting in less buckling. It has been shown that the stress levels in the subchondral bone increase as the polyethylene implant wall thickness is decreased, and that they are lessened by the use of a metal-backed implant. A metal-backed implant also decreases the stresses in the polymethylmethacrylate, and allows a thinner polyethylene liner to be used.

Uncemented implants

There is little reliable information on the use of uncemented implants. However, the performance of metal-backed prostheses using polymethylmethacrylate appears to apply to uncemented implants as well. In porous-coated implants it has been shown that the proportion of surface area in which bony ingrowth occurs is low and that the majority of fixation is by fibrous tissue. If additional screw fixation is used, then immediate rigidity is ensured. Improved fixation occurs with the use of up to three screws, but the use of further screws does not appear to confer any further benefit.

Studies of porous-coated implants have shown that, if additional screw fixation is used, the greatest areas of bony ingrowth occur at the sites of the screw fixation. Threaded implants have also been used but it has been shown by finite element analysis that loads are concentrated mainly on the first and last threads and that bony ingrowth does not occur in any predictable manner. Technical insertion of these cups may be difficult and, to date, results have been disappointing.

It appears that a metal-backed implant, with a polyethylene liner that is cemented in place with a uniform cement mantle of at least 2–3 mm, offers the optimal features. Preservation of the subchondral bone plate is important, and full bony coverage of the acetabular component is desirable.

KNEE REPLACEMENT

Historical perspective

The idea that function of a joint may be improved by surgical alteration of the articular surfaces has attracted interest since the nineteenth century. Verneuil, in 1860, suggested interposing soft tissues in an attempt to reconstruct the joint surface. Subsequently various materials were tried including chromicised pig bladder, fascia lata, nylon and cellophane, and the search for a resurfacing material continues to this day. Resection arthroplasty enjoyed some popularity around the same period. Unfortunately, this procedure restored range of motion and reduced pain, often at the expense of stability. If insufficient bone was resected, then fusion frequently occurred spontaneously. As a result, these procedures tended to be reserved for salvage procedures in infected and deformed joints.

Interpositional arthroplasty was attempted in a modified form by Campbell (1924) who sought to reproduce in the knee the acceptable results seen at the hip with the mould arthroplasty. This was achieved by use of a femoral mould arthroplasty, but results were not good and this method of treatment has not been widely accepted.

Design of total knee prostheses

Although good functional results have been reported early with fixed hinges and unicompartmental arthroplasty, resurfacing prostheses have produced the most reproducible results. These designs have not been without problems, such as polyethylene wear, deformation of tibial inserts, loosening and instability. In addition, there is a longer learning curve compared with insertion of linked prostheses. Reproducibility is related not just to surgical expertise but also to design and instrumentation. Condylar knee replacement has been developed to include meniscal bearing designs, but these are relatively expensive and have experienced problems of instability and 'meniscal' dislocation.

Modern knee prostheses fall into two general types. They are either surface replacements or constrained designs. Surface replacements are either unicondylar or bicondylar. The bicondylar prosthesis may be subdivided into cruciate retaining, cruciate excising or cruciate substituting. Constrained prostheses may be rigid or loose, the loose prostheses employing a floppy hinge.

Current concepts in condylar prosthetic designs have resulted in only minor differences between various prosthetic implants. Generally the arthroplasty design is dependent on cruciate ligament function, and the design must be more anatomical with a flatter articular surface (*Figure 17.9*). With less constrained influence, geometry becomes less important.

Stresses that result in transfer to the bone–cement interface

An important trade-off in the design of a knee prosthesis is the relative shape of the prosthetic implant: the more congruent the articulation between femoral and tibial components, the lower the stresses on the polyethylene and the lower rate of wear (Bartel et al, 1986). With flatter articular surfaces allowing a greater roll-back, higher stresses are applied to the polyethylene and the cruciate ligaments. It has been argued that the cruciate should be excised to allow a full soft tissue release and exposure of the posterior capsule. Technically it is easier to produce a cut across the top of the tibia, rather than leaving bone around the attachment of the posterior cruciate. However, if insertion of the prosthesis results in a loose joint, posterior subluxation may occur if the posterior cruciate is not present. It has been argued that increased horizontal forces applied to the tibial component following posterior cruciate excision may result in implant loosening.

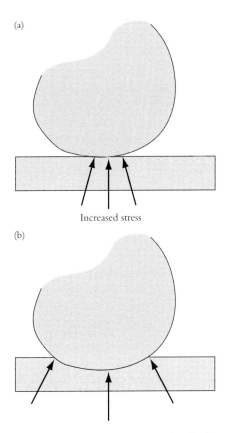

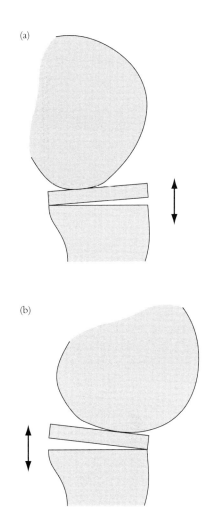

Figure 17.9   Increased stresses within a flat tibial component.

Cruciate retention

Surgeons who support cruciate ligament retention argue
that tension of the posterior cruciate ligament allows
normal rolling and gliding of the femur on the tibia and
that posterior instability does not occur. In addition, it is
argued that the horizontal forces are reduced by the
ligaments rather than transferred to the tibial implant and
the bone–cement interface. Finite element analysis has
suggested that in cruciate sacrificing and substituting
prostheses the stresses during flexion of the knee are less,
particularly when climbing stairs. This results in forward
leaning of the trunk, which is believed to be a compensatory mechanism in the absence of this ligament.

There are difficulties in reproducing the tension in the
original posterior cruciate ligament following prosthetic
joint replacement; if the ligament is too tight it will cause
excess roll-back of the femur, and if it is too loose it will
not function (Andriacchi and Galante, 1988). It has been
shown that reduction in the contact area between the

Figure 17.10   See-saw effect on the tibial component
during flexion–extension of the knee.

femoral and tibial component in posterior cruciate-
retaining prostheses leads to higher surface stresses in the
polyethylene, with increased rates of failure and wear. A
see-saw effect (as shown in *Figure 17.10*) is also seen with
the rolling movement of the femur, which alters point
contact from anterior in extension to posterior in flexion.
This tends to tilt the tibial implant, providing additional
stresses of the bone cement implant and it is considered
that this may cause loosening.

Bone defects

It is common in total knee arthroplasty to encounter
problems with bone deficiency. Cement, cement and
screws, or bone grafts have been used to compensate for

such defects, and bone grafting has traditionally been the method of choice for approaching these problems. More recently, prostheses have been designed with modular wedges and extended intramedullary stems to deal with femoral or tibial bone deficiency. The metal pieces are frequently attached to the implants with screw fixation. However, it has been suggested that metallic debris may occur as a result of micro-motion between the components. This is known as fretting. Although these implants have now entered common usage, long-term follow-up studies are not yet available.

Patella resurfacing

Most surgeons would agree that patella resurfacing is necessary in rheumatoid arthritis, although controversy exists in the treatment of osteoarthritic patients. Most patella components are dome-shaped, which is not ideal because polyethylene shows greater wear when manufactured into a convex surface. Deformation of these components has been common, and has led to the development of oval and sombrero shapes, which appear to be more satisfactory. It is agreed that metal backing of the patella component gives rise to problems, owing to wear of the thin polyethylene component or dissociation from its base (Hsu and Walker, 1989). It is suggested that patella resurfacing should be avoided if the patella articular surface is nearly normal. However, if the patient is obese or if the patella is small or badly destroyed, a prosthetic surface replacement is acceptable.

SHOULDER REPLACEMENT

Historical perspective

Although arthroplasty of the shoulder had been attempted for many years it has been the implant developed by Neer (1955) that has revolutionised shoulder surgery. Initially this proximal humeral replacement was designed for patients who had complex fractures of the head of the humerus, but later experience of arthritic conditions extended its indications. Some further designs involving constrained prostheses of the shoulder have been largely unsuccessful because they appear to over-constrain the shoulder with respect to its normal arcs of motion.

Biomechanics

Difficulties with shoulder arthroplasty have stemmed from the relatively unconstrained design of the normal joint. Biomechanically it is a complex joint which relies on dynamic muscular and ligamentous constraints. It is still poorly understood. It has been suggested that the centre of rotation of the glenohumeral joint is in close proximity (less than 6 mm) to the centre of the humeral head, and that normal motion consists of sliding, rolling and spinning. Spinning should correctly be considered a combination of rolling and sliding.

Motion

The articulating part of the humeral head is approximately one-third that of a sphere, allowing an arc of motion of approximately $150°$. The normal humeral head is somewhat retroverted by $30–40°$, and the articular surface has an upward tilt of $45°$. The humeral head articulates with the glenoid, which has an arc of $75°$ in the frontal plane. There is normally a slight upward tilt and retroversion of the glenoid, but this does not normally pose any significant problem to reconstruction. Motion of the arm involves both glenohumeral and scapulothoracic motion, often known as scapular thoracic rhythm. To achieve maximum arm elevation, external rotation of the humerus is necessary. To replicate normal shoulder motion an implant must replicate normal articular surface curvatures. If, however, the soft tissues are inadequate due to degenerative disease, the implant will be unstable, and in these cases a more constrained prosthesis may be appropriate. This has implications, however, in the type of design that may be used and in the ranges of motion that may be expected.

Constraint

Within the shoulder there are both static and dynamic constraints, with the static elements consisting of the articular surface, capsule and negative pressure. The dynamic stability of the shoulder is important and brought about primarily by the rotator cuff (Reeves et al, 1972). Indeed, even with a deficient rotator cuff and a dynamic imbalance, the activity of the rotator cuff will still tend to centre the humerus on the glenoid surface. Surgically it is important to try to restore the rotator cuff to a normal tension, anteriorly and posteriorly, and for

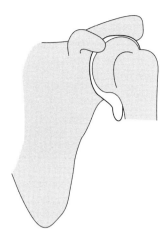

Figure 17.11 Effect of the resultant joint force lying outside the glenoid surface.

there to be appropriate rehabilitation following the surgical procedure.

Forces around the shoulder joint

Forces around the shoulder have been studied extensively and it has been shown that with simple arm elevation a force approximately that of body-weight occurs across the glenohumeral joint at 90° of abduction. Even with a weight as small as 5 kg, this force rises to 2.5 times body-weight, and the force changes depending on the direction of arm elevation. It has been shown that if the resultant vector of force is extrinsic to the glenoid surface (*Figure 17.11*) then the joint is potentially unstable. It has similarly been shown that, should supraspinatus not be working and the deltoid is acting alone to initiate abduction, a poor mechanical advantage results. This demonstrates that it is important to restore the rotator cuff in shoulder surgery. In individuals who have limited abduction of the arm, significant loading occurs at the superior part of the glenoid with associated wear. It has been shown that for every 1 mm increase in component thickness approximately 5% increase in the loosening moment occurs (Walker, 1982). If the radius of curvature of the glenoid component is reduced, this moment decreases proportionately.

Fixation

Glenoid component fixation has remained an area of controversy and it has been shown that the stability of the joint is directly related to the magnitude of axial compression applied (Fukuda et al, 1988). This is greater in more constrained designs, but these designs are also associated with a greater incidence of failure due to surface stresses in the polyethylene. It has been shown that component fixation strength of the glenoid is greatest with a three-pronged implant than with an asymmetrical keel, and that a symmetrical keeled implant has the least resistance to axial displacement.

ELBOW REPLACEMENT

Historical perspective

Coonrad (1982) has described four overlapping eras in elbow replacement, beginning with resection arthroplasty reported by Ollier in 1885 and interpositional arthroplasty as described by Jones in the same year. Interpositional arthroplasty developed to include flaps of muscle, fascia or adipose tissue interposed between the joint surfaces. Other materials were tried, including gold foil, tin, zinc, silicone, linoleum, decalcified bone, chromicised pig's bladder, celluloid and rubber. As a consequence of the rather poor results, elbow arthroplasty moved towards the replacement of one side of the joint or the other. There are occasional reports in the literature from the 1950s and 1960s of some limited success from hinged prostheses, until Dee in 1972 developed a metal-to-metal hinged prosthesis cemented *in situ*.

Lack of understanding of the joint mechanics led to a high rate of failure, and appreciation of the need for biomechanical information about the elbow joint has led to two main types of prosthesis being recognised today. These are the semiconstrained metal-to-polyethylene hinge or snap-fit prostheses and unconstrained metal-to-polyethylene resurfacing prostheses.

Design and biomechanics

In the early 1970s a 25% loosening rate in totally constrained elbow prostheses stimulated interest in the biomechanics of the elbow joint. It has been shown that 2.6 times body-weight may be transmitted across the joint during lifting. Other authors demonstrated that forces across the joint are greater in extension than in flexion, and that there are significant shearing and torsional forces.

The elbow joint possesses two degrees of freedom:

flexion and extension, supination and pronation. The distal end of the humerus through the trochlea and capitellum articulate respectively with the proximal end of the ulna and the head of the radius. The elbow joint has three articulations: radiohumeral, ulnahumeral and radioulna. Generally surgeons consider the elbow joint to be a hinge joint; however, more complex studies show that the elbow does not function simply as a hinge and that position of the axis of flexion alters through the flexion arc. It has been suggested that this motion is in fact helical. Studies have shown that variations of up to 8° in the axis of rotation may occur. These data have supported the development of semiconstrained elbow joint designs and, more recently, it has been shown that the semiconstrained designs closely replicate normal motion. However, for practical purposes, the ulnahumeral joint could be assumed to act as a hinge, except at the extremes of flexion and extension.

Implant selection

Reconstructive surgery at the elbow is now emerging as a suitable primary and secondary salvage procedure for joint disorders. Clearly, the choice of implant is based on the extent and aetiology of the disease process, the needs of the patient and the experience of the surgeon. The aim, along with other implant arthroplasties, is relief of pain. Effectively there are two choices for implant arthroplasty at the elbow joint: firstly, resurfacing implants and, secondly, semiconstrained implants. The potential for instability is higher with the resurfacing implants and loosening is a greater concern with the semiconstrained prosthesis. Both resurfacing and semiconstrained prostheses reduce stresses on the bone–cement interface by allowing more toggle during flexion and extension. It has been shown that to undertake normal activities of daily living a functional arc of motion from 30 to 130° is required with 100° of rotation split between pronation and supination (Morrey et al, 1981).

Total arthroplasty of the elbow has been used with great success in rheumatoid disease, although with the earlier stages of the disease less radical procedures may be required. The use of implant arthroplasty for post-traumatic arthritis has been more controversial because there are higher risks of implant loosening. However, with badly damaged joint surfaces, implant arthroplasty may be a worthwhile option. Clearly if high functional demands are to be placed on the joint, as in younger patients, then joint replacement may not be the procedure of choice and interpositional or distraction arthroplasty may be preferable.

Resurfacing arthroplasty

Design

Resurfacing implants are designed using the ligaments and muscles around the joint to replicate motion that is more normal. The implant surfaces aim in addition to replicate the condylar and sigmoid notch surfaces and contours. Many of these designs involve excision of the radial head, and most involve a metal humeral component and a concave high molecular weight polyethylene component within the sigmoid notch. Although components for the ulna include all polyethylene and metal-backed polyethylene components, it is the metal-backed component that is currently most popular because it seems to reduce cold flow deformation of the polyethylene. Unfortunately, excision of the radial head and loss of the radiocapitellum joint increases the valgus torque on the elbow (Morrey et al, 1991); ideally a resurfacing implant should include radiocapitellum replacement, although experience would suggest that radial head components fail early. Clinically there does not seem to be an advantage to a system that replaces the radial head.

Technical considerations

There have been problems at the elbow joint, particularly with fixation of the components and cement restriction. Cementing techniques at the elbow remain in their infancy.

Complications

Due to the fairly small soft tissue envelope around the elbow there is less protection to a total arthroplasty at this joint than there is in the lower limb and, as a result, complications in the total replacement of the elbow have been higher than at other major joints (Morrey and Bryan, 1982). These have included dislocations, infections, malalignments, component failure, neurological damage and disruption of the triceps. Although the results of this procedure approach those of implant arthroplasty elsewhere in the body, it would seem that incremental improvements in design and fixation may allow resurfacing implants to obtain a more optimal result.

Semiconstrained elbow replacement

Design

Semiconstrained elbow replacements give greater joint stability than unconstrained implants. Original hinged implants, which were fully constrained, provided immediate stability but resulted in loosening at the bone–cement interface. This is due to the change in the valgus-carrying angle during normal flexion and extension of the elbow. Semiconstrained designs seek to overcome this by allowing out-of-plane laxity of 8–10° at the articulation to account for varus, valgus and axial rotation whilst conferring a similar degree of stability to more constrained implants (O'Driscoll et al, 1992). Semiconstrained prostheses allow a greater range of motion than unconstrained implants, and permit reconstruction even in the presence of severe destructive arthritis or following trauma.

An optimal elbow prosthesis should aim to replicate as accurately as possible the axis of rotation, and the surgical technique should preserve as far as possible the soft tissue ligamentous constraints. Biomechanical studies have suggested that, under load, the resultant joint force at the ulnohumeral joint can range from one to three times body-weight. Flexion strength is maximal at 90° of flexion and minimal when the elbow is fully extended. Failure to appreciate the high loads applied to the elbow joint may have accounted for the high loosening rates in early prostheses, where motion was transferred directly through the joint to the bone–cement interface.

It would appear that intramedullary stem fixation may not be adequate to withstand the stresses generated during normal motion. An anterior flange on the distal part of the humeral component may help to reduce axial rotation and lessen the rate of loosening.

Complications

The out-of-plane laxity of a semiconstrained prosthesis has reduced the rate of loosening. This has been supplemented by the use of injecting systems for cement insertion, which has improved the bone–cement interface. Specifically, wear may occur in the bushing of semiconstrained prostheses, leading to deposition of polyethylene debris. Osteolysis, as seen at the hip, is not seen frequently. Bone resorption may result following loosening or cement fragmentation. The optimal thickness of the cement mantle in the humerus and ulna is not known.

REFERENCES

Andriacchi TP, Galante JO. Retention of the posterior cruciate in total knee arthroplasty. *J Arthroplasty* 1988; **3**(Suppl): S13–19.

Bartel DL, Bicknell VL, Wright TM. The effect of conformity, thickness and material on stresses in ultra-high molecular weight components for total joint replacement. *J Bone Joint Surg [Am]* 1986; **68-A**: 1041–1051.

Campbell WC. Mobilisation of joints with bony ankylosis: an analysis of 110 cases. *JAMA* 1924; **93**: 976–983.

Carter DR, Vasu R, Harris WH. Stress distributions in the acetabular region. II. Effects of cement thickness and metal backing of the total hip acetabular component. *J Biomech* 1982; **15**: 165–170.

Charnley J. Total prosthetic replacement of the hip. *Physiotherapy* 1967; **53**: 407–409.

Coonrad R. History of total elbow arthroplasty. In: Inglis AE (ed.) *Total Joint Replacement of the Upper Extremity*. St Louis: CV Mosby, 1982: 75–90.

Council Directive 93/42/EEC. The Council of the European Communities directive concerning medical devices. *Official Journal of the European Communities* 1993; **L169**: 1–43.

Crowninshield RD, Brand RA, Johnston RC, Pedersen DR. An analysis of femoral prosthesis design: the effects of proximal femur loading. *Ninth Open Scientific Meeting of the Hip Society*. St Louis: CV Mosby, 1981: 111–119.

Fukuda K, Chen CM, Cofield RH, Chao EY. Biomechanical analysis of stability and fixation strength of total shoulder prostheses. *Orthopedics* 1988; **11**: 141–149.

Gluck T. Autoplastik-transplantation implantation von Fremdkorpern. *Klin Wochenschr* 1890; **27**: 421–427.

Hsu HP, Walker PS. Wear and deformation of patellar components in total knee arthroplasty. *Clin Orthop* 1989; **246**: 260–265.

McKee GK, Watson-Farrar J. Replacement of arthritic hips by the McKee–Farrar prosthesis. *J Bone Joint Surgery* 1966; **48B**: 245–259.

Morrey BF, Bryan RS. Complications after total elbow arthroplasty. *Clin Orthop* 1982; **170**: 204–212.

Morrey BF, Askew LJ, An KN, Chao EY. A biomechanical study of functional elbow motion. *J Bone Joint Surg [Am]* 1981; **63A**: 872.

Morrey BF, An KN, Tanaka S. Valgus instability of the elbow: a definition of primary and secondary constraints. *Clin Orthop* 1991; **265**: 187–195.

Murray DW, Carr AJ, Bulstrode CJ. Which primary total hip replacement? *J Bone Joint Surg [Br]* 1995; **77B**: 520–527.

Neer CS II. Articular replacement for the humeral head. *J Bone Joint Surg [Am]* 1955; **37A**: 215–218.

O'Driscoll SW, An KN, Korinek S, Morrey BF. Kinematics of semi-constrained total elbow arthroplasty. *J Bone Joint Surg [Br]* 1992; **74B**: 297–299.

Reeves B, Jobbins B, Flowers M. Biomechanical problems in the development of a total shoulder endoprosthesis. *J Bone Joint Surg [Br]* 1972; **54B**: 193-197.

Smith-Petersen MN. Arthroplasty of the hip, a new method. *J Bone Joint Surg [Br]* 1939; **21B**: 269–288.

Verneuil A. De la création d'une fausse articulation par section ou résection partielle de l'os maxillaire inférieur, comme moyen de rémedier a l'ankylose vraie ou fausse de la machoire inférieure. *Arch Gen Med* 1860; **15(series 5)**: 174-181.

Walker PS. Some bioengineering considerations of prosthetic replacement for the glenohumeral joint. In: Inglis AE (ed.) *Symposium on Total Joint Replacement of the Upper Extremity*. St Louis: CV Mosby, 1982: 25.

18

Biomaterials for Orthopaedic Applications

Elizabeth Tanner

INTRODUCTION

The importance of materials to humankind may be seen from the names given to the prehistoric ages. Once our ancestors left their caves the ages were known by the materials that they used – Stone Age, Iron Age. Prehistoric humans initially used materials in their naturally available form, such as flints that could be prepared with sharp edges to make arrow heads, but with time they discovered how to heat and melt metals. This enabled the metals to be cast and then worked and heat treated, improving their mechanical properties from the 'as cast'. This science is known as metallurgy when confined to metals, or materials science when all types of materials are included.

Materials have been used in the human body since the nineteenth century when Gluck (1890) made ivory hip replacements and Parkhill (1897) made his external fracture fixator of silver plated steel. Since then, most orthopaedic implants have been made from either commercially pure titanium or one of three alloys: stainless steel 316L, Co–Cr–Mo alloy or Ti–6Al–4V. These all have substantially higher mechanical properties than the bone that they are replacing or augmenting. Joint replacements are commonly held in bone with bone cement, polymethylmethacrylate, which has lower stiffness and lower fracture toughness than bone, and one of the bearing surfaces is often made from ultra-high molecular weight polyethylene (UHMWPE) with yet lower stiffness. More recently new alloys and composites have been developed with stiffnesses nearer those of bone.

When assessing new materials for use within the body, we need to consider whether they are both biologically and mechanically compatible with the structure that they are supporting or replacing. The biocompatibility requirement is to prevent rejection and the mechanical compatibility requirement is to optimise load transfer between the natural and artificial materials. To understand how artificial materials interact mechanically with natural materials, it is necessary to understand the engineering and biological behaviour of the natural and artificial materials.

The important mechanical properties of materials are the stiffness, known as the Young's modulus, or how much stress is required to produce a given displacement, and the failure behaviour. A material that is loaded to its ultimate, or maximum, strength and then fails immediately is considered to be brittle. However, if on loading a material can reach a stress, the yield stress, where it starts to give or extend for only a small increase in stress, this behaviour is called yield and the material is described as being ductile. If this type of material is used for an implant that is accidentally overloaded, it will bend but not break. A further difference between materials is what happens once a crack starts. Will it go easily through the material or will the material be able to stop the crack? This is called the fracture toughness of the material, and the difference may be seen in a child who undergoes a 'greenstick' fracture where the bone is sufficiently tough to stop the fracture and in an adult's bone.

Engineering terms have been used in this chapter, so a glossary has been included at the end. Some of the references are to books that will expand on the materials science, biomaterials and biomechanics discussed in this chapter, providing further reading.

REPLACEMENT MATERIALS

When considering bone or ligament replacement materials, it is advantageous to have a material that has similar

Table 18.1 Mechanical properties of currently available implant materials and of bone.

Material	E (GPa)	UTS (MPa)	Bend strength (MPa)	K_{IC} (MNm$^{-3/2}$)	G_{IC} (Jm^{-2})	Vicker's hardness	Fatigue limit (MPa)
Alumina	365						
Hydroxyapatite	85	40–100				450	
A–W glass ceramics	118		215	2.0		680	
Tricalcium phosphate	90–120	40–120		1.2			
Bioglass 45S5	30–35		40–60				
Cobalt chromium alloy	230	430–1028					250–670
With porous coating				~100	~50 000		150
Ausentic stainless steel	200	207–1160		~100	~50 000		190–700
Ti–6%Al–4%V	105	780–1050		~80	~10 000		500–625
With porous coating							200
Cortical bone	7–25	50–150		2–12	600–5000	~40	
Cancellous bone	0.1–1.0					~40	
Polymethylmethacrylate (PMMA–bone cement)	3.5	70		1.5	400		
Polyethylene	1	20–30		0.4–4.0	~8.000		
Carbon fibre	200–700	400–5000					

mechanical properties to the materials being replaced (Bonfield, 1987). This prevents high stress concentrations, which occur where load is transferred between two materials with dissimilar mechanical properties because the load transfer occurs over a small area, particularly when subjected to shear stresses (as happens at the interface between a stemmed prosthesis and the supporting bone), and produces a more natural mechanical situation. The materials that are currently available to manufacture orthopaedic implants can be divided into metals, polymers, ceramics and composites (*Table 18.1*).

Metals

A metal consists of atoms arranged in an organised pattern, or crystal structure. With a pure metal all the atoms are identical, but with an alloy some of the atoms are replaced with atoms of a different element. The organised crystal structure continues for a finite distance when the same crystal structure will be encountered, but in a different orientation. Each of these volumes with uniform crystal orientation are called grains; typical grain sizes range from a few micrometres (10^{-6} m) to tens, or occasionally even hundreds, of millimetres

(10^{-3} m). The size and shape of the grains are altered by both working (or deforming) and heat treatment, and have major effects on the failure properties of the metal, with smaller grains usually giving higher strength but not affecting the Young's modulus. Metals, in general, have a high Young's modulus, are tough (that is they are able to resist the growth of microscopic cracks into fractures) and are ductile (that is they have a high extension to failure). This means that they will yield before breaking. They usually have good fatigue resistance: cyclical loads, as produced on a hip replacement during walking, will not produce failure. These properties make metals important for load-bearing applications.

With the exception of commercially pure titanium, pure metals are rarely used, and two or more elements will be alloyed together. In an alloy the mixing is on the atomic scale so that within a grain of stainless steel there will be typically 18% chromium atoms, 6% nickel atoms and the remainder iron and any trace element atoms randomly mixed but in an organised structure (*Figure 18.1*). The alloying atoms may either be substituted into the place normally occupied by the atoms of the main element (substitutional alloying) or, if small, may fit between the larger atoms (interstitial alloying).

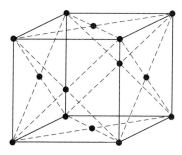

Figure 18.1 Schematic diagram of the face-centred cubic structure of austenite stainless steel used in orthopaedic applications.

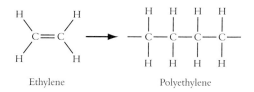

Ethylene   Polyethylene

Figure 18.2 Polymerisation of ethylene to form polyethylene.

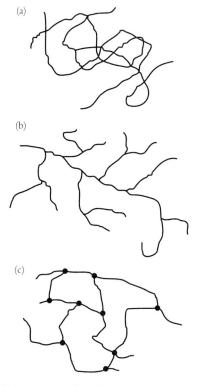

Figure 18.3 Types of polymer chains: (a) linear, (b) branched and (c) cross-linked. From Young (1981) with permission.

Polymers

Polymers have a substantially lower modulus and higher strain to failure than metals, but deform at significantly lower stresses. They are formed of long-chain molecules, produced by polymerisation or the joining of molecules; for example, polyethylene is produced from ethylene molecules (*Figure 18.2*), using the appropriate conditions to initiate the polymerisation and with catalysts to control the rate of polymerisation. Depending on the rate of polymerisation the polymer chains formed may be linear, branched or cross-linked (*Figure 18.3*), so affecting the properties of the polymer. Chain lengths also affect the properties; thus the average molecular weight and its distribution are important (Young, 1981). Typical applications of polymers range from acetabular cups to sutures.

Ceramics

Ceramics, like metals, have an organised crystal structure, but the atoms are different and the atoms of each element have a given position in the crystal structure. Ceramics may have a simple chemical formula like alumina (Al_2O_3) (*Figure 18.4*) or complex like hydroxyapatite ($Ca_{10}(PO_4)_6(OH)_2$). Ceramics can have the highest modulus of all the materials under consideration, reaching 365 GPa for alumina, but are brittle and consequently difficult to manufacture and extremely difficult to shape once manufactured. Being brittle, when ceramics fail they do so catastrophically. Ceramics are now being used for femoral heads and as coatings on implants.

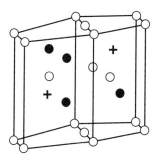

Figure 18.4 Schematic diagram of the closed packed hexagonal structure of alumina showing the oxygen atoms (○), aluminium atoms (●) and the empty holes (+). From Ashby and Jones (1986).

Composites

Composites are mixtures of metals, polymers or ceramics at the microscopic level, as opposed to alloys which are mixtures at the atomic level. By combining the different properties of the different phases the composite can be tailor-made to achieve properties that would not be available from any of the starting materials. Composites can be manufactured on microscopic or relatively macroscopic levels. Micrometer-sized particles of a hard filler in a polymer give a particulate reinforced composite which will have identical mechanical properties in all directions, and the individual microscope particles are not visible to the naked eye. Fibre-reinforced composites use fibres that may be up to several millimetres in diameter and can run the full length of the structure. This will give a material with different mechanical properties when measured along the fibre direction compared with those across it. Fibre-reinforced composites can be used to make light but extremely strong structures with the directions exhibiting maximum stiffness and strength carefully tailored for the application, like the monocoque driver cockpit of a Formula One racing car.

Biological reaction to artificial materials

There are materials properties of interest to materials scientists, other than the stiffness, strength, toughness, fatigue resistance and corrosion resistance, but for orthopaedic applications these are the most important properties (Park and Lakes, 1992). When a material is put into the human body it can provoke one of three types of response: toxic, bioinert or bioactive (Park and Lakes, 1992). Toxic materials provoke an inflammatory or disadvantageous response, resulting in the body trying to reject or remove the material or to isolate it from the body by producing a thick and increasing fibrous capsule around the material. Bioinert materials provide a limited response and a thin fibrous capsule will be formed around the implant. Bioactive materials provoke an advantageous response from the body; the definition of 'advantageous' will depend on the application of the material.

Additionally the reaction of the body to a material will depend on the size and surface texture of the material. Thus polyethylene as an acetabular cup is inert but polyethylene wear debris can lead to osteolysis. We also need to consider the action of the body on the material. In engineering terms the human body is a hostile environment for most materials, being filled with saline solution, which will corrode most metals. The cells within the body will react on any implant placed within the body and infection will alter the pH. The implant material may release materials from itself or it may absorb body fluids, both of which may alter the size and properties of the implant. Some of the responses can be advantageous (e.g. drug release) or disadvantageous (e.g. fluid absorption into the ball of the Starr–Edwards heart valve leading to its failure). Secondly, the forces within the body can be extremely high: in the hip joint, normal walking loads can reach four to five times body-weight and, in the case of a patient who slips or trips, up to nine times body-weight (Bergmann et al, 1993). Additionally, these loads are applied many times a year, in the case of gait up to two million cycles per annum (Wallbridge and Dowson, 1982), while in the cardiovascular system a pulse rate of 60 leads to over 31.5 million cycles per annum. Thus any material implanted into the body has to survive in an extremely hostile environment, compared with many engineering applications, without the opportunity for maintenance.

The specifications for materials for use in orthopaedic implants and the implants themselves are defined by various standardisation organisations; in the UK the British Standards Institution (BSI) defines British Standards (BS), and in the USA the American Society for Testing and Materials (ASTM) produces its own, but virtually identical, set of standards. Within the European Community the standards institutions of the different countries have combined (CEN for non-electrical standards and CENELEC for electrical standards) to produce European Standards (EN) and in most cases the BS and EN standards are identical, although the numbers are different. From January 1995 the CE mark, which may be familiar from children's toys, could be applied to medical implants and it has to be applied from 1998. This certifies that the object has been tested to the appropriate standard, etc. The devices are categorised into one of four classes:

- I – low risk (e.g. walking sticks and first-aid bandages)
- IIa – medium risk, covering most electromedical devices
- IIb – high risk: long-term invasive devices which includes most joint replacement devices
- III – highest risk, which are mainly devices in contact with the central nervous system

For all types of devices post-marketing surveillance is required, with the manufacturer notifying their national authority within 10 days of any serious incidence. The UK system is run by the Medical Devices Agency of the Department of Health.

METALS

The stiffness of metals depends on their chemical composition, but the other mechanical properties depend on metallurgical conditions. The yield stress, ultimate tensile strength and fracture toughness all increase with decreasing grain size and porosity. 'Working', or deliberately deforming a metal beyond yield, can increase the strength, toughness and fatigue resistance but, at the same time, will reduce the strain to failure.

Stainless steel

Considering the metals currently used within the body, stainless steel is ten times as stiff as bone, is highly ductile, has good fatigue resistance and is tough. Stainless steel for medical applications is normally 18% chromium, 13% nickel, 2.5% molybdenum, all by weight, and the remainder is iron, with various contaminant levels permitted but all being less than 1%.

Owing to the nickel content, stainless steel is not suitable for patients with nickel sensitivity. It is reasonably corrosion resistant, although potential exists for crevice corrosion to occur between screws and the plate in internal fixation. Stainless steel has the advantage for internal fixation plates of being ductile, that is it may be plastically deformed (shaped) relatively easily in theatre without too deleterious long-term effects on its mechanical properties. Additionally, being ductile, it may be 'cold worked', increasing its yield stress and ultimate tensile strength. Its fatigue properties are reasonably good, although fatigue fractures were sometimes seen with the early Charnley prostheses. In these prostheses the lateral aspect of the implant was flat and anteroposterior loads, as occur in rising from a seat or walking up or down stairs, resulted in a torsion load to the stem of the prosthesis. With the flat-backed prosthesis this torque, particularly if the proximal cement had loosened, led to a stress concentration on the anterior–lateral corner of the prosthesis, initiating a crack that propagated through the implant. When the lateral aspect was curved, this stress concentration did not occur (Charnley, 1975). The British Standard for stainless steel for orthopaedic use is BS 7252 part 1 whereas the ASTM standards are F55-82 and F56-82 depending on the shape in which the material is supplied.

Titanium and titanium alloys

Commercially pure titanium, that is titanium which is over 99% pure, is corrosion resistant, has a lower Young's modulus (approximately half that of steel), but has a lower fatigue resistance. Similarly the alloy Ti–6%Al–4%V, which was originally developed for the aerospace industry, has a low modulus, is reasonably corrosion resistant, has higher strength than commercially pure titanium and can be used in a variety of engineering applications. Both of these materials, however, are very notch sensitive: although the fatigue resistance is adequate for orthopaedic applications, when notched the fatigue strength is substantially reduced.

Yue et al (1984) considered the effect of applying a Ti–6%Al–4%V porous coating on to the same material core, by sintering at 1250°C for 3 hours in a vacuum, on the fatigue life of hour-glass-shaped rotating–bending–fatigue test specimens manufactured according to ASTM E-466. Whereas the Ti–6%Al–4%V alloy has a fatigue limit of approximately 625 MPa (that is the stress below which the material may be cycled continuously without breaking), the effect of the porous coating was to reduce this to approximately 200 MPa. This was due to fractures initiating at the junction between the porous coating and the core material growing into the bulk material.

Thus the use of these materials as the structural element of an implant that is subsequently porous coated is potentially problematic but careful heat treatment can prevent most of these problems. Also, care should be taken not to produce notches in the implants during surgery. Titanium and titanium alloys, being relatively soft materials, produce a large amount of wear debris, and these wear particles appear black within the body. Wear particles are considered to be a potential cause of implant loosening and are discussed later in this chapter.

The standards for commercially pure titanium are BS 5272 part 2 and ASTM F67-88, whereas those for the alloy are BS 5272 part 3 and ASTM F136-84.

Cobalt–chromium–molybdenum (Co–Cr–Mo) alloy

This alloy consists of 27–30% chromium, 5–7% molybdenum and the remainder cobalt, and is also known by its Howmedica trade name of Vitallium. It has a similar Young's modulus to stainless steel (230 GPa versus 210 GPa). The ultimate strength is higher and it has a higher fatigue limit than some stainless steels. The major advantage that Co–Cr–Mo has over stainless steel and titanium alloys is its substantially better wear properties when used as an articulating surface in joint replacement. It also does not contain nickel, which is useful for patients with nickel sensitivity. It is harder and thus more difficult to machine and its constituent elements are more expensive than stainless steel. The standards defining Co–Cr–Mo alloy are BS 7252 part 4 and ASTM F75-87.

CERAMICS

Ceramics used in the body can be divided into two types, the bioinert and the bioactive, based on the body's response to the material. Bioinert ceramics are generally those used within standard engineering applications, and bioactive ceramics are generally based on calcium phosphates.

Bioinert ceramics

The major bioinert ceramics are alumina (Al_2O_3), shown in *Figure 18.4*, and zirconia (ZrO_2). Alumina has been used for the femoral heads and acetabular cups of total hip replacements in Paris since the late 1970s (Sedel et al, 1990). The major problem with alumina is its low fracture strength and fracture toughness. When alumina cups and femoral heads are used, the mating of the two components has to be extremely accurate; to achieve this the cups and the femoral heads are paired at the factory. With poor size matching, catastrophic failure of the cups can occur, particularly with impact loading of the joints. As ceramics have poor tensile properties, care has to be taken with the fit of the femoral head on the trunion, otherwise tensile stresses are set up in the femoral head leading to fracture of the ceramic component.

The fracture toughness of ceramics can be increased substantially by reducing the grain size. Sedel's current implants have grains that are $3.4 \pm 0.8\,\mu$m in diameter,

approximately one-tenth of these used in the early 1970s. This substantially reduced the fracture of the ceramic components. Even so, of the 187 patients in their series, there were two fractures of the socket and three of the femoral head. One of the femoral head fractures was in a case where the surgeon noticed a mismatch between the head and the acetabular component at implantation; another occurred where a 22-mm rather than 32-mm diameter head was used. Sedel concludes that, to prevent femoral head fracture, a minimum head diameter of 32 mm is necessary and, to prevent socket fracture, the minimum outside diameter of the acetabular cup should be 50 mm. Thus ceramic-on-ceramic implants cannot be used in patients with small acetabula.

The other use of bioinert ceramics is as ceramic-on-polyethylene in joint replacements. The smooth surface finish that can be produced on ceramics and their hard surface make them hard-wearing, low friction materials (Dowson, 1989). When wear occurs in ceramics, grains fall out from the surface leaving a gap. However, when wear occurs on metals, particularly third body wear where there is an additional particle between the two surfaces, a track is gouged out. As metals undergo plastic deformation, ridges are produced on either side of the gouge which produce further wear, particularly with multidirectional movement as occurs in hip replacements. Fisher discusses wear on joints in greater detail in Chapter 16. In ceramic-on-polyethylene joints, owing to the lower modulus and potential for creep of the polyethylene, the matching of the two components is not as critical. The other advantage of not having ceramic–ceramic contact is that shock loading is attenuated, reducing the risk of fracture. Zirconia femoral heads, including those toughened with yttria, are starting to be used, as zirconia has higher strength and toughness than alumina. Some of the early zirconia components had radioactive contamination, but this problem has now been solved.

Bioactive ceramics

The bioactive ceramics are the calcium phosphates and related materials, the bioactive glasses. The most commonly used calcium phosphate is hydroxyapatite ($Ca_{10}(PO_4)_6(OH)_2$) (HAP), which has a similar composition to bone mineral, a carbonated form of hydroxyapatite. In HAP the calcium to phosphorus ratio is 1.67, similar to that in bone. Compared with alumina and other engineering ceramics, HAP has a very low strength and toughness (see *Table 18.1*). It is insoluble within body fluids unless the environment is acidic, as within osteoclastic resorption pits. It is rarely used as a bulk material in any weight–bearing application.

Porous HAP is available as synthetically manufactured material, chemically transformed coral or thermally transformed cancellous bone. With a porous graft material the pores need to be open (i.e. interconnecting) to permit bone ingrowth.

Synthetically manufactured porous materials generally need to have low density for open pores to be formed, and low density leads to low strength, compared with the bulk material, in all forms. Coral can be chemically transformed into hydroxyapatite while retaining its natural structure. This requires the choice of a coral with appropriate structural properties of a common variety (i.e. not covered by the Convention on International Trade in Endangered Species (CITES) and obtained from a sea containing low amounts of heavy metal ions. Even with chemical transformation the heavy metal ions will remain in the coral and at hundreds of parts per million can make a normally bioinert or bioactive material incompatible. Thermally transformed cancellous bone will have an appropriate structure and can have reasonable mechanical properties, but these will be extremely dependent on the region of bone from which it is taken (Hing et al, 1995).

All three forms have different structures; all have poor mechanical properties but encourage bone deposition on the HAP surfaces, thus being good graft materials. When first implanted, the grafts must be protected from high stresses until the individual struts have been covered with bone, which reinforces and toughens the brittle ceramic. A use of porous bulk HAP is for the treatment of bone cysts where the space left after the excision of a benign bone cyst is filled with porous HAP to encourage bone regrowth into the space (Inoue et al, 1991).

The major use of HAP is as plasma–sprayed coatings on orthopaedic implants, in particular joint replacements. Bone bonds to a bioactive coating provided there is limited motion at the interface. HAP is normally used as a thin layer, approximately $50 \mu m$ thick, applied in the regions where bone contact with the implant is required. This means that, for proximal femoral replacements, it is only the proximal region that is sprayed in most cases, although a few designs of implants are fully coated. The thickness of the layer is a compromise between being

sufficiently thick to prevent too rapid resorption of the hydroxyapatite while being sufficiently thin to prevent problems of the fracture of bulk hydroxyapatite. In a recent study of members of the British Orthopaedic Association, it was found that 10% of the respondents were using HAP-coated proximal femoral stems and 8.8% were using hydroxyapatite-coated acetabular cups, compared with only 0.4% using HAP-coated knee replacements (Ballantyne VB, personal communication, 1993).

The length of time required to produce a biological response to HAP is considered to be fairly slow and the addition of tricalcium phosphate (TCP) can be used to increase the response rate. TCP has a calcium/phosphate ratio of 1.5 and is soluble in body fluids, leading to a pool of calcium and phosphate ions in the region of the dissolving TCP. These pools of calcium and phosphate ions are thought to increase the biological response to the implant. To benefit from the combination of the long-term presence of the HAP and the short-term dissolution of the TCP, one of the clinically available coatings for orthopaedic implants is 70% HAP and 30% TCP, although only limited long-term clinical data are available on this coating.

The benefits of a bioactive coating as a method of attaching bone to an implant can be seen by considering the results of Geesink et al (1988) who showed, in the femoral cortex of dogs, that a smooth titanium implant has a maximum interfacial shear strength of 0.6 MPa, but when coated with HAP the strength of the interface was $49.1 \pm 2.3\,MPa$ at 6 weeks, and had increased to $63.9 \pm 1.7\,MPa$ by 6 months. This increased interfacial strength should improve stress transfer between the implant and the bone, and discourage the formation of a fibrous capsule.

Other biologically active materials are the biologically active glasses or bioglasses. Whereas HAP has a defined crystal structure with organised positions for the individual atoms, in a glass there is no defined crystal structure as it is an amorphous material. There are two major series of bioglasses: (1) those developed by Hench in Florida, Bioglass^{R} (Hench and Wilson, 1993), and (2) the bioglasses of the Cerabone^{R} A-W (alpha-wollastonite) series developed by Kokubo et al (1985). These two materials are similar; the difference is in the ratio of the different starting materials. In most bioactive glasses the active materials are SiO_2, Na_2O, CaO and P_2O_5. In the most commonly used Bioglass^{R}, 45S5, these are 45% SiO_2,

24.5% Na_2O, 24.4% CaO and 6% P_2O_5 by weight. In Cerabone® A-W, the composition by weight is 44.7% CaO, 34.0% SiO_2, 6.2% P_2O_5, 4.6% MgO and 0.5% CaF_2.

Bioglass® is prepared by standard sol–gel glass manufacturing methods. When bioactive glasses are placed in body fluids the surface chemistry produces a reaction leading to a hydroxycarbonate apatite (HCA) layer on the surface of the bioglass to which bone can bond. Within 1 hour in rat bone it has been found that the HCA layer is 0.8 μm thick, with a layer of SiO_2 below it. Once the SiO_2–HCA layers have been formed, they are able to adsorb biological factors. This is followed by attachment and differentiation of stem cells and then the generation and mineralisation of bone matrix. After this material has been implanted into bone, the shear strength of the interface may reach 15–25 MPa after 1 month, compared with an inert glass giving a value of less than 0.5 MPa (Kokubo et al, 1985).

Bioglass® has been used clinically as a middle ear prosthesis. It can be drilled with standard surgical equipment, but it must still be remembered that the material is brittle. Cone-shaped devices made from 45S5 Bioglass® have been used in patients who have lost a tooth to prevent alveolar ridge resorption. Another use is as a curved plate which is inserted to repair orbital floor fractures by reconstructing the floor and repositioning the eye. Due to their low mechanical properties bioglasses are commonly used in particulate form to provoke a beneficial biological response around the particles. These may also be mixed with autologous bone chips for alveolar ridge augmentation (Hench and Wilson, 1993).

AW Glass Ceramic, or Cerabone® A-W is a composite containing crystalline phases within an amorphous glass phase (Kokubo et al, 1985). This produces material with higher mechanical properties than glass. Again, an HCA layer is formed on the surface of Cerabone® A-W on immersion in physiological fluids and bone may bond to this layer. When implanted into rat bone, by 8 weeks 60% of hydroxyapatite is covered with bone, whereas nearly 90% of Cerabone® A-W is covered with bone and these amounts of bone cover do not appear to alter thereafter.

Kokubo et al (1985) have attempted to ascertain which elements are required for this response, and it appears that a CaO, SiO_2 phase is necessary for the formation of an HCA layer. When Cerabone® A-W was pushed out from rabbit cortical bone, the interfacial shear strength reached over 20 MPa at 3 months and remained there at 6 months (Tanner et al, 1990). As the mechanical properties of Cerabone® A-W are higher than those of Bioglass®, it may be used in load-bearing applications. Cerabone® A-W vertebral prosthetic devices have been used in patients with spinal metastases leading to paraplegia. An entire vertebrae may be removed and replaced with a Cerabone® A-W prosthesis. It has also been used in patients with burst fractures of vertebrae and, although the paraplegia was not totally resolved in all cases, it was reduced, as were the pain levels. Cerabone® A-W prostheses have also been used in the iliac crest after extensive autogenous bone grafts have been taken and particulate Cerabone® A-W has been used to fill bone defects.

POLYMERS

Polymers have been used in orthopaedics since Sir John Charnley made his original acetabular cups from polytetrafluoroethylene (PTFE) and then replaced them with UHMWPE, when he realised the low wear resistance of PTFE.

Polyethylene

As can be seen from *Table 18.1*, polyethylene has a very low stiffness compared with bone, but is very ductile with an extension to failure of 300% (i.e. it can quadruple its length before breaking). The major problems with UHMWPE are the biological response to both the bulk material and particles, and creep. An acetabular cup, or a tibial plateau, has both constant and cyclical loads, and the static elements of these will lead to the component, which originally fitted, deforming. Bone does not bond to polyethylene, leading to a low strength interface and bone spicules have been reported as wearing polyethylene (Dannenmaier et al, 1985). It has been extensively reported that, in hips that are loose, polyethylene particles, which may be seen with polarised light microscopy, can be seen throughout the fibrous capsule surrounding a loosened implant and not just in the joint space (Howie, 1990; Li and Burstein, 1994). UHMWPE can be used as a bearing surface only where it is providing the concave component of a joint replacement as, when used in a convex configuration, the wear rate increases substantially.

Polyacetal

Polymethylene oxide, also known as polyacetal, which is manufactured under the trade name Delrin, has been used for some joint replacements but produces significantly higher rates of failure than UHMWPE and has thus been discontinued for joint replacements (Bradley et al, 1992, 1993).

Bone cement

The other major polymer used in joint replacement is polymethylmethacrylate (PMMA) or bone cement. A major difference between polyethylene and PMMA is that polyethylene is used already polymerised, whereas PMMA is polymerised *in situ*. Already polymerised PMMA is available, when it is known by the trade name Perspex. For surgical use, partially polymerised polymer beads and methylmethacrylate monomer are mixed with a catalyst and any radio-opacifier used.

As the surgeon is responsible for the mixing (s)he needs to be aware of the problems of *in situ* polymerisation, which is not necessary for polyethylene and other already polymerised components. The mixing process can lead to air entrapment, and these air bubbles act as stress concentrations and potential points for crack initiation. Crack initiation is where, under fatigue loading, a microscopic crack starts on the surface of the pore and under load grows into the bulk material. Thus air bubbles will substantially reduce the strength and fatigue life of the cement; entrapped blood and fat will have similar effects. Secondly, a chemical process occurs when the cement is polymerised and this is exothermic: substantial amounts of heat are generated, potentially leading to thermal necrosis of the bone surrounding the implant. Thirdly, the standard opacifier is barium sulphate, which will abrade polyethylene if the barium sulphate gets between the joint surfaces. Finally, methylmethacrylate monomer is toxic, causing a reduction in blood pressure if there is too much unreacted monomer in the cement which can be absorbed into the bloodstream when introduced into the patient. In an attempt to reduce the exotherm and toxicity, a polyethylmethacrylate (PEMA)-based bone cement was developed by Braden, as reported by Revell et al (1992). This monomer has reduced toxicity and the polymer a lower exotherm, but unfortunately has higher creep behaviour so is unsuitable for clinical use (Weightman et al, 1987).

Biodegradable polymers

More recently, biodegradable polymers have been produced, principally polylactic acid and polyglycolic acid. The major use for these currently is as resorbable sutures. This is because they have limited mechanical properties and fairly high rates of resorption, typically for a suture less than 1 week, although with increasing amounts of polylactic acid and decreasing amounts of polyglycolic acid, this time is increased. Vasenius et al (1989) have developed bulk polylactic acid pins for the fixation of certain low-stressed fractures, for example of the distal fibula.

COMPOSITES

Composites are macroscopic mixtures of materials where the beneficial elements of each material are combined to produce material with intermediate-type properties, for example glass-reinforced plastics (GRP) where the glass has high stiffness, but very low strength due to the easy propagation of cracks through glass, but the plastic is tough, stopping the cracks. In GRP, the glass is in the form of fibres that stiffen the plastic and, if an individual fibre should break, the crack will be stopped by the tough plastic. The behaviour of the composite will depend on the properties of the individual phases and the way they are combined together.

Fibre-reinforced composites will be anisotropic with highest mechanical properties in the direction of the reinforcing fibres and lower stiffness and strength perpendicular to these, as the fibres are usually the materials with the higher properties. Fibres for load-bearing applications are commonly carbon fibres or glass fibres, but polymer fibres can be manufactured by melt spinning, drawing or hydrostatic extrusion. In polymer fibres, the polymer chains are generally oriented along the long axis of the fibres, making the materials substantially stiffer than the bulk material by a factor of 10 or even 20. Particulate-reinforced composites are generally isotropic, unless in the process of manufacture the matrix has become oriented.

With most composites, the weak element is the interface between the two phases. It is rare in orthopaedic composites to find any chemical bond between the two phases, thus the interface is dependent on the mechanical interlock between the two phases, which is generally poor. This is particularly important when a tensile stress is being applied across the interface, that is in any direction in a particulate-reinforced composite or perpendicular to the fibre direction in a fibre-reinforced composite. In all composites, uniform distribution of the two phases is important and it is generally deleterious to have contact between the individual particles of a particle-reinforced polymer as these agglomerates act as crack initiation points. The elements may be put into a composite for either a mechanical or a biological reason; a stiff element will reinforce a more flexible material or a biologically active element will increase the body's response to an inert material.

Fibre-reinforced composites

A variety of composites have been developed for orthopaedic applications. The first reported one was carbon-reinforced carbon (CRC), a material originally developed for Concorde's brake pads, which was investigated for hip replacements. The modulus of CRC is close to that of bone, but this system failed owing to the poor quality control available at the time. One benefit of carbon is that it is biologically extremely compatible with the body. In CRC, the carbon fibres are held within a carbon matrix, with the fibres providing stiffness due to the high orientation of the atom chains within the carbon fibres.

Bradley et al (1980) attempted to produce carbon-reinforced polymer internal fixation plates, where the carbon fibres were held within a polymer matrix, again providing a material that was mechanically compatible with bone. These devices were abandoned as the polymer resin could not be shaped in theatre, thus permitting the internal fixation plates to be used only on straight bones, consequently confining them to the radius and ulna. These plates were used with conventional stainless steel screws.

Taurio and Törmälä (1991) attempted to manufacture implants where polylactic acid fibres were wrapped around an hydroxyapatite core; thus the polylactic acid fibres were holding the core together. This was found to have insufficient compressive or impact strength to be used clinically.

Particulate-reinforced composites

Bonfield and co-workers (Abrams et al, 1984) developed a series of hydroxyapatite-reinforced polymers for bone replacement. The hydroxyapatite was in a particulate form, producing an isotropic material. The benefit of the hydroxyapatite is to stiffen the polyethylene and to provide a biologically active component. The polyethylene toughens the brittle hydroxyapatite and increases the modulus of the composite. Although 40 volume per cent hydroxyapatite was used, similar to the 50 volume per cent hydroxyapatite in bone, because of the isotropy of the composite and much larger reinforcing particles (approximately 1000 times larger than those in bone), the modulus achieved was only 4.5 GPa and the ultimate tensile strength was only just over 20 MPa. Thus, the material was insufficiently strong for load-bearing applications. However, the bond strength between the bone and hydroxyapatite–polyethylene composite is significantly stronger than that between bone and polyethylene alone (Tanner et al, 1990). This material has been used successfully for orbital floor fractures where the bone bonds to the material (Tanner et al, 1994) and is entering clinical trials as an ear implant material.

CONCLUSIONS

In current clinical practice there are materials that work, but within limitations, and these limitations need to be understood by the surgeons who use them. Metals are capable of withstanding the loads and fatigue cycles required of them, but stress relieve the bone, which can eventually lead to loosening. Ceramics can give excellent wear properties but can fracture catastrophically. Bioactive ceramics can cause bonding of the bone to the implant, thus stabilising an implant, but do not have sufficient mechanical properties to be used as bulk materials. Non-resorbable polymers are not stiff enough for load-bearing applications, except as articulating surfaces, and can produce biologically disastrous wear particles. New composites show promise but still have problems that need to be solved before they can enter extensive clinical use.

The ideal artificial material for orthopaedic applications has still to be developed, although new materials are currently being investigated around the world. The salesperson will appear to expand the benefits of their product, but the clinician considering using a new material needs to be cautious and to consider the potential problems as well as the potential advantages before using a new material.

REFERENCES

Abrams J, Bowman J, Behiri JC, Bonfield W. The influence of compounding route on the mechanical properties of highly loaded particulate filled polyethylene composites. *Plast Rubber Proc* 1984; **4**: 261–269.

Ashby MF, Jones DRH. *Engineering Materials 1: An Introduction to their Properties and Applications*. Oxford: Pergamon Press, 1980.

Ashby MF, Jones DRH. *Engineering Materials 2: An Introduction to Microstructure, Processing and Design*. Oxford: Pergamon Press, 1986.

Bergmann G, Graichen F, Röhlmann A. Hip joint loading during walking and running measured in two patients. *J Biomech* 1993; **26**: 969–990.

Bonfield W. New trends in implant materials. In: Pizzofernato A, Ravaglioli A, Lee AJC (eds) *Biomaterials and Clinical Applications*. Amsterdam: Elsevier Science, 1987: 13–21.

Bradley GW, Freeman MAR, Tuke MA. All polymer total knee replacement. *Am J Knee Surg* 1992; **5**: 3–8.

Bradley GW, Freeman MAR, Tuke MA, McKellop HA. Evaluation of wear in an all polymer total knee replacement. Part II: Clinical evaluation of wear in a polyethylene on polyacetal total knee replacement. *Clin Mater* 1993; **14**: 127–132.

Bradley JS, Hastings GW, Johnson-Nurse C. Carbon reinforced epoxy as a high strength low modulus material for internal fixation plates. *Biomaterials* 1980; **1**: 38–40.

Charnley J. Fracture of femoral prostheses in total hip replacement: a clinical study. *Clin Orthop* 1975; **111**: 105–120.

Dannenmaier WC, Haynes DW, Nelson CL. Granulomatous reaction and cystic bone destruction associated with high wear rate in a total knee prosthesis. *Clin Orthop* 1985; **198**: 224–230.

Derby B, Hills DA, Ruiz C. *Materials for Engineering: A Fundamental Design Approach*. Harlow: Longman Scientific and Technical, 1992.

Dowson D. Bio-tribology of natural and artificial joints. In: Mow VC, Ratcliffe A, Woo SLY (eds) *Biomechanics of Diarthrodial Joints*, Vol. II. New York: Springer, 1989: 305–345.

Geesink RGT, de Groot K, Klein CPAT. Bonding of bone to apatite-coated implants. *J Bone Joint Surg* 1988; **70B**: 17–22.

Gluck T. Auto-plastik-transplantation implantation von Fremdkorpern. *Klin Wochensc* 1890; **27**: 421–427.

Gordon JE. *The New Science of Strong Materials, or why you don't fall through the floor*, 2nd edn. London: Penguin, 1976.

Hench LL, Wilson J. *An Introduction to Bioceramics*. Singapore: World Scientific, 1993.

Hing KA, Best SM, Tanner KE, Revell PA, Bonfield W. Mechanical assessment of porous hydroxyapatite before and after osseointegration. In: Hench LL, Wilson J (eds) *Bioceramics 8*. Oxford: Butterworth–Heinemann, 1995: 75–80.

Howie DW. Tissue response in relation to type of wear particles around failed hip arthoplasties. *J Arthroplasty* 1990; **5**: 337–348.

Inoue O, Ibaraki K, Shimabukuro H, Shingaki Y. Solo implantation of porous cuboidal hydroxyapatite for the treatment of simple bone cysts. In: Bonfield W, Hastings GW, Tanner KE (eds) *Bioceramics 4*. Oxford: Butterworth–Heinemann, 1991: 245–254.

Kukubo T, Ito S, Shigematsu M, Sakka S, Yamamuro T. Mechanical properties of a new type of apatite containing glass ceramic for prosthetic applications. *J Mater Sci* 1985; **20**: 2001–2004.

Li S, Burstein AH. Ultra high molecular weight polyethylene: the material and its use in total joint replacements. *J Bone Joint Surg [Am]* 1994; **76A**: 1080–1090.

Park JB, Lakes RS. *Biomaterials: an Introduction*. New York: Plenum Press, 1992.

Parkhill C. A new apparatus for the fixation of the bones after resection and in fractures with a tendency to displacement. *Trans Am Surg Assoc* 1897; **180**: 3–6.

Revell PA, George M, Braden M, Freeman MAR, Weightman B. Experimental studies of the biological response to a new bone cement. Part 1: Toxicity of *n*-butylmethacrylate monomer compared with methylmethacrylate monomer. *J Mater Sci Mater Med* 1992; **3**: 84–87.

Sedel L, Kerboull L, Christel P, Meunier A, Witvoet J. Alumina on alumina hip replacement. Results and survivorship in younger patients. *J Bone Joint Surg Br* 1990; **72B**: 658–663.

Tanner KE, Doyle C, Bonfield W. The strength of the interface developed between biomaterials and bone. In: Heimke G, Soltèsz U, Lee AJC (eds) *Clinical Implant Materials*. Amsterdam: Elsevier, 1990: 149–154.

Tanner KE, Downes RN, Bonfield W. Clinical application of hydroxyapatite reinforced polyethylene. *Br Cer Trans* 1994; **93**: 104–107.

Taurio R, Törmälä P. Coral based and sintered hydroxylapatite blocks reinforced with fibrous cage-like polylactide composite: a comparative study. In: Bonfield W, Hastings GW, Tanner KE (eds) *Bioceramics 4*. Oxford: Butterworth–Heinemann, 1991: 287–294.

Vasenius J, Vainionpää S, Vihtonen K et al. Biodegradable self-reinforced polyglycolide (SR-PGA) composite rods coated with slowly degradable polymers for fracture fixation: strength and strength retention *in vitro* and *in vivo*. *Clinical Materials* 1989; **4**: 307–317.

Wallbridge N, Dowson D. The walking activity of patients with artificial hip joints. *Engineering in Medicine* 1982; **11**: 95–96.

Weightmann B, Freeman MAR, Revell PA, Braden M, Albrektsson BEJ, Carlson LV. The mechanical properties of cement and loosening of the femoral component of hip replacement. *J Bone Joint Surg [Br]* 1987; **69B**: 558–564.

Young RJ. *Introduction to Polymers*. London: Chapman and Hall, 1981.

Yue S, Pillar RM, Weatherley GC. The fatigue strength of porous-coated Ti–6%Al–4%V implant alloy. *J Biomed Mater Res* 1984; **18**: 1043–1058.

GLOSSARY: ENGINEERING TERMS

Anisotropic – having different properties in different directions.

Brittle – a material in which it is easy to initiate and propagate a fracture.

Creep – time-dependent deformation of a material, i.e. under a constant load the material will continue to deform.

Ductile – a material that can undergo a high extension before fracturing.

Fatigue – loading of a material where the load is applied and then removed continuously. Microscopically small cracks in the material open and close with each cycle and, if the stresses are sufficiently large, will eventually lead to fracture of the whole object.

Force or load – measured in newtons (N), which is the force exerted by 1 kg when accelerated by $1 \, \mathrm{m \, s^{-2}}$. On Earth, the force exerted by 1 kg is 9.81 N.

Fracture toughness (K) – a measure of the energy needed to propagate a fracture through the material.

Isotropic – having the same properties in all directions.

Strain (σ) – extension per unit length, normally engineering strain or extension per unit original length, measured as a percentage or microstrain (10^{-6}).

Strength – maximum load a material will sustain without failing. The strength of a material will depend on the type of load being applied.

Stress (ε) – force per unit area usually measured in MPa ($10^6 \, \mathrm{N \, m^{-2}}$).

Ultimate tensile strength (UTS) – maximum stress that may be applied to a material before failing.

Viscoelastic – having mechanical properties that are time dependent. In general, if a viscoelastic material is loaded quickly, it appears to be stiffer than if loaded slowly. Also if a viscoelastic material is held at a constant load, the extension will increase with time (creep).

Yield stress (σ_y) – the initial part of a stress–strain curve is straight for a metal; the yield stress is where the deviation from linearity occurs. Once a metal is loaded beyond its yield stress, plastic or non-recoverable deformation occurs.

Young's modulus (E) – ratio of stress to strain in the linear region of a stress–strain curve, also called modulus of elasticity, normally measured in GPa ($10^9 \, \mathrm{N \, m^{-2}}$).

19

Kinematic and Kinetic Analysis of Function

Denis RW May

INTRODUCTION

This chapter is concerned with the forces and displacements in the human body that enable us to walk and to perform our daily living activities. The study of displacements and movements is known as **kinematics** and the study of forces that of **kinetics**. Both of these studies require separate scientific techniques for analysis and measurement.

Kinetics can be further divided into two subgroups. The analysis of stationary or very slow moving forces is called **statics** and the study of moving forces is known as **dynamics**.

Analysis of function in human movement is very important in many fields of study, from the tactile and manipulative coordination required for microsurgery and scientific nanotechnology, through the ultimate efficiency, performance and endurance of athletes, to the surgical reconstruction of diseased and dysfunctioning joints and the assistive devices required to enable very severely disabled and multideficient patients to have an acceptable quality of life and reasonable degree of mobility and independence.

The study of human locomotion crosses a great many, sometimes very disparate, disciplines, from the biological and medical disciplines of kinesiology, physiology, neurology, anatomy, rheumatology and orthopaedics, through the scientific and engineering studies of biomechanics, kinematics and kinetics, and electronics, instrumentation, computing and data acquisition, to mathematical modelling, statistical analysis and interpretation of results.

Most work in this field has studied locomotion (gait analysis), but other joints have also been investigated.

DEFINITION OF TERMS

When a force is applied to a body and it moves, the force is said to do **work**. Work is force multiplied by the distance moved. In moving, bodies have **energy**. This is known as kinetic energy. Kinetic energy has the formula $KE = \frac{1}{2}mV^2$ and is measured in **joules**. **Potential energy** also exists by virtue of position or state, $PE = mgh$. During walking, therefore, in mid-stance, when the centre of gravity of the body is at its highest level, the body has maximum potential energy, which can be converted into kinetic energy for forward propulsion.

Force can, therefore, take many forms. Tractive or tension forces are pulling forces. Propulsive or compressive forces are pushing forces. Shear forces cause bodies to slide over one another.

The **centre of gravity**, or centre of mass of a body, is that point through which the whole weight of the body can be supposed to act.

A force can also tend to turn a body. This turning effect is called a **moment of force** and is equal to the force times the perpendicular distance about which it is turning. A moment is measured in newton metres.

When a body is moving it is said to have **momentum and inertia**. The momentum of a body is the mass times the velocity at which it is moving. The inertia of a body is that tendency for it to continue in its existing state of motion. Moment of inertia is given the symbol $I = Mk^2$ where k is the **radius of gyration** of that body. For a pendulum swinging on a light string, the radius of gyration and centre of gravity are the same point. For other more complex bodies, such as the swinging shank of a leg, these points are separate and the radius of gyration point is often called the **centre of percussion**.

Kinematics is the study of movements or displacements. This is usually in isolation to the sets of forces that are causing these movements. **Displacement**, either **linear** or **angular**, is change of position and is usually measured in **metres** or, if angular, in **degrees** or **radians**. **Velocity** is rate of change of displacement and is measured in metres per second, or if angular, radians per second and is, therefore, the first time derivative of distance $v = ds/dt$. **Acceleration** is the rate of change of velocity and is measured in metres per second squared or, if angular, radians per second squared and, therefore, $a = d^2s/dt^2$ is a second time derivative of distance. **Aggravation** is the rate of change of acceleration and is, therefore, the third time derivative of distance. All these studies can be related mathematically to enable us to build up a fascinating picture of how each of us walks and moves.

HISTORICAL BACKGROUND

Early pioneering work on gait analysis was conducted by the Weber brothers in 1836. They observed and measured many of the movements required during walking and running. These included the inclination of the head and trunk, alternations of the swinging and stance phases of walking. They described in great detail the difference between walking and running, and investigated the effects of muscle function involved in walking and propulsion.

Marey, in 1882, was the first to use photography for the analysis of motion. This inspired Maybridge to set up a sequential array of cameras, which enabled him to study how humans walk and move; he continued his studies on horses and other animals, and even studied how birds fly.

Once cinephotography was established, this led to the classical studies of Braun and Fischer in 1895 which even today, 100 years later still dominate the study of human locomotion. The fundamental studies of human locomotion in relation to the design of artificial limbs conducted at the University of California in Berkeley in the mid 1940s (Eberhart et al, 1947), stimulated the design of more modern developments, such as the design of the Kistler force plate and kinematic measuring systems such as Vicon and Selspot.

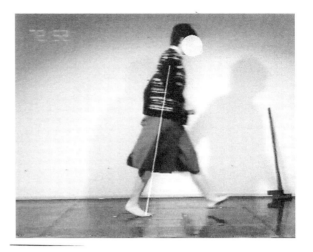

Figure 19.1   Video Vector Generator showing the ground reaction force in magnitude and direction superimposed on the video of the subject walking.

Vicon, manufactured by Oxford Metrix, Oxford, UK, employs networked television cameras to collect fields of data. The cameras are equipped with synchronous infrared strobes and are capable of tracking up to 30 markers simultaneously.

The Video Vector Generator developed at Oswestry, UK, converts the force data obtained from a Kistler force plate into a force vector line image, which is superimposed on the image of the patient walking. Therefore, for the first time an instrument visually couples the ground reaction forces with the kinematic analyses of patients walking (*Figure 19.1*).

EXPERIMENTAL TECHNIQUES

Bernstein et al (1903) established the following criteria as a minimum requirement in the recording of body movement. He suggested the method should provide for an uninterrupted progression; it should not interfere with or influence in any way the performance of the activities; and it should lend itself to an easy interpretation and evaluation of the data obtained.

For kinematic studies of gait, most investigations utilise a special walkway with or without an associated video system to record the position of markers attached to the subject.

Today, various systems are available commercially. Full motion analysis based on powerful software has been written to run in the Microsoft Windows environment on IBM or PC compatibles. One such system is the Coda MPX30 system from Charnwood Dynamics, UK. The secret of this system lies in the design of the special cameras, which do not have lenses. Instead, the infrared light from light emitting diode (LED) markers passes through a flat window upon which is a random pattern of black lines, rather like a bar-code. The intelligent markers are small infrared LEDS, which flash in response to control signals from the Coda scanner. Optically telemetered electromyographic systems are also available, providing up to 16 channels of electromyographic signals which can be acquired synchronously with movement and data analysis. This allows phasing activities of the muscles to be seen as the patient is walking and to be recorded on videotape if required.

The conducting floor pathway

The **temporal factors** of gait have been measured using a standard gait analysis walkway with a specially designed conducting floor. This walkway was a raised platform about 20 m long to allow a series of uninterrupted steps to be taken. Metal foil strips bonded to the soles of the subject's shoes formed the contacts, and the circuit was so arranged that, when standing with one foot on the floor, the conducting path was open, until the heel of the other foot made contact. The circuit then closed and remained so during the double support phase. At the instant either foot was removed from the floor, for example during the swing phase, the circuit was again interrupted. In this way accurate measurements of timing and distance were recorded. The conducting path is usually thin aluminium foil and the same techniques are often used for footprint analysis. In this way measurements of walking base width, and of toe in–toe out angles, have also been made.

The glass walkway

The glass walkway is a raised platform long enough to enable the subject to reach an easy, comfortable and natural gait in the middle or working section from either direction. The working section has a glass floor, usually constructed of 100-mm armour-plated glass under which is placed a mirror inclined at 45°. A camera placed about 14 m away can photograph the side and the bottom of the subject with a minimum of parallax and perspective error.

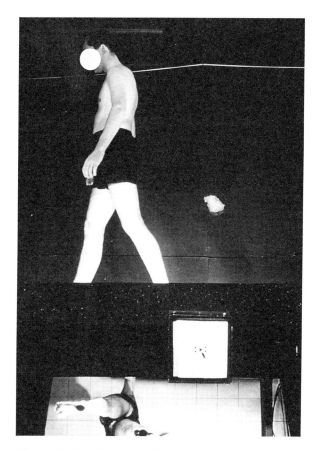

Figure 19.2 The glass walkway, showing a worm's eye view of foot contact areas and pelvic rotations during walking.

A clock is placed in the field of view of the camera to synchronise the time–motion relationships. *Figure 19.2* depicts such a glass walkway; the 'worm's eye view' shows contacts of the feet with the glass plate and pelvic rotations during walking.

Interrupted light techniques

To achieve greater accuracy in the measurement of component velocities, flicker photometry has been used. Illuminated targets were fixed to the estimated joint centres of the leg and the subject walked in a darkened room in front of the open lens of a camera. The field of view of the camera was interrupted at a specified frequency by a revolving slotted disc with a synchronous motor. In this way the time interval could be obtained with much greater precision and thus the numerical

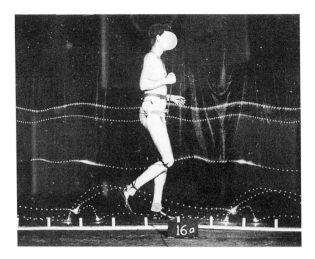

Figure 19.3 Interrupted light techniques showing a subject walking on a level plane, the light being illuminated at intervals of one-sixtieth of a second.

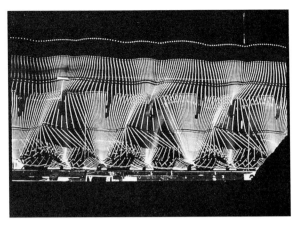

Figure 19.4 Stick diagram showing the kinematics of walking including the upper and lower extremities.

differentiation approximated more closely. *Figure 19.3* shows a subject during normal level walking with the lights illuminated at time intervals of one-sixtieth of a second, and illustrates the sinusoidal movements of walking.

KINEMATIC MEASUREMENTS

Measurement of displacements

Several methods have been used in the past to measure the motion of the lower extremity. All the methods, however, rely ultimately in the production of a **stick diagram**.

Stick diagrams

The centre of rotation of each joint is marked and a photographic record of the walking activity obtained. The centres of each joint for a given instance of time are joined together with straight lines. The successive position of sequential time intervals are reproduced in a single plate over a complete walking cycle. This results in a series of segmental lines and is called a stick diagram.

Figure 19.4 shows a stick diagram of an above-knee amputee walking. Markers are placed on the head, shoulder, elbow and wrist to illustrate the kinematics of

the upper extremity and the hip, on the lateral aspect of the knee and on the lateral malleolus to illustrate the kinematics of the lower extremities.

Pin studies

To determine accurately the path of motion of the true skeleton, as opposed to the position of markers on the skin, target pins have been attached firmly to the bone. Stainless steel pins are inserted under local anaesthesia into the cortices of the bones. The regions usually selected are the tuberosity of the ileum, the abductor tubercle of the femur and the tibial tubercle. Great care must be exercised in the placement of the pins, and *Figure 19.5* shows a photograph of the bifurcated target pin for locating the great trochanter of the femur. For example, a pin cannot be located directly into the greater trochanter of the femur as this would severely limit the function of the iliotibial tract, thus causing the patient to walk with gross abnormality.

Measurement of angular displacement

The angle of the limb segments at any point in time during the walking cycle can, of course, be computed by accurate measurement of the stick diagrams. This is most laborious, however, and **electrogoniometry** is often used for measurements of hip, knee and ankle during the walking cycle. Unless a **telemetric device** is used, this has the disadvantage of trailing wires during ambulation.

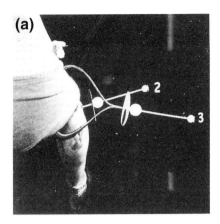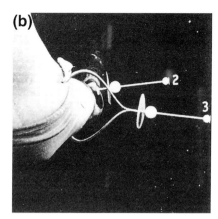

Figure 19.5 Pin studies illustrating the rotation of the tibia with respect to the femur at the knee joint when (a) flexed and (b) fully extended.

Measurement of velocities

The velocities of the segments of the limb can be calculated from the stick diagrams by numerical differentiation. Using the approximation $V = \frac{ds}{dt} \approx \frac{\delta s}{\delta t}$. Errors can occur, however, owing to the differences of small quantities.

Measurement of accelerations

The accelerations of leg segments can be calculated from the stick diagram by a second numerical differentiation; again, quite large errors can occur because of the differences of small quantities. May (1972) used numerical methods up to and including tenth-order central differences to achieve higher accuracy.

Electrical transducers that are sensitive to acceleration and that are small in size and have a small mass have been used. Seismic mass accelerometers have also been developed and been used in conjunction with normal as well as prosthetic and orthotic devices.

Data obtained from these experiments have been fairly limited because of the difficulty of analysing the results. The accelerometer must be placed very accurately at the centre of percussion of the leg segments; otherwise, the acceleration sensed will be the vector sum of the vertical and horizontal translatory accelerations as well as the angular and centripetal components. The exact locations of the centre of percussion of the thigh and the shank *in vivo* are quite difficult to measure, and the accelerations of the shank are modified by the transducer itself. Furthermore, very complex data recording and read-out

equipment are required for these techniques and in the past this has limited much of this work.

KINETICS

Kinetic studies of the leg deal with the forces acting in the segments during the phasic motions of gait. Two separate systems need to be analysed: the **external reaction forces** and the **internal forces**.

Measurement of reaction forces

Various methods have been evolved to measure the floor reactions during walking. Most techniques use some form of strain gauge sensing transducer. Usually two identical systems are used, one for each foot, separated by an average step length.

The force plate

The force plate is a strain-gauged unit placed in the floor of the walkway or inclined ramp, or which forms part of a step in a staircase. It consists of a rigid upper platform which is supported on beams and designed such that the deflection of the latter indicates the centre of the pressure of the foot. For example, determination of the magnitude, direction, and point of application of the resultant forces of the foot on the floor is accomplished by measuring the resultant vertical force, the fore and aft shear forces, the lateral force and the torque about the centre of the plate.

Pylon studies

External and ground reaction forces have also been estimated using **instrumented pylons**. These are prosthetic and orthotic devices which have strain gauges attached to them, and in this way measure **bending** as well as **direct axial forces** on the subjects.

The instrumented leg

This is a special device basically for a below-knee amputee with a **patella tendon-bearing prosthetic** limb. These devices usually measure the bending moments and direct axial forces about the knee and ankle. Success, however, has been fairly limited owing to cross-coupling effects of one transducer on the other, and hence difficulty in interpreting the results.

Measurement of internal forces

Internal muscle forces are generally much larger than the associated external load, and these play a major factor in determining loads on the skeleton. The most convenient method for assessing **muscle activity** is the use of **electromyography**. The changes of electrical potential that occur when muscle fibres contract are recorded and examined. Wire or needle electrodes may be inserted into the muscle bulk, and signals obtained as such are much stronger than those obtained from surface electrodes. The needle or wire, however, does produce discomfort and this tends to change the mode of gait of the subject. For this reason, surface electrodes applied to the skin over the active muscles are generally preferred. If the skin is abraded and the electrodes applied with electrojelly, the external impedance is reduced virtually to that of the wire or needle electrode.

Figure 19.6 shows summary curves of the electromyographic activity of the major muscle groups of the lower extremity as a percentage of maximum activity and against the percentage of the walking cycle. This is the method usually employed as there are no direct correlations between muscle activity and moment or muscle force about the joint.

The magnitude of the internal forces acting within the skeletal system during walking has not been well docu-

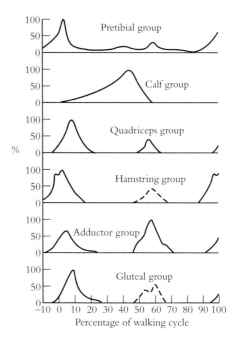

Figure 19.6   Summary curves showing the electromyographic activity of the major muscle groups of the lower extremity during walking.

mented in the literature. **Implanted telemetry** is perhaps the only and the best way forward. The methods adopted so far for measurement with forces relate to patients with implants. Using telemetry, Bergman et al (1993) recorded the hip joint forces in two patients with total hip replacements and recorded a maximum loading condition of about 870% of body-weight during stumbling. In the same paper, the **torsional moments** around the stem of the implants were recorded as 40.3 Nm and 24 Nm for each of the two patients. These measurements, of course, incorporate the gross external ground reaction forces and the internal muscle stabilising forces across the joints.

Strain gauges have been applied directly to bone. This technique is invasive and has been applied only in a research environment; it is not suitable for routine clinical use.

Energy cost studies

Many different methods have been employed in the past to assess **energy expended** by humans during walking, rest and other muscular activity. Common methods include **direct calorimetry** (McArdle et al, 1986),

indirect calorimetry and **heart rate monitoring**. There are basically two applications of indirect calorimetry: closed- and open-circuit spirometry.

The closed circuit is often used in laboratory settings. It is called a closed circuit because the subject breathes continuously from a prefilled spirometer of oxygen while the exhaled carbon dioxide is absorbed by potassium hydroxide.

In open-circuit spirometry the subject inhales ambient air. Analysis of the different composition of inhaled and exhaled air provides a simple measure of oxygen consumption. Open-circuit spirometry uses either a lightweight portable spirometer or the Douglas bag. The Douglas bag collects a volume of expired air over a given time. It is later analysed for oxygen and carbon dioxide composition. This method usually makes use of a treadmill or a cycle ergometer. A mouthpiece to inhale and exhale ambient air is also used. *Figure 19.7* shows the set-up for energy cost studies at the Robens Institute. The equipment used is a Woodway motorised treadmill (A), three Douglas bags attached to a trolley (B), which were connected via tubing to a mouthpiece (C) which incorporates a two-way high-velocity low-resistance breathing valve. A pump (D) connected to a digital air volume meter (E) is used to pump all the air out of each bag after use, and at the same time measures the volumes. The oxygen and carbon dioxide gas analysers are shown (F).

The energy cost of walking can significantly limit both the speed of walking and the potential range. Bard and Ralston (1959) have shown that, at a normal walking speed of about 1.3 m per s, average minimum energy consumption is about 0.8 calories per metre per kilogram of body-weight. If we walk faster or slower, more energy is consumed. These authors have also observed that the walking speed that minimises energy consumption is the same as the comfortable, natural, walking speed the subject would normally adopt. Nelms (1982) has shown that there is a linear relationship between heart rate and oxygen consumption. MacGregor (1981) has described a method of combining the parameters of heart rate and speed of walking to produce a single index that can be used as an indicator of locomotor efficiency.

This so-called physiological cost index (PCI) is defined as follows:

$$PCI = \frac{\text{Heart rate, walking} - \text{heart rate, resting}}{\text{Walking speed}}$$

The same author reports that in normal subjects the PCI ranges from about 0.11 to 0.51 beats per metre.

ORGANISATION OF THE HUMAN LOCOMOTOR MECHANISM

We all walk by rotation of the long bones about the joints, actuated by the muscles and controlled by the autonomic nervous system. The human skeleton is the fundamental structural framework and the bones, joints, muscles, ligaments and tendons make up the system.

Bones are classified as long (e.g. femur), short (e.g. phalanx), flat (e.g. scapula) and irregular (e.g. ileum). The long bones are generally annular in cross-section, providing an excellent strength to weight ratio. They are hydraulically stabilised by fluid in the medullary canal and generally consist of cancellous or spongy bone at the articulating ends and of hard, compact, cortical bone in the middle, where the bending stresses are highest. The articulating ends are covered with a viscoelastic structure – cartilage. This is about 2–3 mm thick and provides an exceptionally efficient articulation for shock absorption and load-bearing.

Joints are classified as fixed (e.g. cranial) semi-fixed (e.g. vertebrae) and free (e.g. knee and finger). Free joints are described by their shape, for example hinged (finger joints), saddle (ankle) and ball and socket (hip). The free joints allow movement and are lubricated by sinovial fluid enclosed by a protective capsule.

Ligaments join the bones together and provide constraints to unwanted movements; they offer stability to

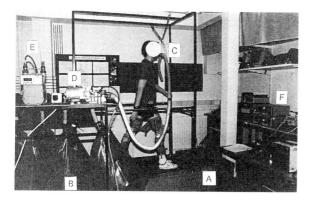

Figure 19.7 Energy cost studies showing the set-up of the equipment used for oxygen consumption. See text for details.

the system, which is generally flexible and which increases with stiffness as the amount of flexion of the joint increases.

Muscles work in a complex fashion to articulate and stabilise the joints. Anatomy books classify the knee as a hinged joint. It is, in fact, far more complex than this, providing sliding, gliding, rolling and twisting, and is probably the most complex joint in the body. It consists of three separate joints. The patellofemoral joint and the medial and lateral tibiofemoral joints. The femur and tibia of the knee both have bicondylar surfaces, being convex for the femur and concave for the tibia. These condylar surfaces have good general congruity and, when the meniscus is included, the regions of actual contact become quite extensive and capable of distributing high loads. The medial compartment is usually more highly loaded than the lateral compartment.

The length of the radius of curvature of the femoral condyle shortens from the position of full extension to full flexion, resulting in a locus of instantaneous centres of rotation which curves distally and posteriorly. The rate of change of curvature is different for the medial and lateral compartments, resulting effectively in a twisting of the knee during flexion and extension. This is particularly significant at full flexion and full extension. *Figure 19.8* illustrates the kinematics of motion of the knee with idealised mechanical simulation for a knee simulator.

USE OF MUSCLES IN STANDING AND WALKING

In standing, the legs are constrained in a straight position by the muscles. The knee is often fully extended, and hyperextension is prevented by the ligamentous structures. In walking, pelvic drop is limited by the contralateral hip abductors. The leg hangs and the swing is controlled by the extensors and flexors of the knee and hip to position the foot to take weight. Momentum and push-off from the other leg carries the body over ready for the next step.

Standing

In the upright position, the hip and knee joints are almost fully extended and the foot is approximately at right angles to the leg.

These joints are constrained in such position by the muscles and ligamentous structures. Extension of the hips is prevented by tension in the iliofemoral ligament at the anterior of the joint. Excessive extension is prevented by contraction of the soleus muscles on two sides, which also play a part in preventing lateral bending of the lumbar trunk.

Flexion of the knees is prevented by contraction of the vastae muscles and the rectus femorus, in which case the latter also prevents hyperextension of the hip. However, the knee is usually fully extended and gravity tends to cause further extension. This hyperextension is resisted by the ligaments of the knee. The foot is fixed by contact with the ground, and the tibia and fibula are kept from dorsiflexion with respect to the ankle by the contraction of the soleus. The tibialis anterior and peroneus longus may also play a part in maintaining the arches of the foot, and the body-weight is transmitted through the forefoot and heel to the ground.

Walking

When the left foot is lifted from the ground to make a step, the support for the pelvis is lost on that side; body-weight must, therefore, be transferred more to the right (Trendelenburg sign) and the tendency for the pelvis to drop must be corrected. This is accomplished by concentric contraction of the gluteus medius and the tensor fasciae latae of the right. Not only do they prevent the drop, but they actually raise the left side, so helping the foot to clear the ground as the leg swings forward.

Having tilted the pelvis, these muscles remain in isometric contraction to maintain the new position. The left femur is flexed by the concentric contraction of the soleus and rectus femorus. The shank hangs from the knee under gravity. Flexion is controlled mainly by the quadriceps. On the right, the psoas and quadriceps are stabilising the hip and knee.

The next stage is accompanied by a forward swinging of the body produced by contraction of the extensors of the right ankle. At the same time, the left limb is projected forward by extension of the knee under the action of the quadriceps. The calf group slows the shank down to bring the foot into a position where body-weight can fall upon it and momentarily the weight rests on both feet, the so-called 'double support phase'. Momentum, however, carries the body forwards and upwards on the left foot, and this is assisted by push-off of the right limb.

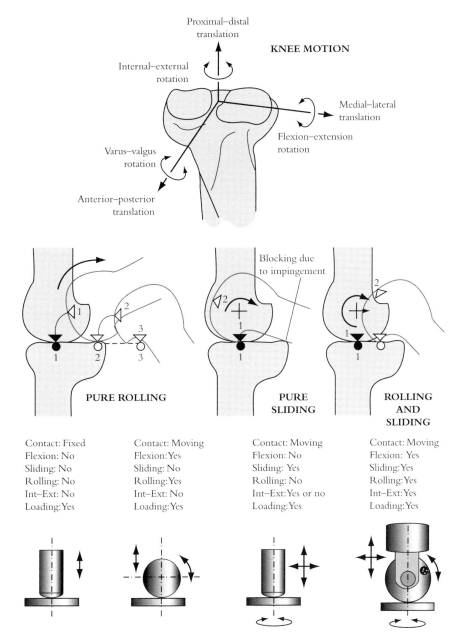

Figure 19.8 Kinematics of the motions of the knee. *Top:* Displacement of the tibia relative to the femur can be described using a right-hand set of axes. Three translations and three rotations can define motion. *Middle:* Knee flexion consists of rolling combined with sliding: motion for pure rolling (left); motion for pure sliding (centre); motion for combined rolling and sliding (right). *Bottom:* Kinematic mechanical simulation used for knee simulator, meniscal bearing simulator and pin-on-plate. From Lilley (1994), with permission.

This push-off involves a number of actions. There is lateral rotation of the hip produced by the piriformis obturators, gluteus maximus and the hamstrings. Extension of the knee is maintained by the quadriceps. The weight is transferred to the toes and coincident contraction of the plantar flexors of the ankle and toes lift the body-weight forward. The arch is maintained by the tibialis posterior so as to form a rigid lever. The push-off complete, the left leg assumes support of the body as described above, and the right leg takes the next step.

COMPLEXITY OF NORMAL GAIT

Many attempts have been made to describe normal gait, but it is important to appreciate that variations occur dependent on very many factors. Walking may be rapid or slow, it may be vigorous or slovenly, youthful or aged. It varies with the roughness or smoothness of the terrain and inclination of the surface. It is dependent on the lighting and visibility, whether the environment is known to the ambulator and whether or not that environment is hostile. Gait differences are brought about by footwear and other items of clothing, and can be also varied by conscious control to bring about profound changes. The mere consideration of anatomy and physiological processes involved in the act of normal walking would be incomplete without making due allowance for conscious thought, proprioception and the vast fields of conditioned reflexes that are brought into play.

Yet each individual has a characteristic gait that can make him or her immediately recognisable by both sound and sight. We can all recognise our friends and relatives by observing them from a distance in silhouette or listening to sequential footfalls. We all have our own particular idiosyncrasies of gait, whether it be the way we hold our head, the orientation of our trunk, or the way we swing our arms and legs. All these gait characteristics can be analysed and various phases defined. This process is termed gait analysis.

Gait analysis

Gait analysis is the qualitative and quantitative measurement of the translations and rotations of various segments of the body with respect to each other, and to fixed axes in space and the time rate of change of such motions in normal and pathological locomotion. These include such factors as arms swinging, trunk movements and changes in head orientation, as well as the major movements of the lower extremity.

Qualitative gait analysis is used at the practical or clinical level to observe deviations from normal. It is used to obtain basic parameters from the normal mechanisms upon which the designs of assistive devices can be based.

Quantitative gait analysis

Precise measurement of pace and stride length, the times of various phases of movements and the associated forces acting is the aim of gait analysis. These measurements can be divided into four basic groups: **spatial factors**, **temporal factors**, **kinematics** and **kinetics**.

Spatial factors include distance measurements such as stride and step lengths, walking base widths and limb alignment factors such as toe-in or toe-out.

Temporal factors include the times taken for the different phases of walking. These include velocity of walking, step rate (cadence), time of contact between feet and ground, stance phase times, double stance time, swing phase time and, in running, the periods of flight. Measurements can be made in a variety of ways from a simple stopwatch timing device through to specialist kinematics already outlined briefly.

Kinematics of locomotion studies the displacements, velocities and accelerations, both linear and angular, of the segments without any reference to the forces that are causing these movements.

Kinetic studies deal with the forces acting on the limb segments during the phasic motions of gait. Two separate systems need to be analysed: the external forces or the reaction forces, and the internal forces. It can be argued that all skeletal bones are involved in locomotion studies. In practice, however, it is necessary to look only at the gross movements of the lower extremity.

MAJOR EVENTS OF THE WALKING CYCLE

The walking cycle is basically divided into two distinct phases: the stance phase, when load is applied to the leg in question, and the swing phase, when load is applied to the contralateral leg and the leg in question is pendulating or swinging through.

Wide agreement, internationally, has arrived at a series of major events, whereby the whole of the walking cycle is divided into a percentage axis, beginning with heel contact of the left foot at 0%. *Figure 19.9* shows the major events that occur successively during the walking cycle.

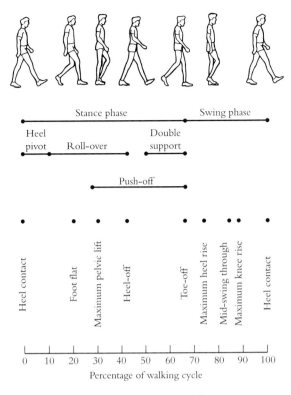

Figure 19.9 Major events of walking.

The exact position along the percentage axis, of course, varies with cadence and with the individual, but the graph shows typical values for a normal subject walking at a cadence of about 90 steps per minute.

Heel pivot occurs during the first 10% or so of the walking cycle, followed by the **roll-over period** which lasts from about 10 to 42%. During this period **foot flat** occurs at about 20%, and **maximum pelvic lift** at about 30%. The **push-off** period starts at about 28% and finishes at approximately 65%; this is also the **toe-off** position. **Heel-off** occurs a little before mid-push-off at about 42%. The **double support phase**, when momentary load is on both legs, begins at about 50% and ends with toe-off at 65%. The stance phase thus ends with toe-off and the swing phase commences at about 65% and continues until the left heel again contacts the ground at 100%. **Maximum heel rise** occurs at about 72%, followed by **mid swing through** at about 84%. **Maximum knee rise** occurs at about 88% followed by heel contact at 100%, which initiates the stance phase of the walking cycle.

For normal adult walking, the stance phase is usually about twice as long as a swing phase. The exact position of these events along the percentage axis will vary according to the individual and their particular gait characteristics. Perhaps it is not surprising, however, how little variation there is. An individual may have push-off at, say, 60–65% and maximum pelvic lift from 28 to 32%, even comparing an athletic sportsperson to an old enfeebled geriatric. Major walking cycle changes always indicate some gait pathology. The major events also depend on age and the stage of walking development reached.

The development and decline of locomotion

Bipedal gait has evolved over many millions of years. Each child has to learn to walk and learn that evolutionary process in a matter of the first couple of years of life. The average child steps purposefully at 9 months, can walk with some support at 12 months, walks unsteadily but unaided by about 15 months and will experience rudimentary running at about 18 months. The ability of the child to walk, run, accommodate stairs and ramps, even carrying loads, is similar to that of an adult by 5 years of age. *Table 19.1* shows typical locomotor function according to age.

Birth to 1.3 years is classified as the infant group, where crawling and simple support is the general form of mobility. In the younger child, from 1.3 to 5 years, mobility is characterised by highly flexed abducted thighs with little hip function. The child uses a typical bow-legged, flat-footed type of walk with little ankle function. This toppling gait has the major mobility coming from the knee, and passive movements occur at the metatarsophalangeal joints as the centre of gravity is displaced. Voluntary, purposeful, activity of the metatarsophalangeal joint does not start until around 3 years of age.

The gait of older children is much more varied. They often slouch along, dragging their feet and kicking stones. They jump, hop, skip and run. Such extremes of activities pose tremendous strength, weight and durability problems to the engineer designing assistive devices to aid such cases.

In the adolescent group, maturity is beginning. The very vigorous rough play activities tend to give way to the still very active but essentially 'normal' type of adult walk.

Table 19.1   Typical locomotor function. From May and Davis, 1974.

Age group (years)	Group	Mobility	Cadence (steps per min)	Speed of walking ($m\ s^{-1}$)	Stride length (m)	Stance phase ratio
0–1.3	Infant	Crawling Simple support	—	—	—	—
1.4–5.0	Young child	Toppling gait	113	1	0.42	0.8
5.1–9.5	Older child	Very high play activity	90	1.3	1.00	0.9
9.6–11.0	Preadolescent	High activity	88	1.5	1.27	1.0
11.1–15.0	Adolescent		85	1.7	1.42	0.8
15.1–18.0	Young adult		80	1.6	1.52	0.5
	Very active adult	Very fast ⎫	120	2	1.83	0.7
	Active adult	Fast ⎪ Normal-	105	1.7	1.65	0.6
18–70	Normal adult	Normal ⎬ type	95	1.4	1.50	0.5
	Sedentary adult	Slow ⎪ gait	80	1.2	1.40	0.5
	Inactive adult	Very slow ⎭	65	1	1.20	0.5
> 70	Geriatric	Concurrent disabilities	<50	<0.7	<1	—

The table shows typical locomotor activity in the various stages of gait development and decline. Cadences in the adult, of course, will be more a function of individual character than age as, indeed, are stride length and speed of walking. The geriatric group will also depend on factors other than age.

Adult walking spans the age range from about 18 to 70 years, and large variations occur that depend on a great many varying factors. Above the age of 70 years, the senile or geriatric gait may be characterised as disabled, possibly with many other concurrent disabilities.

Table 19.1 also gives typical values of cadences according to age and gait development. Normal gait is reasonably symmetrical; pathological gait need not necessarily be so. The cadence of the young child is typically 113 steps per minute. This typically decreases to about 90 steps per minute in the older child, to about 85 steps per minute for the adolescent, and to 80 steps per minute for the young adult where essential adult activity is taking place.

Drillis (1958) and others have conducted statistical surveys of cadence by observing 936 pedestrians walking; the results are shown in *Table 19.2*. Typical velocities of walking in metres per second are also given, together with typical stride lengths.

Another measure of gait is the ratio of swing phase time to stance phase time. In normal gait this varies between 0.5 and 1.0, depending on cadence and age. For example, when the ratio is 0.5, the stance phase is twice as long as a swing phase. For normal active adults the arithmetic mean of walking is about 112 steps per minute, with a standard deviation of 9.8 and a variability of error of about 9%. Very slow walking is about 78–100 steps per minute, very fast being 125–144 steps per minute. Much faster than this, and walking becomes running. One of the definitions of running is when the double support time becomes zero.

Angular displacements of the limb segment

Figure 19.10 shows the angular displacements of the thigh, shank and foot plotted against percentage of walking cycle. The reference angles in *Figure 19.10* are taken with respect to the vertical axis. The continuous line is the graph of the thigh angle, the small dotted line is the graph of the shin angle and the large–chain dotted line the graph of the foot angle.

At **heel contact** in the sagittal plane, the foot is dorsiflexed some 30°, the knee is virtually fully extended and the hip is flexed to about 26°. As **heel pivot** occurs, the foot plantar flexes and becomes flat on the floor at about 20% and stays approximately so until about 42%. During this period the thigh extends uniformly through 90° at about 34%, and hyperextends to a maximum of about −12° at 50%. After this, the thigh flexes through 0° at 62% to a maximum of about 26° at 80%, and stays reasonably constant until **heel contact** at 100%.

The knee is virtually fully extended at **heel contact** and thus the shin has an angle of about 26°. As the thigh extends, the knee flexes slightly: at about 15% the knee is flexed to some 18°. At about 38% the knee is again virtually straight and again uniformly flexes to a maximum of about 60° at 76%. During the whole of this

Table 19.2 Statistical survey of cadence. From May, 1972.

	Class limits	% of total		
Cadence (steps per min)				
Very slow	78.0–100.0	10	Arithmetic mean	112.5
Slow	100.1–107.0	20	Standard deviation	9.8
Normal	107.1–117.6	40	Variability (%)	9.71
Fast	117.7–125.0	20		
Very fast	125.1–144.0	10		
Stride length (inches)				
Very short	42.0–53.0	10	Range (78–42)	36
Short	53.1–56.5	20	Arithmetic mean	60.1
Normal	56.6–63.0	40	Standard deviation	3.96
Long	63.1–67.0	20	Variability (%)	6.58
Very long	67.1–78.0	10		
Speed of walking (feet per s)				
Very slow	2.30–3.70	10	Range (7.2–2.3)	4.9
Slow	3.71–4.30	20	Arithmetic mean	4.76
Normal	4.31–5.20	40	Standard deviation	0.58
Fast	5.21 5.80	20	Variability (%)	12.15
Very fast	5.81–7.20	10		

swing phase period, the orientation of the shin has been decreasing uniformly. At 70% the shank begins to re-extend linearly, through 0° at about 90% to a maximum of 26° at heel contact at a 100%.

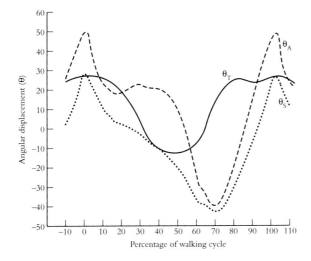

Figure 19.10 Angular displacements of the lower extremity. S, shin; T, thigh; A, ankle/foot.

Vertical translations of the joints

Figure 19.3 illustrates the vertical displacements of the hip, knee and ankle. It can be seen that the hip locus approximates to a sine wave of amplitude in the region of about 40 mm and a period of 50% of the walking cycle with a third harmonic superimposed. If the leg is assumed to be a non-extensible strut pivoting about the ankle joint, the locus of the hip joint would be a series of circular arcs with the lowest turning point at the extremes of hip flexion–extension and the highest point at mid-stance. Taking the leg to be some 97 cm long and moving through a circular arc of some 60° would give a pelvic displacement of amplitude of 100 mm. To avoid pelvic drop, however, the knee is fully extended and the ankle is plantarflexed at the two extremes. At mid-stance the knee is slightly flexed and the ankle is at minimum level, thus effectively lowering the pelvis and reducing the vertical amplitude by more than half, to 40 mm. Vertical movements of the knee have a maximum amplitude of about 75 mm, the largest rise occurring in the swing phase at about 88% of the cycle, whereas that of the ankle has a maximum amplitude of about 165 mm and this occurs at 70% of the cycle.

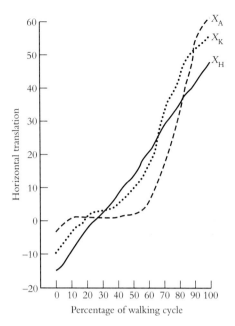

Figure 19.11   Horizontal translations of the hip (H), knee (K) and ankle (A).

Horizontal translations of the joints

Figure 19.11 shows the horizontal displacements of the lower limb joints. The continuous line depicts the hip joint, the small dotted line the knee joint and the large-chain dotted line is of the ankle joint.

Because the purpose of walking is a forward translation of the body, all the graphs show a forward slope along the percentage cycle axis. The reference axis was taken at the point of heel contact of the foot and, hence, at 0% the ankle, knee and hip have minus dimensions. The most linear graph is that of the hip. The oscillating forwards and backwards of the knee and the ankle result in the smooth uniform translation of the body. The small ripples are due to displacement of the centre of gravity of the body from the centre of the hip joints. It can also be noticed that at no time are the three centres on the same vertical straight line, again emphasising that even at mid-stance the knee is slightly flexed.

Angular velocities of the thigh and shank

At heel contact the thigh has virtually no angular velocity. It then progressively revolves backwards about the hip joint and the angular velocity uniformly increases in the negative sense up to about mid-stance. At this point it

reverses and fairly uniformly increases in the positive sense to push-off, from where it again reverses and revolves forwards and slows down for heel contact.

At heel contact, the angular velocity of the shank, like that of the thigh, is approximately zero, but this is in the process of revolving in the forward sense, and immediately after **heel contact** in the **heel pivot** period it speeds up through the **roll-over** phase and then drops when the knee flexes in mid-stance. It then recovers slightly and increases in the negative sense to **push-off**. At push-off the shank rapidly revolves in the positive direction to mid-swing-through and quickly slows up to position the foot for heel contact.

Angular accelerations of the limbs

At heel contact the shank decelerates rapidly to position the foot, and then accelerates quickly into heel pivot and roll-over. During roll-over the shank decelerates and then recovers at about mid-stance to initiate knee flexion, and again reverses to straighten the knee and accelerate up to the initiation of push-off. Here the acceleration dips to allow the foot and the ankle to store energy for push-off, and continues accelerating up to the end of the push-off phase to initiate the swing phase. The acceleration is, of course, maximal when the velocity is zero, and drops off to zero when the velocity is maximal at about mid-swing-through. After this, the angular acceleration rapidly increases in the negative sense to stop the shank and to position the foot for heel contact at 100%.

The coronal plane

In the coronal plane the control of hip abduction–adduction in the stance phase is of great importance. During mid-stance the pelvis drops on the non-supported side. This is limited to about 5° by the action of the supporting hip. Some patients can even lift the pelvis to prevent dropping completely (negative Trendelenburg sign).

The pelvis also sways from side to side, providing a total excursion of some 5 cm. For normal adults, the **walking base width** is of the order of 5–10 cm. For pathological gait and to increase **lateral stability**, this may be increased to 20 cm or more. The side movements of the body and the axial rotations of the leg during mid-stance, while the foot remains flat on the floor, are all accommodated by the mobility of the joints, mostly within the foot itself, particularly the subtalar joint.

The transverse plane

In the transverse plane, rotations of the pelvis, femur and tibia all occur in normal individuals. The magnitudes of these rotations vary from about 3° to 15° for the pelvis, from about 8° to 25° for the femur and from about 15° to 25° for the tibia. Relative transverse rotation of the tibia with respect to the femur varies from about 5° to 12°, with an average of some 9°. Relative transverse rotation of the tibia with respect to the femur varies from about 5° to about 12°, with an average of some 9°. Relative transverse rotation of the femur with respect to the pelvis varies from 5° to about 12° with an average of about 8°

Inward and outward rotations of the segments are related to weight-bearing. Inward rotation takes place during the phase of no-weight to full-weight, and outward rotation takes place during the phase of full-weight-bearing to no load. Again, all of these rotations appear to be absorbed in the articulation of the foot and ankle, and related ligamentous structures.

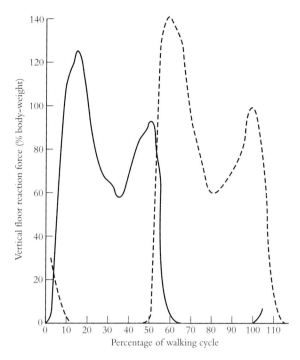

Figure 19.12   Vertical floor reaction force. ——, Left leg; – – –, right leg.

KINETICS OF NORMAL WALKING

Vertical floor reaction forces

Figure 19.12 shows the vertical floor reaction force as a percentage of gross body-weight plotted against percentage walking cycle. The continuous line shows the curve of the left leg and the chain-dotted line that of the right leg. The overlap period of about 50–65% is the **double support phase**.

Both curves exhibit the characteristic double peak but are not identical, and clearly show in this particular case that the right side is dominant. It should be noticed, however, that the time taken for a complete cycle for each leg is very similar. At heel contact, weight is smoothly transferred on to the leg and, due to the inertia of the falling body, reaches a maximum of some 140% body-weight.

Push-off occurs on the contralateral leg, which thrusts the body forwards and upwards, and relieves the supporting leg of some of the load. While the knee flexes at about mid-stance, the load decreases to about 50–60% of body-

weight, even though there is only a single point of contact with the floor. This is due to the inertial effect thrusting the body forwards and upwards, and relieving load from the contacting leg.

As the contralateral leg decelerates for heel contact, the load smoothly increases to about full body-weight and then rapidly decreases to zero for toe-off at about 65%.

Horizontal floor reaction

Figure 19.13 shows the graph of the fore and aft shear components of the floor reaction in the sagittal plane. The continuous line represents the left leg and the dotted line the right leg, and both curves show the negative–positive peaks. The right leg shows the greatest positive peak, indicating that it is dominant in the forward thrust of the body. The overlap represents the double support period and again, timewise, the cycles are similar.

At heel contact the foot is well ahead of the body and the resultant force is directed downwards and forwards. This is reacted at the heel by a negative shear force, preventing the foot from slipping forward. This reaches a

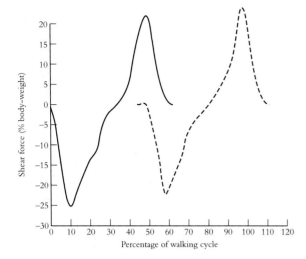

Figure 19.13   Fore and aft shear force. ——, Left leg; – – –, right leg.

maximum of some 25% body-weight at the end of heel contact, at about 10% of the walking cycle. The negative shear force then decreases smoothly until the resultant force is directly above the foot support point at about 46% mid-stance, when it becomes zero. As the body moves ahead of the foot, the shear force increases positively to prevent slipping backwards to a maximum of about 26% of body-weight at push-off, and then rapidly falls to zero at toe-off.

The engine rudder theory of walking

Kinematic analysis of these results, together with the kinetics just discussed, leads one to postulate that one leg is consistently more highly loaded than the contralateral leg, even for normal walking. The difference can be of the order of 15–20%. This dominant leg is referred to as the engine leg because it is pushing and thrusting the subject forward. The contralateral leg is the rudder leg, and this is the leg that is consistently **toeing in** and **toeing out**, guiding the subject around corners.

This phenomenon has also been observed by Chodera and Levell (1972) in analysing footprint patterns during walking. They state that, in the 320 experimental runs that were conducted from more than 40 subjects, not one person was shown to walk in a straight line. They also reported that one leg was consistently toeing in and toeing out.

The coronal plane

In the coronal plane the lateral shear forces are considerably smaller. Starting at zero at heel contact, the shear force increases smoothly to a maximum of about 5% body-weight in mid-stance and then decreases uniformly to zero at toe-off.

In the transverse plane, Eberhart and co-workers (1947) have measured axial torque, starting at about zero at heel contact, and smoothly increasing to about −4.5 Nm at 15–20% of the walking cycle. It reduces to zero at mid-stance and then progressively increases to about 9–11 Nm at 40–50% just before toe-off.

Anthropometry

Measurements of the various segments of the lower extremity are expressed in terms of two basic parameters: the total weight of the subject and the functional length of the thigh. The latter is the distance between the hip centre and the lower articular border of the femur. The data used are those of Braun and Fischer (1895) and are as follows:

Length:
   Thigh = L_T
   Shin   = $0.97\,L_T$
Centre of gravity:
   Head, arms, trunk above the mid-hip centre
$$h_H = 0.69\,L_T$$
   Thigh from hip centre $h_T = 0.44\,L_T$
   Shank from the tibial plateau $h_S = 0.63\,L_T$
Radius of gyration:
   HAT $k_H = 0.58\,L_T$
   Thigh $k_T = 0.31\,L_T$
   Shank $k_S = 0.40\,L_T$
Moment of inertia:
   Thigh $I_T = 0.0115\,W L_T^2$
   Shank $I_S = 0.0128\,W L_T^2$
Weight:
   HAT $W_H = 0.6\,W$
   Complete lower limb $= 0.2\,W$
   Thigh $W_T = 0.12\,W$
   Shank $W_S = 0.08\,W$

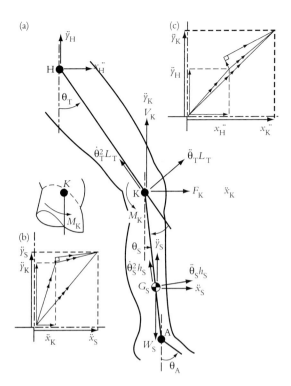

Figure 19.14   Knee dynamics: space and vector diagrams. See text for explanation of notation.

DYNAMIC ANALYSIS OF THE LOWER EXTREMITY

This section is included to illustrate a method of computing the dynamic joint stiffness of the knee. It is not intended to be a rigorous mathematical model. To simplify the equations of motions of the hip, thigh, knee and shank during the swing phase period of walking, without introducing significant errors, the foot, ankle and shin are treated as a rigid body and collectively called the shank.

Classical Newtonian mechanics are used to derive the differential equations of motion of the lower extremity in terms of the leg segment constants and their translations in space.

Referring to *Figure 19.14*, the following notation is used:

$F =$ The horizontal component of resultant force positive in the positive X direction.

$V =$ The vertical component of resultant force positive in the positive Y direction.

$W =$ The weight of the body positive in the negative Y direction.

$M =$ The moment about the joint centre.

$I =$ The moment of inertia of the body about the centre of gravity.

$m =$ The mass of the body.

$x =$ Linear displacement positive in the positive X direction.

$y =$ Linear displacement positive in the positive Y direction.

$\theta =$ Angular displacement with respect to the Y co-ordinate.

$\dot{x}, \ddot{x} =$ The corresponding linear velocity and acceleration positive in the positive X direction (the first and second time derivatives).

$\dot{y}, \ddot{y} =$ The corresponding linear velocity and acceleration positive in the positive Y direction (the first and second time derivatives).

$\dot{\theta}, \ddot{\theta} =$ The corresponding angular velocity and acceleration (the first and second time derivatives).

$L =$ Length along the mechanical or polar axis.

$h =$ Distance of the centre of gravity 'G' of body from joint centre.

$k =$ Radius of gyration of body about the joint centre.

$K =$ Subscript refers to knee joint.

$H =$ Subscript refers to hip joint.

$T =$ Subscript refers to thigh.

$S =$ Subscript refers to shank.

Taking moments about the centre of gravity of the shank:

$$M_K - V_K h_S \sin \theta_S - F_K h_S \cos \theta_S = I_S \ddot{\theta}_S \qquad (1)$$

Resolve forces in the Y direction:

$$V_K - W_S = \frac{W_S}{g} \ddot{y}_S \qquad (2)$$

Resolve forces in the X direction:

$$F_K = \frac{W_S}{g} \ddot{x}_S \qquad (3)$$

From equation (2) we have:

$$V_K = \frac{W_S}{g} \ddot{y}_S + W_S \qquad (4)$$

Substituting (3) and (4) in equation (1) gives:

$$M_K = I_S \ddot{\theta} + \frac{W_S}{g} \ddot{y}_S h_S \sin \theta_S + W_S h_S \sin \theta_S$$
$$+ \frac{W_S}{g} \ddot{x}_S h_S \cos \theta_S$$

but

$$\ddot{y}_K = \ddot{y}_S - \dot{\theta}_S^2 h_S \cos \theta_S - \ddot{\theta}_S h_S \sin \theta_S$$

and

$$\ddot{x}_K = \ddot{x}_S + \dot{\theta}_S^2 h_S \sin \theta_S - \ddot{\theta}_S h_S \cos \theta_S$$

Therefore:

$$M_K = \frac{W_S}{g}(h_S^2 + k_S^2)\ddot{\theta}_S + \frac{W_S h_S}{g}(g + \ddot{y}_K) \sin \theta_S$$
$$+ \frac{W_S h_S}{g} \ddot{x}_K \cos \theta_S \tag{5}$$

Now, from a similar position about the hip, we have:

$$\ddot{y}_K = \ddot{y}_H + \dot{\theta}_T^2 L_T \cos \theta_T + \ddot{\theta}_T L_T \sin \theta_T \tag{6}$$
$$\ddot{x}_K = \ddot{x}_H - \dot{\theta}_T^2 L_T \sin \theta_T + \ddot{\theta}_T L_T \cos \theta_T \tag{7}$$

Therefore:

$$M_K = \frac{W_S}{g}(h_S^2 + k_S^2)\ddot{\theta}_S + \frac{W_S h_S}{g}[(g + \ddot{y}_H) \sin \theta_S$$
$$+ \ddot{x}_H \cos \theta_S] + \frac{W_S h_S}{g} L_T[\dot{\theta}_T^2 \sin(\theta_S - \theta_T) \tag{8}$$
$$+ \ddot{\theta}_T \cos(\theta_S - \theta_T)]$$

The anthropometric and gait analysis data are fed into these equations and the effective dynamic joint stiffness of the knee is computed for three different speeds of walking.

Equation (8) shows the knee moment in terms of the motions of the shin and thigh segments. The first term in this equation is a function of the motion of the shin; it is a linear function of the angular acceleration of the shank and is independent of its position in space. The second term describes the linear motions of the hip joint; for good dynamic cosmesis, these accelerations should be small. Thus, the second term is usually small, exceptions being the first and last step in any sequence and any sudden changes in cadence. The last term describes the cross-coupling effect of the thigh and shin on the system, and gives the differential equation of control of the knee joint in the walking cycle. It shows that the knee moment is dependent on the angular acceleration of the shank, and the square of the angular velocity of the thigh, and is a function of the orientation of the shank with respect to the thigh.

Substituting the gait analysis and anthropometric data into equation (8), we obtained the dynamic joint stiffness three-dimensional plot as shown in *Figure 19.15*.

The function of the knee in the swing phase can be interpreted physically as follows. Consider a constant cadence plane, immediately after toe-off: when the knee is fully or very nearly fully extended the moment resisting knee flexion is minimal so that the knee can be

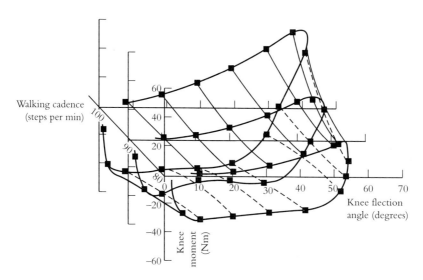

Figure 19.15   Three-dimensional plot of dynamic joint stiffness of the knee. See text for details.

easily flexed and allow the toe to clear the ground. As the angle of flexion increases, the resisting moment must increase smoothly and progressively to retard the shank and prevent excessive heel rise. After full flexion the shin must not hesitate or impart any sensation that the leg is left fully flexed in space. Hence, a positive extending moment from the quadriceps is required to initiate re-extension of the knee. As the shank extends, the knee moment must again increase progressively to damp the knee and obviate terminal impact at full extension.

The dynamic joint stiffness of the knee curve can be interpreted for energy by considering the areas under various parts of the curve. Energy loss results whenever the moment opposes motion (dissipative), and energy is gained by the shank when the moment and motion are in the same sense. Following the closed loop in clockwise direction, it can be seen that the major part of the cycle is dissipative, except for the small area of positive work just after full flexion. A small amount of positive work (about $0.4\,J$) is required to initiate shank extension. Calculating the areas, it is found that the ratios are approximately $-8 : +1 : -24$. This means that most of the energy must be dissipated in retarding the extending shank and preventing hyperextension of the knee just before heel contact. It can be seen that the positive work required to re-extend the knee occurs at an angle in excess of $50°$ of knee flexion. It is for this reason that patients with total knee replacement or patellectomy can walk perfectly normally on the level, even with an extensor lag of some $20–30°$, and the corresponding deficiency in quadriceps function and efficiency.

PATHOLOGICAL GAIT

We have seen that there is considerable variety in normal gait, depending on the individual. There is, however, a clearly identified normal pattern of walking, and normal ranges can be defined for most of the parameters already discussed.

The locomotor system often produces abnormal patterns of movement or force application. Many of these abnormalities can be simply identified by eye, which the clinician routinely does in the clinic when following up their patients. Some of the common gait deviations are described below.

Abducted gait

The heel swings through in a line laterally displaced from the normal walking line of progression. This is accompanied by excessive lateral displacement of the pelvis and is often associated with toeing in.

Lateral bending of the trunk

The trunk bends towards the supported side when the leg is in the stance phase. This is usually to bring the load line more over the hip centre of the support side.

Circumduction

The leg swings out following an outward curve path as it swings through. This is usually to increase ground clearance.

Medial whip

The heel moves medially towards the contralateral leg as the leg leaves the ground at toe-off.

Lateral whip

The heel moves laterally at toe-off.

Lumbar lordosis

There is excessive curvature of the lumbar spine. The pelvis tilts downwards and forwards when the leg is in the stance phase. This is usually caused by a flexion contracture of the hip or to change the load line to bring it in front of the hip joint.

Hip hiking

Hip hiking is a gait modification which lifts the pelvis on the swinging leg side, again to increase the toe clearance in mid-swing.

Steppage

Steppage is a simple swing phase modification incorporating excessive hip and knee flexion and used mostly in drop foot.

Vaulting

In vaulting, the ground clearance of the swinging leg is increased by vertical displacement of the entire body by excessive plantar flexion of the contralateral limb.

Foot slap

In foot slap, as weight is transferred to the leg after heel contact the forefoot suddenly strikes the ground. This is due to weakness in the dorsiflexors of the ankle.

Uneven step lengths

The length of the step taken with the affected side is considerably different from that of the contralateral leg.

Uneven timing

The time intervals between successive heel contacts is different.

Uneven arm swing

The amount and direction of the arm swing on the affected side is completely different from that on the sound side.

Uneven heel rise

The heel rise on the affected side is different from that of the contralateral leg.

REFERENCES

Bard G, Ralston H. Measurements of energy expenditure during ambulation. *Arch Phys Med Rehabil* 1959; **40**: 415–420.

Bergmann G, Graichen F, Rohlmann A. Hip joint loading during walking and running measured in 2 parts. *J Biomechs* 1993; **26**: 969–990.

Bernstein N, Poher L. *Investigation of the biodynamics of locomotion*, P Flüger's Arch. Physiol. Vol. 2. 1903 (in Russian).

Braun W, Fischer O. *Der Gang des Menschen*. Leipzig: S Hirzl, 1895.

Chodera JD, Levell RW. Footprint patterns during walking. In: Kennedy RM (ed.) *Perspectives in Biomedical Engineering*. Glasgow: University of Strathclyde, 1972: 81–90.

Drillis RJ. Objective recordings and biomechanics of pathological gait. *Ann N Y Acad Sci* 1958; **74**: 86.

Eberhart HD, Elftman H, Inman VT. *Fundamental Studies of Human Locomotion*. Berkeley: University of California, July 1947.

Lilley P. *An investigation of wear in lower limb endoprostheses*. PhD Thesis, Kingston University, 1994.

MacGregor J. The evaluation of patient performance. *Physiotherapy* 1981; **67**: 30–33.

Marey J. Sur la reproduction par la photographie de divers phases de vol des oiseaux compt. *Rendu* 1882; **94**: 683.

May D, Davis B. Gait and the lower limb amputee. *Physiotherapy* 1974; **60**: 166–171.

May D. *Analysis of Design Criteria in the Development of the Lower Extremity*. PhD Thesis, University of Surrey, 1972.

McArdle WD, Katch FJ, Katch VL. *Exercise Physiology: Energy, Nutrition and Human Performance*. Philadelphia: Lea and Febiger, 1986.

Nelms SD. Measurement of work. In: Harrison GA (ed.) *Energy and Effort*. London: Taylor and Francis, 1982: 1–25.

Weber W, Weber E. *Mechanik des Menschlichen Gehwerkzevge*. Gottingen: Mieterich, 1836.

Index

Note: page numbers in **bold** indicate tables and numbers in *italics* indicate illustrations